f26.45.

Ophthalmic Photography

AF756157

WITHDRAWN

Ophthalmic Photography

EDITED BY
JOHNNY JUSTICE, JR.
C.R.A., F.O.P.S.

Formerly Assistant Professor of
Ophthalmology, Cullen Eye Institute,
Baylor College of Medicine,
Houston, Texas

Little, Brown and Company
Boston

Copyright © 1982 by Johnny Justice, Jr.

First Edition

This book is a revised and expanded version of a previous publication, Ophthalmic Photography, edited by Johnny Justice, Jr. *International Ophthalmology Clinics* 16(2): 1976.

All rights reserved. No part of this book may be reproduced in any form or by any electronic or mechanical means, including information storage and retrieval systems, without permission in writing from the publisher, except by a reviewer who may quote brief passages in a review.

Library of Congress
Catalog Card No. 81-84194

ISBN 0-316-47731-1

Printed in the United States of America

HAL

To the advancement of ophthalmic photography and to those members of the Ophthalmic Photographers' Society, who, through the establishment of dynamic and creditable programs in education and certification, have fulfilled the goals of its founding members

Contents

Preface

Since the advent of fluorescein angiography, there has been a marked increase in the demand for qualified ophthalmic photographers. The purpose of this book is to present various ophthalmic photographic techniques in order that the novice as well as the experienced ophthalmic photographer and the interested ophthalmologist can approach these techniques in a practical manner.

In response to this need for trained ophthalmic photographers, the Ophthalmic Photographers' Society was founded in 1969. Originally a small group of 10 people, it is now an international group with more than 500 members. The society has local and national courses that lead to certification. This program was developed by a few hardworking persons who had the foresight to appreciate its necessity.

In February 1981, after 23 years of association with medical institutions such as Duke University School of Medicine, the Bascom Palmer Eye Institute at the University of Miami School of Medicine, the Jefferson Medical College and the Wills Eye Hospital of Philadelphia, and the Cullen Eye Institute at Baylor College of Medicine, Houston, I decided to enter the exciting world of private enterprise. In addition to starting my Ophthalmic Photography and Ultrasonography Service, I have joined Akorn, Inc., and Kowa, Optimed, Inc., as a consultant.

I would like to thank the innumerable ophthalmologists, ophthalmic photographers, and friends who have played a major role in the development of my career as an ophthalmic photographer and ultrasonographer. I am especially indebted to Doctors Edward W. D. Norton, J. Donald M. Gass, and David Paton.

Grateful acknowledgment is extended to Adrienne Jacobson and Carol P. Justice, C.R.A., for their help in the preparation and editing of the manuscript.

Finally, I wish to express my appreciation to the contributing authors. Without their enthusiasm and expertise, this book would not have been possible.

J. J.

Contributing Authors

Lee Allen, F.O.P.S., F.A.S.O.
Associate Emeritus, Department of Ophthalmology, The University of Iowa College of Medicine; Ophthalmic Photographer, Artist, and Ocularist, University of Iowa Hospitals and Clinics, Iowa City, Iowa
Chapter 14

Thomas Behrendt, M.D.
Professor of Ophthalmology, Jefferson Medical College; Attending Physician, Thomas Jefferson University Hospital, Philadelphia
Chapter 10

William M. Bourne, M.D.
Assistant Professor, Mayo Medical School; Consultant in Ophthalmology, Mayo Clinic, Rochester, Minnesota
Chapter 19

Bruce J. Busse
Formerly Ophthalmic Photographer, The Abraham Lincoln School of Medicine, and Illinois Eye and Ear Infirmary, Chicago
Chapter 7

Earl A. Choromokos, F.O.P.S.
Assistant Professor of Ophthalmology, University of Cincinnati College of Medicine, Cincinnati, Ohio
Chapter 18

Kenneth W. Christopherson, B.S., C.R.A.
Instructor of Ophthalmology, and Director of Ophthalmic Photography and Diagnostic Services, Cullen Eye Institute, Baylor College of Medicine, Houston, Texas
Chapter 13

David D. Donaldson, M.D.
Associate Professor of Ophthalmology, Harvard Medical School; Surgeon, Massachusetts Eye and Ear Infirmary, Boston
Chapter 12

Reva Hurtes
Librarian, Bascom Palmer Eye Institute, University of Miami School of Medicine, Miami, Florida
Chapter 1

Johnny Justice, Jr., C.R.A., F.O.P.S.
Formerly Assistant Professor, Department of Ophthalmology, Cullen Eye Institute, Baylor College of Medicine, Houston, Texas
Editor; Chapters 2, 3, 4, 6, 16, and 25

Sadao Kanagami
Department of Ophthalmology, Jichi Medical School, Tochigi, Japan; Ophthalmic Photographer and Consultant, Kanto Teishin Hospital, Tokyo, Japan
Chapter 5

Richard A. Levacy, M.D.
Ophthalmologist, Beaumont, Texas
Chapter 6

Csaba L. Martonyi, F.O.P.S.
Assistant Professor of Ophthalmology, The University of Michigan Medical School; Director of Ophthalmic Photography, University of Michigan Hospital, Ann Arbor, Michigan
Chapter 17

Mizuo Matsui, M.D.
Professor of Ophthalmology, Nihon University Medical School; Director, Department of Ophthalmology, Surugadai Hospital, Tokyo, Japan
Chapter 16

Michel Mehu
Chief Ophthalmic Photographer, Albany Medical College of Union University, Albany, New York
Chapter 9

David Mittelman, M.D.
Assistant Professor of Ophthalmology, Loyola University of Chicago Stritch School of Medicine; Director of Pediatric Ophthalmology, Loyola University Medical Center, Maywood, Illinois
Chapter 7

Paul R. Montague
Senior Ophthalmic Photographer, The University of Iowa College of Medicine, Iowa City, Iowa
Chapter 24

Jamie Nicholl, B.F.A., C.R.A.
Ophthalmic Photographer, Wills Eye Hospital, Philadelphia
Chapter 20

Oleg Pomerantzeff, D.Eng.
Senior Scientist and Head, Department of Physics, Eye Research Institute of Retina Foundation, Boston
Chapter 11

Stephen N. Schindler, M.D.
Resident, Cullen Eye Institute, Baylor College of Medicine, Houston, Texas
Chapter 6

Jerry Sewell, B.S.
Assistant Professor of Ophthalmology, Louisiana State University School of Medicine in New Orleans, Louisiana
Chapter 22

Eileen Slipakoff
Senior Fundus Photographer, Department of Ophthalmology, Thomas Jefferson University Hospital, Philadelphia
Chapter 10

Arthur Smialowski, F.R.P.S.
Formerly Director, Bascom Palmer Eye Institute, University of Miami School of Medicine, Miami, Florida
Chapters 8 and 21

Joseph W. Soper, F.C.L.S.A.
Clinical Assistant Professor of Ophthalmology, Baylor College of Medicine; Director, Contact Lens Clinics, Baylor Affiliated Hospitals, Houston, Texas
Chapter 15

Terrance L. Tomer, F.O.P.S.
Director of Diagnostic Photography, Wills Eye Hospital, Philadelphia
Chapter 20

W. A. J. van Heuven, M.D.
Professor, and Head of Retina Division, Department of Ophthalmology, Albany Medical College of Union University, Albany, New York
Chapter 9

Barrett P. Walker, B.S.
Formerly Associate, Department of Ophthalmology, Emory University School of Medicine; Emory University Clinic, Atlanta, Georgia
Chapter 23

Ophthalmic Photography

Evolution of Ophthalmic Photography

R. HURTES

In striving for scientific precision, medicine has always sought accurate methods to document clinically witnessed disease processes. The eye is the only organ in the body that may be precisely examined in situ; because of its accessibility and transparency, pathologic processes as well as normal physiology can be observed in living tissue. The invention of the ophthalmoscope in 1850 and the slit lamp in 1911 brought ophthalmology to the level of an exact science by providing a unique opportunity for clinical observation beyond all other branches of medicine.

It seems strange that the eye should be compared so often to a camera when it was the eye that sparked the imagination for the development of the camera. Christopher Scheiner, a German Jesuit, proved in 1625 that the eye forms images directly from light. He removed the opaque sclera from the back of an animal eye, held the eye in front of his own, and pointed it at an object. To his delight, the inverted image of the object was visibly projected onto the retina of the animal eye. Actually, Father Scheiner had only confirmed the proposal made by Leonardo da Vinci a century earlier. Leonardo demonstrated his theory of how the eye sees by using two adjacent rooms, one well lighted and the other dark. He made a tiny hole in the wall between the rooms and, while standing in the dark room, held a piece of paper close to the small aperture. When the paper was adjusted to the proper distance from the hole, inverted images of objects in the lighted room were projected onto the paper. Leonardo did not invent the *camera obscura,* but he was the first to understand its principles and their relationship to the eye.

The seventeenth century was a creative period in the field of optics, and many studies were made of animal and human eyes. During this period, Lippershey invented the telescope and Galileo refined it. Another very important development was the formulation of the laws of refraction by thinkers such as Snell, Descartes, Hooke, and Newton. From these foundations, photography was to grow almost two centuries later.

Photography was born in 1826 when Nicéphore Nièpce photographed a sunlit garden from his window in Gras, France. The expo-

I would like to express my appreciation to Dr. Edward W. D. Norton, Dr. Joel Glaser, Mr. Jean-Marie Parel, and Miss Rose Beck for reading this chapter and offering suggestions for improvement, and to Mr. Joseph Goren for reproducing the figures.

sure time required for this first photograph was 8 hours! Thus it was proved that light images could be recorded and kept permanently.

Since 1888, when George Eastman developed his "everyman's camera," the Kodak, photography has become a means of documentation in which almost everyone can participate. However, not until 1889, when Eastman developed flexible film to replace the cumbersome glass plates, did photography become an increasingly popular and professional phenomenon. The age of tripods, portable darkrooms, and technical magic was gone, and the age of instant reproduction had arrived.

Since Eastman's time, every new camera has further freed the photographer to concentrate on the subject rather than on photographic techniques, and the act of taking pictures has become swifter and simpler. In ophthalmology, improved and simplified methods of calibration and technique have enabled accurate comparison between photographs taken at different sittings. Thus, photography and ophthalmology joined hands, and a solid union was created.

Fundus Photography

Since the day that physicians could first see into the back of the living eye, attempts have been made to document their observations accurately with elaborate drawings. The details of these drawings were painstakingly obtained through a laborious process for the artist and a fatiguing ordeal for the patient; however, some magnificent works were created. For instance, one should look at the beautiful atlases of Liebrecht [36] and Oeller [48], who painted on canvas with oils to obtain likenesses of their observations as seen through the magic window of the ophthalmoscope. (An interesting footnote is that Liebrecht eventually gave up ophthalmology to devote himself to painting.)

In 1907, Dimmer published the first textbook of fundus photographs (Fig. 1-1), and after his death his student, Pillat, published an atlas [15]. This volume was followed by Bedell's book [4] in 1929, which was the first English-language atlas to contain photographs and the first demonstration of stereophotographs.

Good fundus photographs were difficult to obtain since large portions of the fundus were obscured by the reflexes from ocular tissues caused by the lamp used for exposure of the film. Jackman and Webster [31] took the first human fundus photograph in 1886; however, the optic nerve appeared as an irregular blotch and the arteries and veins were not visible.

Using his own method of photography, Howe [29] in 1887 documented a fundus photograph in which the disc was perfectly distinct and the vessels were so clear that arteries could be distinguished from veins. He described the difficulties encountered in taking the picture

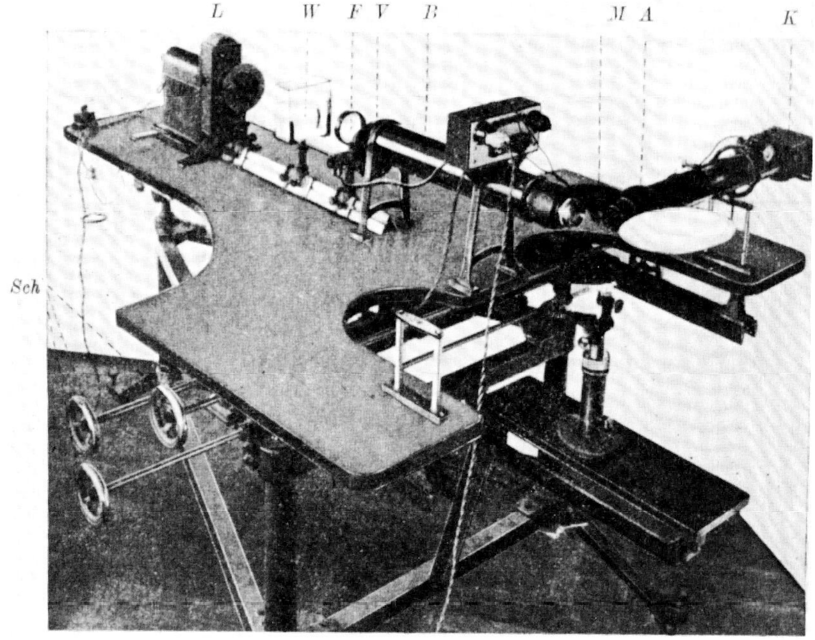

Fig. 1-1. Dimmer's fundus camera. L = *light source;* W = *water cooling system;* F = *fixation point;* V = *shutter apparatus;* B = *illumination system;* M = *metal mirror;* A = *observation system;* K = *camera;* Sch = *knobs to move table.* (*Condensing lens not shown.*) (*From F. Dimmer and A. Pillat,* Atlas photographischer Bilder des Menschlichen Augenhintergrundes. *Leipzig: F. Deuticke, 1927.*)

and the manner in which these difficulties were overcome. First, there was the problem of photographing the red reflection. The plate was made sensitive by an elaborate treatment with the following solution: "erythrosine, 1.5 drachm; ammonia (88°), 1 drachm; alcohol, 6 ounces; nitrate of silver, 1 drachm. Converted into chloride with hypochloric acid, thoroughly washed, and redissolved in ammonia."

The second problem was finding the proper means of projecting the fundus onto the plate with the camera placed in front of the eye. Howe found that the demonstration ophthalmoscope, which enabled two observers to view the fundus simultaneously, was inadequate. He conducted many experiments using lenses of different powers, various sized apertures in concave mirrors, a variety of camera lenses, and daylight and artificial light. He finally adopted the procedure of placing an ordinary Argand gas burner (a lamp with a tubular wick that admits a current of air inside as well as outside the flame) in the focal point (13 inches) of a concave mirror that had an aperture of about 1/2 inch. The light reflected from the mirror passed through a planoconvex lens with a focal distance of about 1/2 inch, and an alum cell was interposed in the line of the ray to protect the patient's eye from the heat. The final difficulty was keeping the patient's eye comfortable when it was exposed to the glare and heat of the lamp; this Howe did with topical cocaine.

Although these procedures were adequate, successful fundus photographs as we know them today were possible only after the invention of the reflexless ophthalmoscope by Thorner in 1899 [57] and its perfection by Gullstrand in 1910 [25]. The success of good photography also depended on the development of a proper light source, one that would give good illumination and also be comfortable to the patient. Nordenson, with the help of Zeiss (Fig. 1-2), modified Gullstrand's ophthalmoscope and developed a fundus camera that used a carbon light source [43, 44]. The general principle of this camera was the basis for all subsequent instruments.

Hartinger, in 1930, replaced the carbon arc light source with a high-intensity incandescent lamp; later, in 1936, he developed the reflexless ophthalmoscopic lens with a small black dot in the middle [28]. In 1953, Hansell and Beeson [26] described a xenon arc tube with which excellent color photographs of the retina could be made. Around that time, Ogle and Rucker [49] made an important contribution to fundus photography with the incorporation of their electronic flash, which was developed at about the same time as the xenon light source. Drews [19] further perfected the electronic flash in 1957. Donaldson [17], with the help of Edgerton, perfected in 1964 a special flashtube for use in his stereocamera which emitted light from the end of the tube, thus allowing greater intrinsic brilliance.

In the earliest years of fundus photography, a major problem (besides the reflexes from light sources and from the eye itself) was movement of the patient's eye during film exposure. Exposure times had vastly decreased from the 8 hours that Nièpce needed to photograph his garden, but even a time of several seconds was too long. Technical advances in light sources; tremendous improvements in film quality, developing techniques, and filter efficiency; and the reduction of exposure time to milliseconds vastly improved the quality of photography. Beginning with Dimmer, who worked for 10 years perfecting his technique, scores of investigators have improved and simplified the procedure for fundus photography.

Until 1972, only a small area (about 30 degrees) of the fundus could be photographed on a single exposure; larger areas were documented by photographing overlapping fields of the fundus and piecing these pictures together to form a mosaic of the larger area. However,

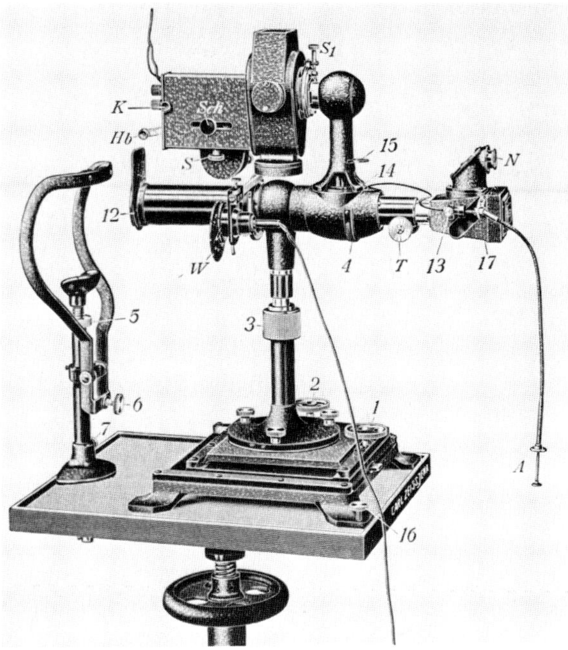

Fig. 1-2. Zeiss-Nordenson fundus camera. (From H. Hartinger, Ein neue reflexfreie Ophthalmoskoplinse für die Zeiss-Nordensonsche Netzhautkammer. Z. Ophthalmol. Optik. *24 : 137, 1936.*)

exciting work may make it possible to photograph the entire retina on one exposure by means of a Japanese-designed optical fiber system placed in a circular fashion into a corneal contact lens. This technique illuminates the entire retina and allows reflection-free observation [51].

Fundus Cinematography

In 1934, Lijo Pavia [37] substituted a motion picture camera for the plateholder in the Nordenson camera and successfully recorded the pulsations of the retinal vessels. Bailey and Swan [3], in 1959, described a simple, practical camera that eliminated the high concentration of light formerly required for cinematography. It consisted of three units: (1) a mounted +20 D condensing lens such as that used in indirect ophthalmoscopy; (2) a paraxial illumination system with a device for changing magnification (the body of a Zeiss dissecting microscope); and (3) the 16-mm Arriflex camera, containing a through-the-lens continuous focusing device. This camera permitted the detection of vessel changes that were not discernible with ordinary direct ophthalmoscopy or with serial single-frame photographs.

Fluorescein Angiographic Photography

A major contribution to the field of fundus photography was that of Novotny and Alvis [47] who, as medical students, published their findings on retinal circulation following injection of a dye. Theirs was not a new concept; Flocks and colleagues had experimented with this technique by injecting trypan blue into the intracarotid arteries of cats. They later documented these findings with cinematography after injecting 2 cc of 10% fluorescein into the femoral vein of a cat [22]. They used a cobalt blue filter and 16-mm daylight Super Anscochrome film processed at an emulsion speed of 100.

Novotny and Alvis injected a bolus of 5 ml of 20% sodium fluorescein into the cubital vein of a human; within a few seconds the dye had circulated through the blood vessels of the retina. Permanent photographic records could now be made of the circulation of blood through vessels in normal and diseased eyes.

For this type of photography, the camera is equipped with two special filters [33], one to allow as much blue-exciting light as possible to reach the fundus by filtering out the green yellow light and another to eliminate the reflected blue-exciting light and, at the same time, allow the passage of the fluorescent light. Ideally, only the fluorescent light from within the retinal and choroidal vessels should reach the film.

Fluorescein angiography has contributed tremendously to our understanding of disease in the ocular fundus; moreover, it has added a new dimension to our understanding of the eye. We are now able to study the physiologic processes of the eye and to correlate new observations with anatomic knowledge. Over the past 15 years, this technique has forced physicians to observe the fundus more carefully than ever and therefore has contributed greatly to our understanding of the normal and diseased retina. Thus angiography has become an important tool for ophthalmologists through the medium of the camera.

Television Ophthalmoscopy

One of the newer developments in ophthalmic photography is the use of television for projecting ophthalmoscopic pictures of the eye [11]. Among the many advances in this area is a device for taping fluorescein angiograms in which a miniaturized television camera, a beam-splitter, and an optical relay are utilized in conjunction with the Zeiss retinal camera [59].

Stereoscopic Fundus Photography

Stereoscopic fundus photography has been attempted since 1909, when Thorner first tried to take two photographs through opposite halves of the pupil by inverting the camera [58] (Fig. 1-3). Many investigators have made an effort to obtain good stereographs, some by moving the

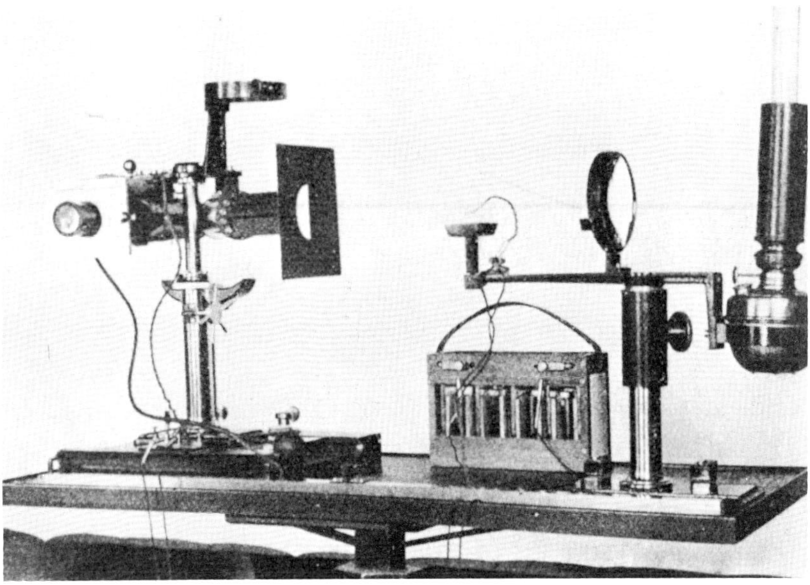

Fig. 1-3. Thorner's stereoscopic fundus camera. (From D. D. Donaldson, A new camera for stereoscopic fundus photography. Trans. Am. Ophthalmol. *62 : 429, 1964.)*

patient's eye very slightly between exposures [45], and others by moving the camera while the eye remained fixated [4] (Fig. 1-4).

Krakau [34] fitted his camera with appropriate prismatic devices for the photographic registration of depth. Allen [1] designed a system in which a cornea-induced parallax was utilized; the camera was directed through one side of a well-dilated pupil for the first exposure and, without any angulation, was moved to a parallel position on the other side of the pupil for the second exposure. The device could be positioned to shift the optical axis of the camera either horizontally or vertically. As is the case with many innovations, Allen's separator was mechanized by Parel and colleagues [50] and by Allen [7] at about the same time independently of each other. Parel's retinal camera consisted of an automatic filter-changing device, a data recording system synchronized with the dye injection and displayed on the film format separately from the fundus image, and the automated stereo system based on Allen's separator. The Allen separator is the basis for today's stereoscopic camera.

Regardless of the efficiency of Allen's technique, however, one must realize that it is still a serial, albeit instantaneous, procedure. In true stereoscopic photography, both views should be recorded simultaneously. To my knowledge, the only person to construct such a camera

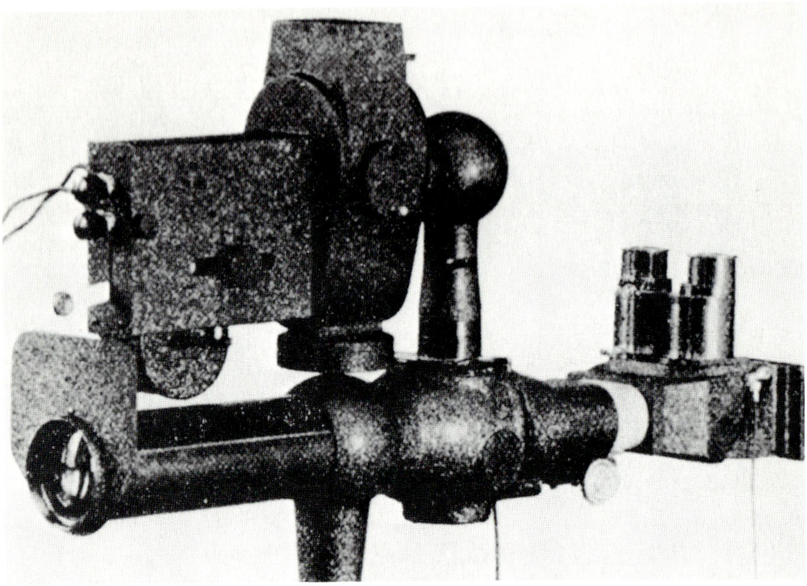

Fig. 1-4. Nordenson's stereoscopic fundus camera with binocular eyepieces. (From D. D. Donaldson, A new camera for stereoscopic fundus photography. Trans. Am. Ophthalmol. *62 : 429, 1964.*)

was Dr. Donaldson [17], who developed in 1964 an instrument based on the principles of indirect ophthalmoscopy (Fig. 1-5). To describe it simply, this camera integrated two fundus cameras using the same primary aspheric objective to take simultaneous photographs, and it incorporated a new electronic flash that provided adequate illumination for 35-mm color film. Binocular fundus images were seen while focusing. The camera was speedy and easy to operate, and the resulting stereogram was free of distortion and had a high degree of definition. The depth effect was absolutely reproducible.

Others have attempted to devise improved stereoscopic techniques. Mikuni and Yaoeda [42] developed a rapid system for taking serial photographs using the Allen separator. Saheb and coworkers [52] constructed a twin prism, mounted on the camera objective to reduce error between exposures, which took instantaneous stereophotographs with constant separation of images. However, this system created certain distortions (as one would expect when light is passed through a prism) and also required an 8-mm pupillary diameter, which would present a distinct obstacle in many patients.

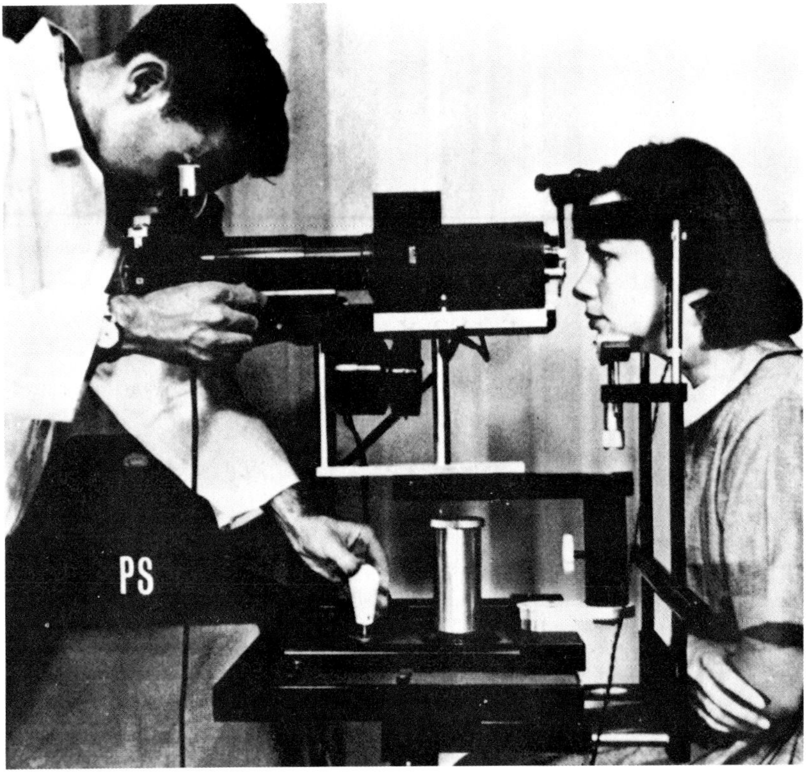

Fig. 1-5. Donaldson's stereoscopic fundus camera. (From D. D. Donaldson, A new camera for stereoscopic fundus photography. Trans. Am. Ophthalmol. *62 : 429, 1964.)*

Photogrammetry

One of the newest and most promising areas of ophthalmic photography is the technique known as *photogrammetry* [9], the art of obtaining reliable measurements by means of photography. The basic concept of this procedure is that if a subject can be photographed, then a method can be found to determine the size, shape, position, and altitude of this subject on the exposed film.

The techniques of photogrammetry developed from a union of several disciplines: photography, surveying, and aviation. Originally, it was used for mapping the surfaces of the earth. The principle of the method is the reconstruction of a three-dimensional model from stereo pairs of photographs and the measurement of certain points on this model. Mikuni and Yaoeda [42] published their method of mathematically plotting the elevations of the optic disc and then constructing a contour map from which a plastic model was made. Crock and Parel [10] utilized this theory employing aerial photogrammetry and an analytic plotter computer.

Photogrammetry has permitted the analysis of disease processes such as papilledema, early disc atrophy and cupping, and tumor growth; it makes possible in-depth, accurate measurement of changes in the volume and surface of the fundus structures. Before this development, fluorescein angiography contributed greatly to our understanding of fundus diseases at a descriptive and qualitative level; with photogrammetry, the information can be analyzed quantitatively. The technique is still in its infancy, and certain problems remain to be solved, such as the high cost of computer time required to analyze the stereophotographs and the means of obtaining good simultaneous stereoscopic photographs.

External Photography

External photographic examination of the eye has been popular since 1900, when Drüner first reported his procedures using routine photography [20]. Later technical improvements and better camera design made color photography possible. Brilliant lighting (flash) made it possible to take rapid photographs on ultrarapid film, thus eliminating defects caused by movement. Drüner described a stereocamera in his paper published in 1900, and later investigators reported several other cameras of this type; Donaldson perfected the technique in 1954 with his camera [16], and Matsui and coworkers further improved on it in 1973 [41].

Cinematography is another valuable means of documenting changes in the external part of the eye, such as circulation of blood in the conjunctival vessels or the flow in the aqueous veins. Motion picture recordings of nystagmus, ocular motor palsies, and other abnormal eye movements and gaze positions have been a boon to teaching services.

Fluorescein angiography of the anterior segment, introduced by Jensen and Lundbaek in 1968 [32], was improved on by many others, most recently by Matsui and coworkers [40, 41]. It was still another technique for documenting the blood circulation in the anterior portion of the eye as well as changes in pathologic processes such as tumors, iris atrophies, and diabetes.

In documenting corneal changes, the objective method of taking keratographs is most helpful in recording changes in patients with keratoconus or changes that occur after corneal transplantation. For this type of photography, a retroilluminated target of concentric rings is placed in front of the cornea and the reflected image is recorded by a fixed-focus camera with the lens mounted at the center of the target [2, 27], (Fig. 1-6).

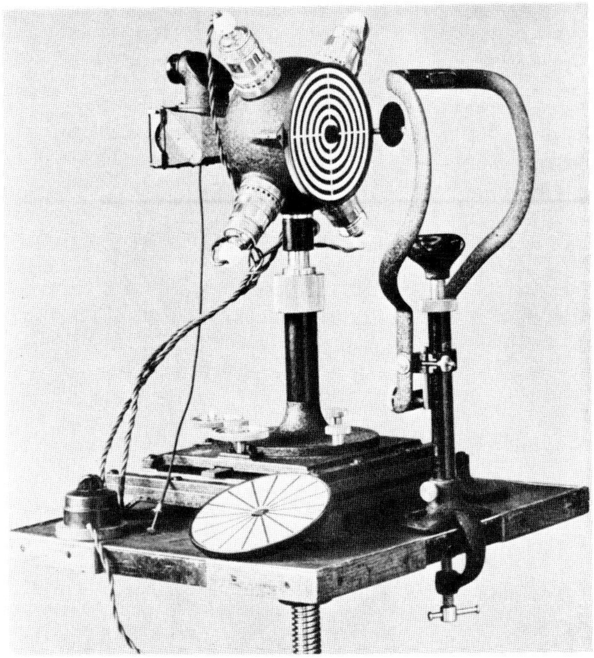

Fig. 1-6. Keratographic camera setup. (From H. Hartinger, Ein neues photokeratoskop. Ber. Dtsch. Ophthalmol. Ges. *48 : 360, 1930.)*

Slit-Lamp Photography

Photography using the beam of the slit lamp was not very successful initially, since the use of this instrument essentially involves a kinetic procedure in which the observer constantly adjusts the focus of the illuminating beam and of the microscope to obtain an in-depth, composite view of the ocular tissues. Thiel [55] met with some success in 1930 (Fig. 1-7), and Sysi [54] in 1949 incorporated a small camera in one of the objectives of the microscope, which allowed a high degree of accuracy (Fig. 1-8).

Finally, Goldmann [24] introduced in 1940 the most satisfactory arrangement, consisting of a camera that moved forward along the extended optical axis of the eye during exposure of the film and worked constantly in association with the slit lamp so that the image of the slit remained in the central field of the camera and in focus with the lens of the camera. Pictures thus obtained gave a sharp optical section through the cornea and the lens.

Many other investigators have further improved Goldmann's technique. Brent used a Leica with 35-mm Ektachrome film and a Haag-

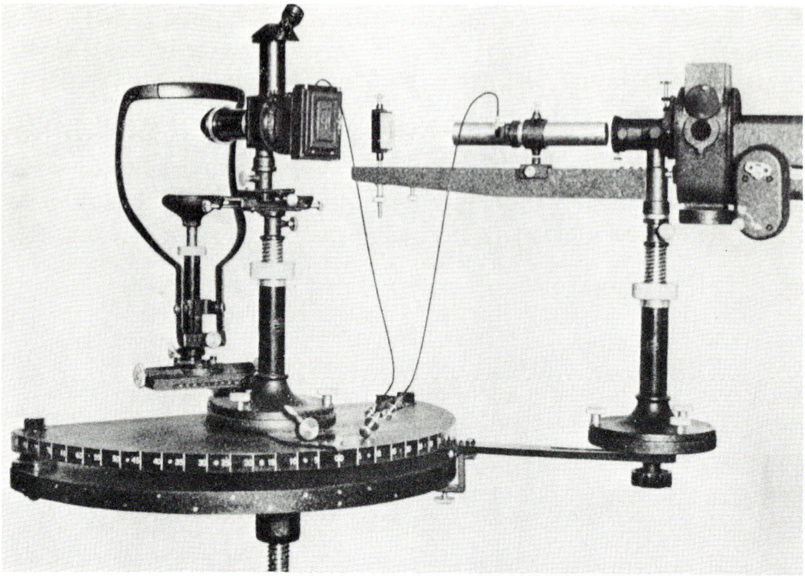

Fig. 1-7. Thiel's slit-lamp camera setup. (From R. Thiel, Photographierte Spaltlampenbilder. Ber. Dtsch. Ophthalmol. Ges. *48 : 355, 1930.*)

Streit slit lamp equipped with a special transformer. Norton [16] converted the slit lamp into a permanent stereocamera, and Zeiss and Nikon developed the photo slit lamp for photographing the slit-lamp beam as well as for standard external photography. The manufacture of the photo slit lamp by Carl Zeiss in 1965 made possible faithful color photography of ocular structures and lesions using all forms of slit-lamp illumination—diffuse, indirect, scleral scatter, retroillumination, and focal illumination with wide and narrow slits. The slit lamp can now be used for both external and fundus photography.

Goniophotography

Goniophotography, photography of the angle of the anterior chamber, was introduced in 1927 by Thorburn, who used a stereocamera equipped with Gullstrand's Pointolite lamp [56]. He was able to obtain only 1.7× magnification, and the exposure time was 3 to 4 seconds! Castroviejo made the procedure more practical in 1935 [8] by using a Leitz Ultrapak microscope with a 3.8 objective and a No. 4 ocular attached to a Leica camera equipped with Panchromatic film. The illuminating lamp was 3½ watts with a straight filament, and the exposure time was 1/20 of a second. Castroviejo was able to get accurate photographs with this equipment, but the structural details were still not clear.

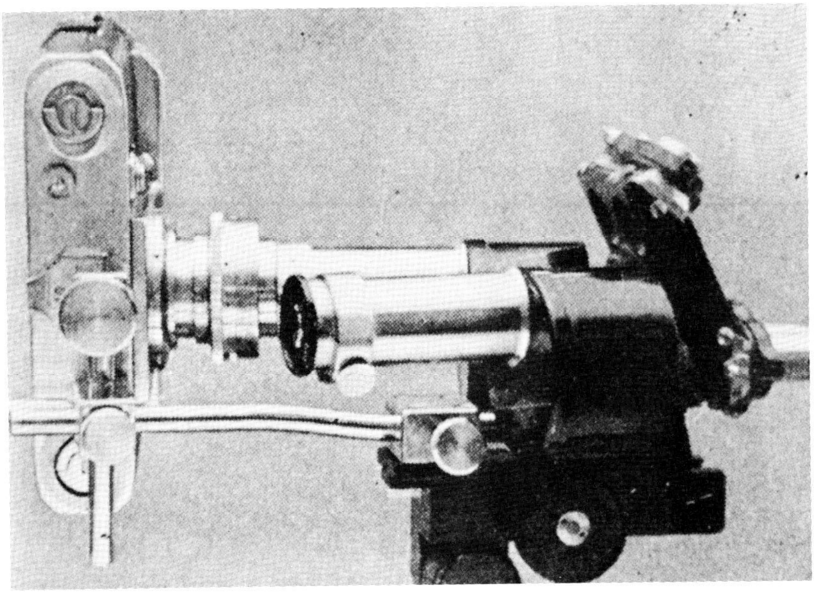

Fig. 1-8. Sysi's slit-lamp camera setup. (From R. Sysi, A simple device supplementary to the slit lamp to photograph parts of the eye. Acta Ophthalmol. *27 : 403, 1949.)*

Sloan and Lichter simplified this procedure using a Koeppe lens, a Heine gonioscope, and a Kowa RC fundus camera with a +8 lens held in front of the viewing system [53]. In 1954, Donaldson reported his technique for stereogoniophotography [16].

Transillumination

The technique of transillumination is well known for diagnosing tumors and detecting subtle clinical abnormalities. Opacities of the eye can be recorded this way, using photography combined with photometry. Goldmann modified his technique to record photometric readings. Dekking employed transillumination as early as 1936 and perfected it in 1948 [14].

For this procedure, the eye is illuminated by a pencil of light, and the image of the cornea or lens is formed in the focal plane of an ocular, where it is thrown onto a photometric field. The brightness of this field can be varied and made to equal the brightness of the image of the structure to be measured. The optical density of the opacity can then be read on the photometer scale. Photographing opacities in the transparent media of the eye as seen against the fundus glow caused by axial illumination was evolved by Douvas and Allen in 1950 [18].

Fincham, in 1955, developed an apparatus consisting of a beam of light directed centrally on a pellicle of optically worked glass which acted as a transparent mirror, while a camera mounted in direct alignment with the eye produced a magnified image of the whole area [21].

Lenticular opacities were similarly recorded by Lubkin with a fundus camera focused at the plane of the lens [39]. Lichter, in 1972, used fiber optic illumination together with a modified Kowa RC 2 fundus camera to obtain photographs of subtle clinical findings such as anterior segment pigment dispersions [35].

Photography with Different Wavelengths of Light

Infrared photography, first introduced by Dekking [13], permits pictures to be taken through opaque media, for instance, corneal opacities. The longer rays of light penetrate such opacities, providing pictures of the iris and the pupil that are invisible to ordinary illumination. This procedure also accentuates pigmentary changes of the iris and permits the pupillary aperture to be photographed in darkness.

Dallow and McMeel [12] recently used an infrared photographic technique to penetrate vitreous and retinal opacities such as hemorrhages and neovascular tissue. With this technique, they could visualize the choroidal vasculature, the optic disc, and the retinal vessels.

Another technique employed red-free light to visualize fundus details not observable with ordinary light. Hoyt and coworkers [30] adapted Voyt's system of direct ophthalmoscopy with special illumination in which the longer red wavelengths were filtered from the white light emitted from a carbon arc. Hoyt used a Zeiss fundus camera equipped with a No. 65 Wratten green filter and Kodak Plus-X film. This technique made subtle nerve fiber layer changes visible and, for the first time, accessible to objective morphologic analysis.

Still another fundus photographic technique in which light from the visible spectrum is employed is called *spectral reflectance photography* [5]. Spectral reflectance refers to the percentage of light reflected from a structure in a given special region. The camera is equipped with interference filters, which differ from absorption filters in reflecting back all wavelengths except those they are designed to transmit. Using this technique, one can visualize details in the fundus that would not be visible to ordinary white light.

Pupillography

Another photographic aid, first advocated by Bellarminoff [6] in 1885, utilized a slit method for recording pupillary movements. To obtain the normal pupil size, however, ordinary light must be used and the exposure time must be short enough to fall within the latent period of the pupillary light reflex. Fuchs [23] first reported in 1903 an apparatus in which the aperture of the camera and the light were controlled and synchronized. The complications of stimulating pupillary contraction by visible light could also be overcome with infrared light. Bellarminoff was the first to employ cinematography of pupillary movements (the pupillogram), but Lowenstein and Loewenfeld [38] developed an improved and efficient technique, and their vast contributions to our understanding of the pupil and of the lesions affecting it are legendary and universally acclaimed.

Conclusion

In 1968, Johnny Justice, Jr. originated the idea of an international society of ophthalmic photographers. In 1969, the Ophthalmic Photographers' Society, which currently has more than 500 members, was founded. As its charter states, "Its members are dedicated to serving ophthalmology out of which this major photographic specialty has grown, and to contributing their talents and expertise to the preservation and enhancement of vision."

The camera has become one of the indispensable tools for the diagnosis and documentation of eye diseases. Through the years, simpler and less expensive photographic techniques have been investigated and reported, and more and more ophthalmologists are equipping their offices with these photographic systems. This is hardly the end of the evolution of ophthalmic photography; many improvements remain to be developed and techniques refined. Nevertheless, a cycle has been completed. The camera exists because men were intrigued by the function of the eye and wished to be able to reproduce on a permanent record that which the eye enabled the brain to record. How appropriate then that ophthalmology has turned the camera into a valuable tool for recording the structures of the eye.

References

1. Allen, L. Ocular fundus photography: Suggestions for achieving consistently good pictures and instructions for stereoscopic photography. *Am. J. Ophthalmol.* 57 : 13, 1964.
2. Amsler, M. Über Photokeratoskopie. *Ber. Dtsch. Ophthalmol. Ges.* 48 : 202, 1930.
3. Bailey, P., Jr., and Swan, K. C. Cinematography of human retinal vessels: A practical clinical and research technique. *J.A.M.A.* 170 : 1373, 1959.
4. Bedell, A. J. *Photographs of the Fundus Oculi.* Philadelphia: Davis, 1929.
5. Behrendt, T., and Wilson, L. A. Spectral reflectance photography of the retina. *Am. J. Ophthalmol.* 59 : 1079, 1965.
6. Bellarminoff, L. Anwendung der graphischen Methode bei Untersuchung der Pupillenbewegungen: Photocoreograph. *Pflügers Arch.* 37 : 107, 1885.
7. Blodi, F. C., Allen, L., and Frazier, O. *Stereoscopic Manual of the Ocular Fundus in Local and Systemic Disease.* St. Louis: Mosby, 1970. Vol. 2, p. 1.

8. Castroviejo, R. Goniophotography of the angle of the anterior chamber in living animals and human subjects. *Am. J. Ophthalmol.* 18 : 524, 1935.
9. Crock, G. Stereotechnology in medicine. *Trans. Ophthalmol. Soc. U.K.* 90 : 577, 1970.
10. Crock, G., and Parel, J-M. Stereophotogrammetry of fluorescein angiographs in ocular biometrics. *Med. J. Aust.* 2 : 586, 1969.
11. Dallow, R. L. *Television Ophthalmoscopy: Instrumentation and Medical Applications.* Springfield, Ill.: Thomas, 1970.
12. Dallow, R. L., and McMeel, J. W. Penetration of retinal and vitreous opacities in diabetic retinopathy: Use of infrared fundus photography. *Arch. Ophthalmol.* 92 : 531, 1974.
13. Dekking, H. M. Infrarot-Photographie des Auges. *Graefe Arch. Ophthalmol.* 130 : 373, 1933.
14. Dekking, H. M. Opacity meter for cornea and lens. *Ophthalmologica* 115 : 219, 1948.
15. Dimmer, F., and Pillat, A. *Atlas Photographischer Bilder des Menschlichen Augenhintergrundes.* Leipzig: F. Deuticke, 1927.
16. Donaldson, D. D. A new camera for medical stereophotography with special reference to the eye. *Arch. Ophthalmol.* 52 : 564, 1954.
17. Donaldson, D. D. A new camera for stereoscopic fundus photography. *Trans. Am. Ophthalmol. Soc.* 62 : 429, 1964.
18. Douvas, N., and Allen, L. Anterior-segment photography with the Nordenson retinal camera. *Am. J. Ophthalmol.* 33 : 291, 1950.
19. Drews, R. C. Fundus photography by electronic flash: I–IV. *Am. J. Ophthalmol.* 44 : 170; 356; 522; 633, 1957.
20. Drüner, L. Über Mikrosteropsie und eine neue vergrössernde Stereoskopcamera. *Z. Wissensch. Mikros.* 17 : 281, 1900.
21. Fincham, E. F. Photographic recording of opacities of the ocular media. *Br. J. Ophthalmol.* 39 : 85, 1955.
22. Flocks, M., Miller, J., and Chao, P. Retinal circulation time with the aid of fundus cinematography. *Am. J. Ophthalmol.* 48(2) : 8, 1959.
23. Fuchs, A. Die Messung der Pupillengrösse und Zeitbestimmung der Lichtreaktion der Pupillen bei einzelnen Psychosen und Nervenkrankheiten. *Jahrb. F. Psychiat. Neurol.* 24 : 326, 1903.
24. Goldmann, H. Spaltlampenphotographie und Photometrie. *Ophthalmologica* 98 : 257, 1940.
25. Gullstrand, A. Neue Methoden der reflexlosen Ophthalmoskopie. *Ber. Dtsch. Ophthalmol. Ges.* 36 : 75, 1910.
26. Hansell, P., and Beeson, E. J. G. Retinal photography in colour. *Br. J. Ophthalmol.* 37 : 65, 1953.
27. Hartinger, H. Ein neues Photokeratoskop. *Ber. Dtsch. Ophthalmol. Ges.* 48 : 360, 1930.
28. Hartinger, H. Ein neue reflexfreie Ophthalmoskoplinse für die Zeiss-Nordensonsche Netzhautkammer. *Z. Ophthalmol. Optik* 24 : 137, 1936.
29. Howe, L. Photography of the interior of the eye. *Trans. Am. Ophthalmol. Soc.* 4 : 568, 1885–1887.
30. Hoyt, W. F., et al. Homonymous hemioptic hypoplasia: Fundoscopic features in standard and red-free illumination in three patients with congenital hemiplegia. *Br. J. Ophthalmol.* 56 : 537, 1972.
31. Jackman, W. T., and Webster, J. D. On photographing the retina of the living human eye. *Phil. Photographer* 23 : 275, 1886.
32. Jensen, V. A., and Lundbaek, K. Fluorescence angiography of the iris in recent and long-term diabetics. *Acta Ophthalmol.* 46 : 584, 1968.

33. Justice, J., Jr., and Sever, R. J. Technique of Fluorescein Fundus Photography. In J. L. Smith (Ed.), *Neuroophthalmology Symposium of the University of Miami and the Bascom Palmer Eye Institute.* St. Louis: Mosby, 1965. Vol. 2, p. 82.
34. Krakau, C. E. T. Papillary protrusion measurements by means of stereophotographs of the fundus. *Acta Ophthalmol.* 34 : 140, 1956.
35. Lichter, P. R. Transillumination photography of the eye. *Am. J. Ophthalmol.* 73 : 927, 1972.
36. Liebrecht, R. L.. *Atlas der Ophthalmoscopie.* Berlin: Hirschwald, 1863.
37. Lijo Pavia, J. L. Fondo de ojo. Su cinematografia cineretinografia. Nuevas adquisiciones como documentacion clinica. *Rev. Otoneurooftal.* 9 : 325, 1934.
38. Lowenstein, O., and Loewenfeld, I. E. Electronic pupillography: A new instrument and some clinical applications. *Arch. Ophthalmol.* 59 : 352, 1958.
39. Lubkin, V. Photography of the red reflex. *Arch. Ophthalmol.* 43 : 718, 1950.
40. Matsui, M., et al. Some improved methods of anterior segment fluorescein angiography: Basic system. *Am. J. Ophthalmol.* 74 : 1075, 1972.
41. Matsui, M., et al. Some improved methods of anterior segment fluorescein angiography: II. Simultaneous photographic system. *Am. J. Ophthalmol.* 76 : 54, 1973.
42. Mikuni, M., and Yaoeda, H. Measurement of elevation of fundus by means of stereophotography. *Acta Soc. Ophthalmol. Jpn.* 71 : 389, 1967.
43. Nordenson, J. W. Om centrisk Fotografering au Ogonbottnen. *Hygea* 77 : 1538, 1915.
44. Nordenson, J. W. Augenkamera zum stationären Ophthalmoskop von Gullstrand. *Ber. Dtsch. Ophthalmol. Ges.* 45 : 278, 1925.
45. Nordenson, J. W. Stereoskopische Ophthalmographie durch einfache Aufnahmen. *Ups. Läk Forh.* 32 : 295, 1927.
46. Norton, H. J. Absolute stereophotography of the slit-lamp optical section. *Am. J. Ophthalmol.* 58 : 797, 1964.
47. Novotny, H. R., and Alvis, D. L. A method of photographing fluorescence in circulating blood of the human retina. *Circulation* 24 : 82, 1961.
48. Oeller, J. N. *Atlas of Ophthalmoscopy.* Translated by A. H. Knapp. Wiesbaden: Bergmann, 1896–1899.
49. Ogle, K. N., and Rucker, C. W. Fundus photographs in color using a high-speed flash tube in the Zeiss retinal camera. *Arch. Ophthalmol.* 49 : 435, 1953.
50. Parel, J-M., et al. Automatic retinal camera for fluorescein angiography. *Med. J. Aust.* 1 : 291, 1968.
51. Pomerantzeff, O., and Schepens, C. L. Wide-Angle Camera. In R. C. Pruett, et al. (Eds.), *Retina Congress, Boston, 1972.* New York: Appleton-Century-Crofts, 1974. P. 115.
52. Saheb, N. E., et al. The use of photogrammetry in evaluating the cup of the optic nerve head for a study in chronic simple glaucoma. *Can. J. Ophthalmol.* 7 : 466, 1972.
53. Sloan, D. B., and Lichter, R. P. Simplified goniophotography. *Am. J. Ophthalmol.* 63 : 1801, 1967.
54. Sysi, R. A simple device supplementary to the slit lamp to photograph parts of the eye. *Acta Ophthalmol.* 27 : 403, 1949.

55. Thiel, R. Photographierte Spaltlampenbilder. *Ber. Dtsch. Ophthalmol. Ges.* 48 : 355, 1930.
56. Thorburn, T. A gonioscopical study of anterior peripheral synechiae in primary glaucoma. *Svensk. Läk. Handl.* 53 : 252; 273, 1927.
57. Thorner, W. A new stationary ophthalmoscope without reflexes. Translated by C. Barck. *Am. J. Ophthalmol.* 16 : 330; 376, 1899.
58. Thorner, W. Die stereoskopische Photographie des Augenhintergrundes. *Klin. Monatsbl. Augenheilkd.* 47(1) : 481, 1909.
59. Yuhasz, A., et al. A new apparatus for video tape recording of fluorescein angiograms. *Arch. Ophthalmol.* 90 : 481, 1973.

2

Ocular Fundus Photography

JOHNNY JUSTICE, JR.

Ocular fundus photography as a clinical aid in the documentation of intraocular diseases has been available since the early part of this century. Since that time, ocular fundus photography has evolved quietly but steadily, primarily through the efforts of Bedell [2], Allen [1], and others [3, 4]. Improved cameras, better films, stereo techniques, and fluorescein angiography have advanced the fundus photograph beyond its documentary role to that of a frequently vital pretherapeutic and posttherapeutic procedure. Thus, with the increasing significance of fundus photography in ophthalmologic care, the importance of instrumentation technology and technique deserves special emphasis. In this chapter, I will discuss the fundus photographer, equipment, care and maintenance of equipment, methodology, artifacts of illumination, stereo fundus photography, film, and processing procedures.

The Fundus Photographer

Fundus photography is now sufficiently specialized to require the full-time concentration of the photographer. A background in photography is important but is not a prerequisite for choosing this occupation. While gaining technical skills, the photographer must also develop familiarity with the clinical pathology of the fundus. The performance of technical duties relates directly to the photographer's understanding of the lesions examined and the ways in which their special peculiarities can be shown photographically. The growth and significance of an ophthalmic photography laboratory depend heavily not only on the skill but, more importantly, on the interest and enthusiasm of the photographer. Many ophthalmologists perform their own fundus photography; however, despite the ophthalmologist's interest in recording and further defining disorders of the retina and choroid, a photographer is usually responsible for the excellence of this service.

Equipment Available for Fundus Photography and Fluorescein Angiography

Several instruments are currently available for fundus photography and fluorescein angiography. I have had the opportunity to use most of them and will attempt to evaluate them in regard to both engineering and, more importantly, the quality of the photographs produced.

Grateful acknowledgment is extended to Carol P. Justice and Ann Bryant, who helped with the manuscript; and to Ditte Jacobsen, who assisted in the preparation of the illustrations for this chapter.

1. The Canon CR-60 Z is a zoom optics fundus camera with the angle of view variable from 20 to 60 degrees. The quality of the optics is excellent. Mechanically, it is rather difficult to operate, but the instrument's major shortcoming is that to obtain uniformly illuminated fundus photographs with a pupil size less than 6 mm is practically impossible.
2. The new Kowa RC-XV is the most exciting fundus camera developed in some time. This instrument was designed by Sadao Kanagami, one of the most experienced ophthalmic photographers in the world. This instrument and the new Kowa Photo Slit Lamp ASL-6 are explained in detail in Chapter 5. It would appear that Kowa has taken the lead in the production of quality instruments for photography in ophthalmology while maintaining reasonable prices.
3. The Nikon Retinapan 45 II has quality optics, and it is possible to vary the magnification from 20 to 45 degrees, although certainly not with the ease that the Canon, Kowa, and Topcon variable magnification instruments permit. Mechanically, it is difficult to operate.
4. The Topcon fundus cameras consist of four different models, the TRC-Fe, the TRC-FE 3, the TRC-FET, and the TRC-WT, a recent model that has a simple switching system for varying magnification from 20 to 45 degrees. Mechanically, their instruments are relatively easy to use, but the quality of the optics does not compare to that produced by Canon, Kowa, Nikon, and Carl Zeiss.
5. The West German Carl Zeiss fundus camera has a long history of success and produces excellent quality fundus photographs. Unfortunately, the decision to discontinue the FF-II power supply was a mistake: The new FF-III power supply has simply not been reliable. Along with the Canon zoom fundus camera, this instrument is significantly more expensive than its competitors.
6. I have had limited experience with the Mamiya, the Olympus, and the East German Zeiss fundus cameras. The quality of the photographs that I have taken and seen appears to be reasonably good, but the Mamiya and Olympus are not available in this country and, although sold on a limited basis, the East German Zeiss instrument does not enjoy a good reputation for service and repair.
7. The Pomerantzeff 120-degree fundus camera is a contact lens camera with great potential; however, I have not had an opportunity to evaluate this unique instrument, which is covered in Chapter 11.
8. The Donaldson simultaneous stereo fundus camera, which is moderately priced, is ideal for color stereo fundus photography but cannot be used for fluorescein angiography. This instrument is described in Chapter 12.

Care and Maintenance

Most fundus cameras are fairly sturdy instruments and require a minimal amount of care and maintenance. The objective lens should be covered by the lens cap when not in use, even during office hours. The entire instrument should be covered at night and on weekends and holidays. In spite of these efforts to maintain a clean instrument, foreign matter on the lens is a constant problem for the photographer. Children have an uncanny interest in touching the objective lens with their fingers, leaving fingerprints and smudges. Cleaning the front surface of the objective lens can be done easily by the photographer. Kodak lens cleaner and a cotton-tipped applicator covered with a good quality lens tissue can be used on a routine basis without any damage to the surface of the lens. However, removal of the objective lens by the photographer to clean its back surface is a serious mistake; this maneuver should be done only by a qualified manufacturer's representative. Dust spots and smudges on the back surface of the lens are particularly noticeable in eyes with a high degree of myopia. The photographer should be able to replace viewing lamps, electronic flash tubes, and fuses when they become ineffective. Power supply problems should be referred to an electronics expert, preferably a manufacturer's technician.

Basic Techniques

Top quality fundus photographs are dependent on many details of production. The most important points for the photographer to follow are:

1. Make sure that the pupil is widely dilated. We use one drop of 1% Mydriacyl followed by one drop of 10% Neo-Synephrine. These are quick-acting drugs of short duration. Usually, the pupils are well dilated in 20 to 30 minutes. Cyclogyl is an excellent cycloplegic for photography; however, in fairness to the patient, it is not recommended because the pupil remains dilated much longer than is necessary. An 8-mm pupil is ideal, but photography, both single frame and stereo, can be carried out with pupils that are considerably smaller.
2. Set the focusing eyepiece on the proper correction (Fig. 2-1). Out-of-focus photographs will result if the focusing eyepiece is not properly set by the photographer. Even if no one else uses the camera, the setting should be checked each time. Consistently sharp photographs are difficult to obtain initially for many young photographers because of their accommodation problem. In these instances a cycloplegic refraction is sometimes helpful. Practice makes perfect and persistence pays dividends.
3. Make sure that the correct camera body with the proper film is

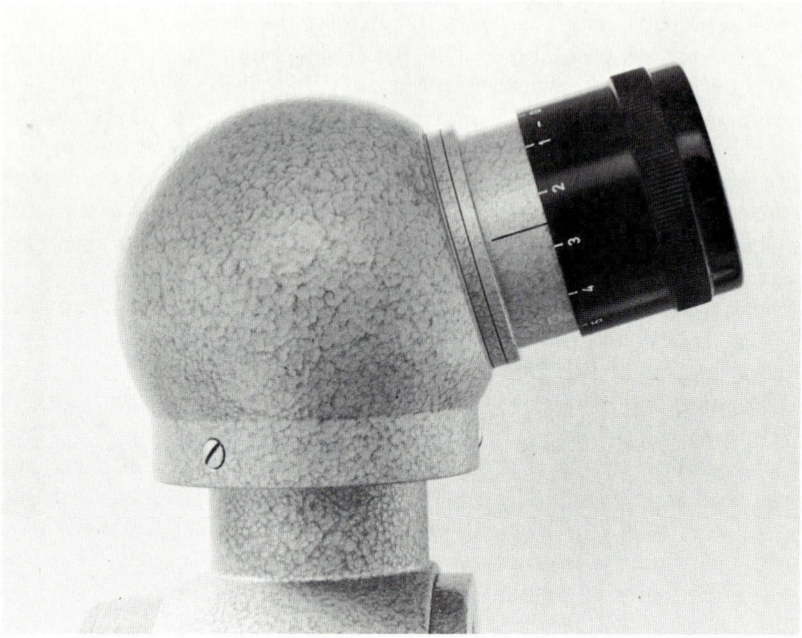

Fig. 2-1. Focusing eyepiece.

attached to the instrument. To avoid mistakes, attach the appropriate film label to the camera back.

4. Check the shutter speed for the proper electronic flash synchronization. Shutter speeds in the range of 1/30 to 1/60 of a second can be used. Faster shutter speeds on most camera backs will result in partially exposed photographs.
5. Insert the synchronization cable in the proper electronic flash connection on the camera body.
6. Take an identification photograph of the patient's name, the date photography is performed, and other pertinent information. All subsequent photographs will pertain to that patient. To avoid errors and angry referring ophthalmologists, all photographs should be appropriately labeled as rapidly as possible after their return from processing (Fig. 2-2).
7. Inform the patient about the procedure.
8. Seat the patient comfortably at the instrument with chin on the chin rest and forehead against the headrest.
9. Instruct the patient to look at the fixation device.
10. Focus the filament of the viewing lamp on the cornea.
11. After properly focusing the filament of the viewing lamp, look through the eyepiece and bring the retinal vessels into focus.

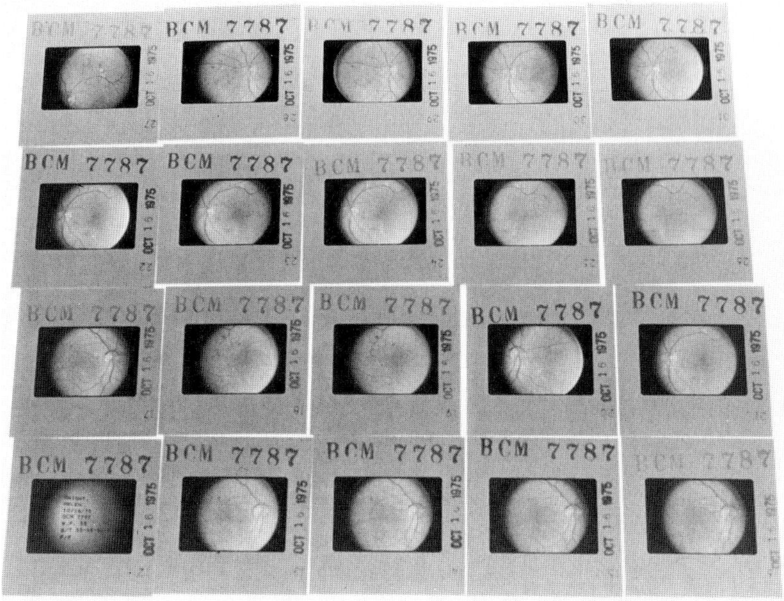

Fig. 2-2. Identification photograph and subsequent fundus photographs.

12. When the image is in proper focus and the specific area of interest is in view, release the shutter.
13. Wind the camera immediately so that it will be ready to take the next photograph.

Artifacts of Illumination

From a technical standpoint, manipulation of the "joystick" is the single most vital aspect of fundus photography. This sensitive control mechanism is most directly related to rather common artifacts of illumination.

If the fundus camera is too close to the eye, a bright, crescent-shaped light will appear at the edge of the photograph (Fig. 2-3A, B). When the camera is too far from the eye, a low-contrast photograph (blue gray) will be produced (Fig. 2-3C, D). Optimal illumination is achieved within a small zone between these two extremes, at a distance from the eye determined by its own optics (Fig. 2-3E, F). To determine the optimal position of the camera, it is useful as a routine matter to focus the projected filament image of the viewing lamp (Fig. 2-4A) directly on the cornea. Then, while the fundus is viewed, small anterior-posterior excursions of the joystick (Fig. 2-4B) will provide the artifact-free viewing needed for final focusing and photographing.

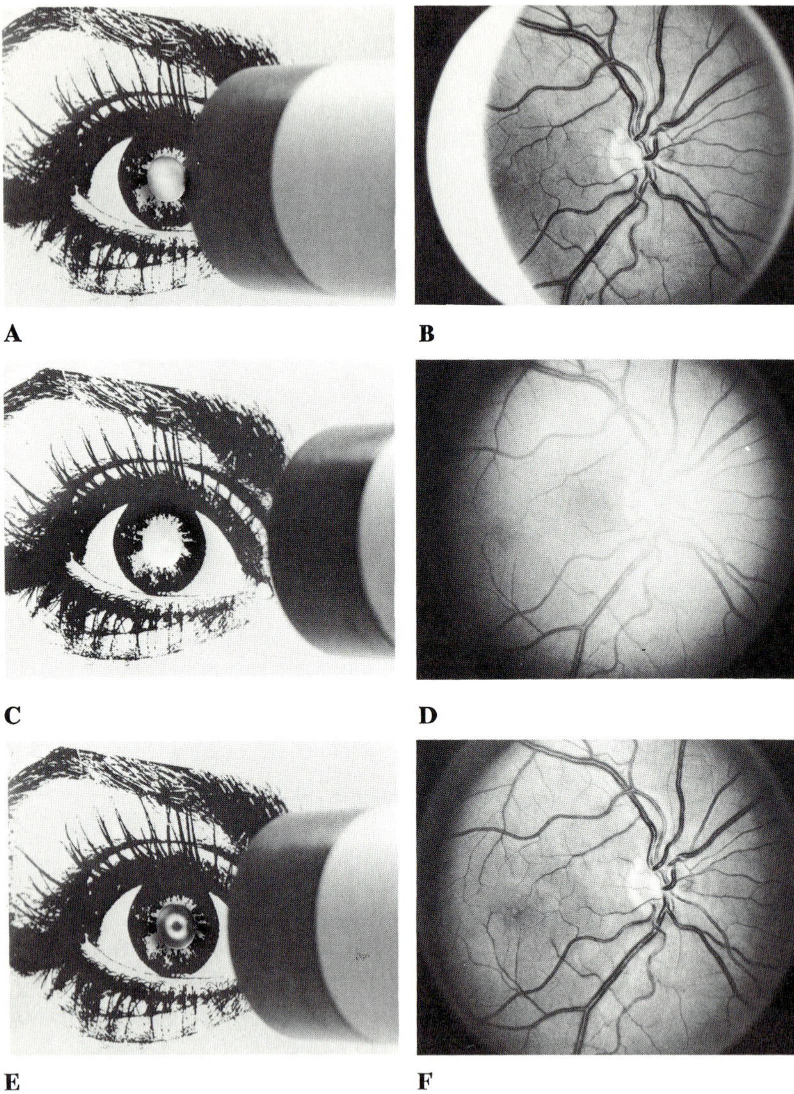

Fig. 2-3. Artifacts of illumination. (A) The camera is too close to the subject; (B) note the crescent-shaped artifact. (C) The camera is too far away from the subject: (D) a low-contrast photograph with blue haze (if color film is used). (E) The camera is at the proper distance and the filament is focused on the cornea: (F) a properly illuminated fundus photograph.

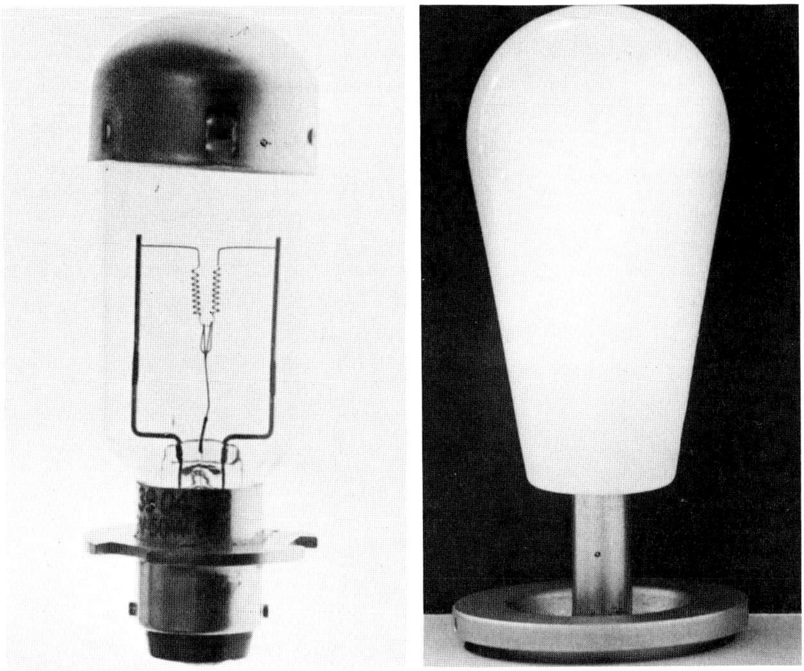

A B

Fig. 2-4. To obtain proper illumination: (A) *Focus filament of viewing lamp on the cornea.* (B) *Small anterior-posterior movements of the joystick will provide artifact-free photographs.*

Stereo Fundus Photography

Stereo fundus photography is the best way of documenting blurred disc margins, optic nerve head cupping, and the degree of retinal elevation from serous or solid detachments. As long as a standard stereo technique is used, comparative serial photographs of this type can be invaluable in the appraisal of change in the appearance of a lesion. Stereo fundus photographs can be obtained by three methods:

1. The cornea-induced parallax method, advocated by Bedell in 1929, produces excellent stereo photographs using standard fundus camera equipment alone. The first photograph is taken through the temporal side of the pupil and the other through the nasal side. A lateral shift of 3.5 mm is recommended for optimal stereopsis, but any lateral shift will create a stereo photograph.
2. A very effective manually operated stereoscopic separator, designed by Allen in 1965, is now available commercially with motor drive. Certain patients with early cataracts, corneal opaci-

ties, or vitreous haze require manual alignment of the camera, as described in the preceding entry.

3. The Donaldson simultaneous stereo fundus camera takes beautiful stereo photographs and is now available. It is described in Chapter 12.

Film and Processing

At one time, I used Kodachrome daylight film, as others in ophthalmic photography do. Unfortunately, Kodachrome film must be developed in a Kodak laboratory. Because of the 5- to 7-day delay in receiving the processed film, I switched to Ektachrome-ER daylight film. This film can be processed either locally or in one's own darkroom. The quality of the photographs is excellent, although the resolution is not quite as good as that obtained using Kodachrome.

Conclusion

This chapter has reviewed fundus photography techniques while emphasizing the important parameters of producing high-quality fundus photographs. The role of fundus photography has extended beyond that of a documentary service to one with specific diagnostic value. Thus, ocular fundus photography relates directly to patient care and is an essential part of the sophisticated armamentarium of any clinical ophthalmologic unit.

References

1. Allen, L. Ocular fundus photography. *Am. J. Ophthalmol.* 57 : 13, 1964.
2. Bedell, A. J. *Photographs of the Fundus Oculi.* Philadelphia: Davis, 1929.
3. Justice, J., Jr. The Basic Techniques of Fundus Photography and Fluorescein Angiography. In K. Shimizu (Ed.), *Proceedings of the International Symposium on Fluorescein Angiography* (ISFA), Tokyo, 1972.
4. Kirkendall, W. M., Snyder, E. B., and Frazier, O. Instant positive photographs and stereograms of ocular fundus fluorescence. *Arch. Ophthalmol.* 75 : 192, 1965.
5. Wong, D. The fundamentals of ocular fundus photography and retinal fluorescence photography. *Photography Applications in Science, Technology and Medicine,* Winter 1968/1969.
6. Wong, D. Fundus photography and fluorescein angiography. *J. Ophthalmic Photography* 2(1) : 15–55, 1979.

3

Fluorescein Angiography

JOHNNY JUSTICE, JR.

Using the basic techniques for fundus photography described in Chapter 2, the photographer or the ophthalmologist can usually make the transition to fluorescein angiography from routine fundus photography with relative ease. If the techniques for obtaining a good fundus photograph are followed, a good angiogram will result. In this chapter, I will discuss filters for fluorescein angiography, methodology, film and developing, and the importance of a rapid angiography service with high-quality angiograms.

Filters

Novotny and Alvis first described a practical method of fluorescein angiography in 1961. Since then, other investigators have published improvements in their technique [6–8]. In 1966, Hodge and Clement's description [4] of the use of an *interference filter,* an excitor filter with a peak transmission of 80 percent at 4700 Å, was the most significant technical contribution since the advent of fluorescein angiography. However, their choice of Ilford 109 (yellow) as a barrier filter allowed too much overlap (pseudofluorescence). Haining and Lancaster [3], in 1968, showed that the advantages of the interference filter are better exploited when both excitor and barrier filters are of this type. Their B-4 excitor and B-5 barrier filters allowed minimal pseudofluorescence. In 1974, Delori [2] described a set of interference filters (excitor and barrier) designed specifically to study choroidal circulation. After using these filters for the past few years, I find that they are excellent for the choroidal circulation and are unsurpassed for retinal vessel fluorescence (Fig. 3-1).

The most exciting feature of this truly excellent set of filters is that the photographer can better visualize fluorescein passage through the retinal and choroidal vessels. This set of filters offers two advantages: (1) Better visualization during angiography allows the photographer to obtain better illumination, thus eliminating the rather common artifacts of illumination that frequently appear during angiography; and (2) active leakage sights can be detected visually, allowing the photographer to give the referring ophthalmologist a preliminary report. Improvement in filter combinations for fluorescein angiography will surely come to the forefront in the future, but at present, the Delori

I would like to thank Ann Bryant for helping with the manuscript, and Robert Simmons, Carol P. Justice, and Ditte Jacobsen for their help with the photographs for this chapter.

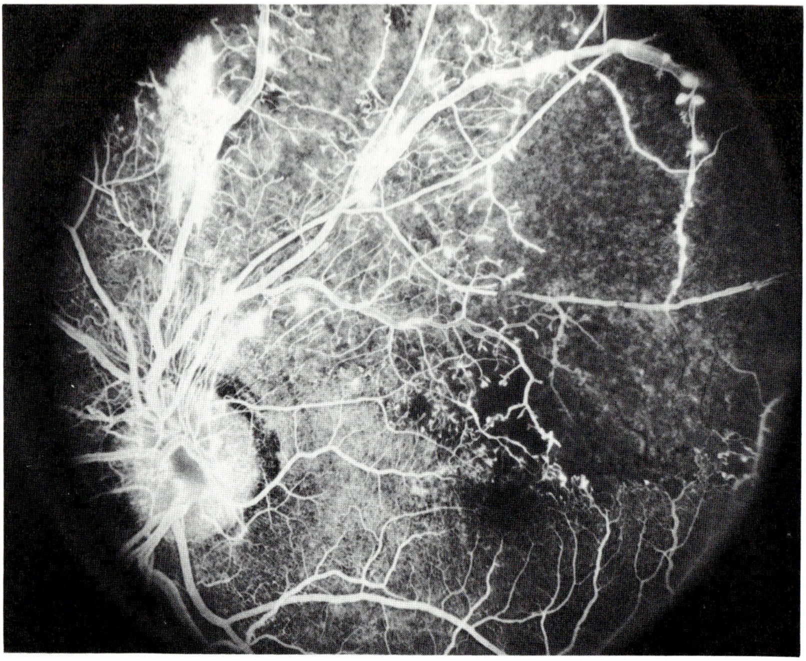

Fig. 3-1. Note the quality of the choroidal and retinal vessel fluorescence; branch vein occlusion with neovascularization and "capillary avascularity."

combination (SE 40 excitor filter and SE 50 barrier filter), available from Spectrotech, Inc., is recommended as an international standard.

Many of the absorption filters used in black-and-white angiography are suitable for color fluorescein angiography [6, 7]. The excitor filter must have a transmission range of 400 to 500 mm with some additional transmission in the red part of the spectrum [1, 5]. The resolution and reproducibility of color fluorescein angiography are not comparable to that of black-and-white angiography.

Methodology

After making the proper choice of excitor-barrier filters for a particular fundus camera, the photographer should routinely follow several steps.

1. Always take stereo color fundus photographs of both eyes (when possible) before undertaking fluorescein angiography. Angiography frequently demonstrates pathologic changes in the fellow eye that may have been overlooked or are not visible ophthalmoscopically. In addition, after fluorescein injection, the leakage of

fluorescein beneath the retina, into the retina, into the vitreous, and into the aqueous obscures fundal detail, thus lessening the quality of stereo color fundus photographs.

2. Explain the entire procedure in detail to the patient. It is especially important that the patient be aware that urine will be discolored for 24 to 36 hours following the fluorescein injection. The skin color is sometimes yellow or jaundiced in appearance. We explain to the patient the possibility of reactions to intravenous fluorescein and have a consent form signed (see Chap. 6).
3. Make sure that the proper camera back with the appropriate barrier filter and appropriate film is properly attached to the fundus camera.
4. Take a photograph of the patient's name, the date the study is performed, and any other information that will be helpful when the study is being reviewed.
5. Seat the patient comfortably at the instrument.
6. Follow instructions (see Chap. 2) for obtaining high-quality fundus photographs.
7. Take a red-free fundus photograph with a green filter (Kodak Wratten No. 58).
8. Before the fluorescein injection, the illumination diaphragm should be changed to the appropriate excitor filter and a control photograph should be taken.
9. Extend the patient's right or left arm across the armrest. The fluorescein should be injected as rapidly as possible into an antecubital vein. In studies completed by the author and Kirk E. Mullen of the Cullen Eye Institute, Houston, Texas and by Terrance L. Tomer and Jamie Nicholl of the Wills Eye Hospital, Philadelphia, it was determined that Ak-Fluor fluorescein dye* (5 cc 10% and 2 cc 25%) produced significantly fewer "reactions" than dye available from other sources. Assuming that the technique of photography is good, the contrast and quality of the angiogram depend primarily on the rapidity of injection and the quality of the film processing.
10. Activate the timer (if available) simultaneously with the injection of dye.
11. Take rapid sequential stereo angiograms at the rate of 1 per second, starting approximately 7 seconds after the injection of fluorescein; continue for about 20 seconds. Then angiograms should be taken every 10 to 20 seconds for 1 minute, then at 5 minutes, 15 minutes, and 30 minutes postinjection, depending upon the pathologic condition under examination.

* Available from Akron, Inc., Metairie, La.

Film and Developing

There are many films and developers available for use in fluorescein angiography (processing and printing are covered in Chap. 8). We use Kodak Tri-X black-and-white film (TX 135-36) and develop it in Kodak D-11 developer, stock solution for 6 minutes at 72°F. An 8- by 10-inch contact print is made on Kodak Ektamatic SC paper and an 8- by 10-inch enlargement is printed of a specific angiogram in order that minute details can be seen in high magnification. The prints are developed by the stabilization technique (Kodak Ektamatic Processor).

Rapid Angiography Service

Obviously, the best angiograms can be obtained if the pupil is well dilated and if there is no opacity in the optical media such as lesions of the cornea, cataractous changes in the lens, or vitreous abnormalities. The application of a topical anesthetic, topical fluorescein, applanation and Schiotz tonometry, or other ophthalmologic testing that disturbs the corneal epithelium is not recommended before or on the same day that fluorescein angiography is being performed. Unfortunately, many patients have to travel long distances to see an ophthalmologist, so the convenience of the patient has to be considered. Consequently, most of the angiograms performed in our laboratory are carried out on the same day as the aforementioned procedures. Although these situations are not ideal, adequate angiography can be performed. If at all possible, however, the patient should be rescheduled for angiography at a later date.

It is our usual routine to send a complete fluorescein angiography report (Fig. 3-2) 2 to 3 days following a fluorescein study. This package includes: (1) a typewritten report, (2) an 8- by 10-inch contact sheet of the entire study, (3) one or more 8- by 10-inch enlargements of specific angiograms, and (4) stereo color fundus photographs.

We usually process films at the end of the day, and a report is dictated the following morning. The reports are typed and usually signed on the same day. The Medical Illustration Department at the Baylor College of Medicine gives 1-day processing on Ektachrome-X color film. Color slides are labeled and stereo slides are mounted less than 48 hours following fluorescein angiography.

Through the years, I have found that the best way to keep ophthalmologists happy with my work is to give them what they want when they want it. An ophthalmologist is looking for quality and speed, and it is the responsibility of the photographer to deliver these.

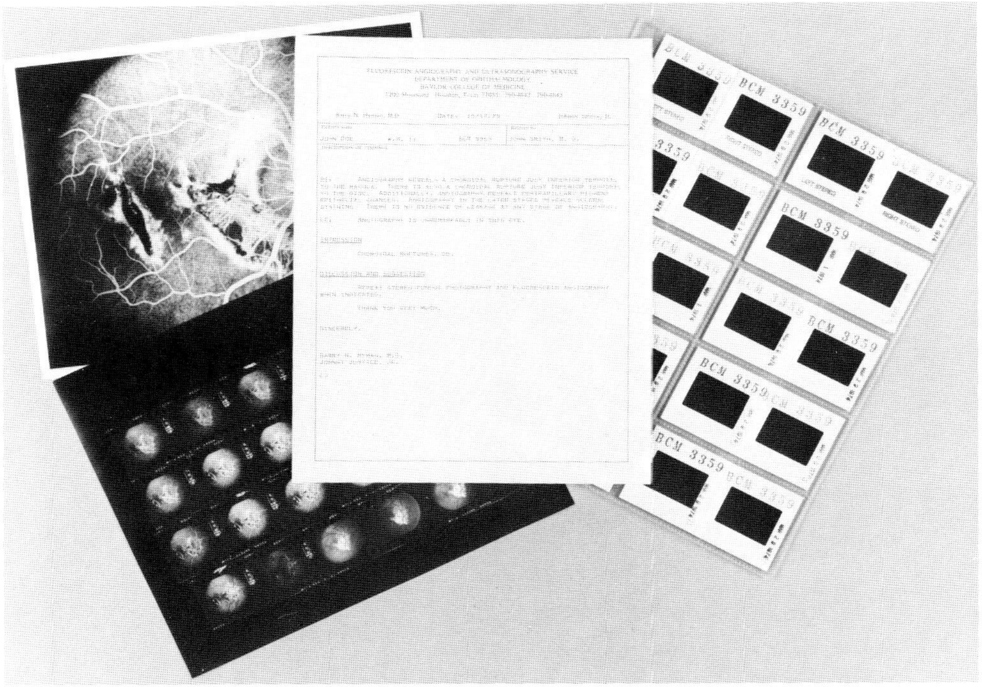

Fig. 3-2. Complete fluorescein angiography report: a typewritten report, an 8- by 10-inch contact sheet, an 8- by 10-inch enlargement of a specific angiogram, and stereo color fundus photographs.

References

1. Allen, L., and Frazier, O. The Results of Test on Broadband Filter Combination for Fluorescein Angiography. In K. Shimizu (Ed.), *Proceedings of the International Symposium on Fluorescein Angiography* (ISFA), Tokyo, 1972. Pp. 48–59.
2. Delori, F., Ben-sira, I., and Tremtee, C. Improved filters for fluorescein angiography. Presented at AAOO, October, 1974.
3. Haining, W. M., and Lancaster, R. C. Advanced techniques for fluorescein angiography. *Arch. Ophthalmol.* 70 : 1, 1968.
4. Hodge, J. V., and Clement, R. J. Improved method for fluorescence angiography of the retina. *Am. J. Ophthalmol.* 61 : 1400, 1966.
5. Hÿvarinen, L., and Hochheimer, B. F. Filter systems in fluorescein angiography. In W. M. Haining (Ed.), Recent Advances in the Technical Aspects of Fluorescein Angiography. *Int. Ophthalmol. Clin.* 14(3) : 49, 1974.
6. Justice, J., Jr. The Basic Techniques of Fundus Photography and Fluorescein Angiography. In K. Shimizu (Ed.), *Proceedings of the International Symposium on Fluorescein Angiography* (ISFA), Tokyo, 1971. Pp. 60–68.
7. Justice, J., Jr., and Sever, R. J. Technique of Fluorescein Fundus Photography. In J. L. Smith (Ed.), *Neuro-Ophthalmology. Symposium of the University of Miami and the Bascom Palmer Eye Institute.* St. Louis: Mosby, 1965. Pp. 82–83.
8. Machemer, R., Norton, E. W. D., Gass, J. D. M., and Chormokos, E. Pseudofluorescence—A problem in interpretation of fluorescein angiograms. *Am. J. Ophthalmol.* 70 : 1, 1970.
9. Schatz, H., Burton, T. C., Yannuzzi, L. A., and Rabb, M. F. *Interpretation of Fluorescein Angiography.* St. Louis: Mosby, 1978.

4

Basic Interpretations of Fluorescein Angiography

JOHNNY JUSTICE, JR.

During the past 20 years, fluorescein angiography has provided much new information concerning intraocular diseases. In the early 1960s, investigators at the Bascom Palmer Eye Institute established fluorescein angiography as a helpful adjunct in the evaluation of intraocular disorders. Since that time, investigators throughout the world have contributed enormously to the wealth of new information that has been derived from fluorescein angiography.

Stereo fluorescein angiography provides anatomic information that is sometimes not apparent either by direct examination or by stereo fundus photography. This technique is particularly valuable in the diagnosis, treatment, and follow-up of patients with intraocular diseases.

Basic Angiographic Anatomy

We are primarily concerned with the retinal and choroidal circulatory systems, which are separated by the retinal pigment epithelium and Bruch's membrane. The increased intensity of the pigment epithelium in the macular region is the primary reason that this area is dark in a normal angiogram. Of secondary importance is the presence of intraretinal yellow pigment (xanthophyll) in the macular region, which absorbs some of the exciting light.

The Normal Angiogram

The choroidal vessels, some capillaries of the optic nerve head, and any cilioretinal vessel present usually fill approximately one full second ahead of those in the proximal branches of the central retinal artery (Fig. 4-1B). Following the injection of fluorescein into an antecubital vein, normal arm-to-retina circulation is usually in the range of 8 to 16 seconds depending on cardiac output, which is an extremely variable factor. After perfusing the retinal arteries (Fig. 4-1C), the dye passes into the capillary bed and then drains in a laminar fashion at the margin of the veins (Fig. 4-1D). The midvenous phases can demonstrate several laminar columns of dye (Fig. 4-1E). The veins become uniformly fluorescent in a later phase of filling (Fig. 4-1F). Gradually a decrease in background fluorescence follows (Fig. 4-1G). Usually there is no leakage of fluorescein from the retinal vessels. The

I would like to thank Ann Bryant and Carol P. Justice for their help with the manuscript, and Ditte Jacobsen for her help in the preparation of the photographs for this chapter.

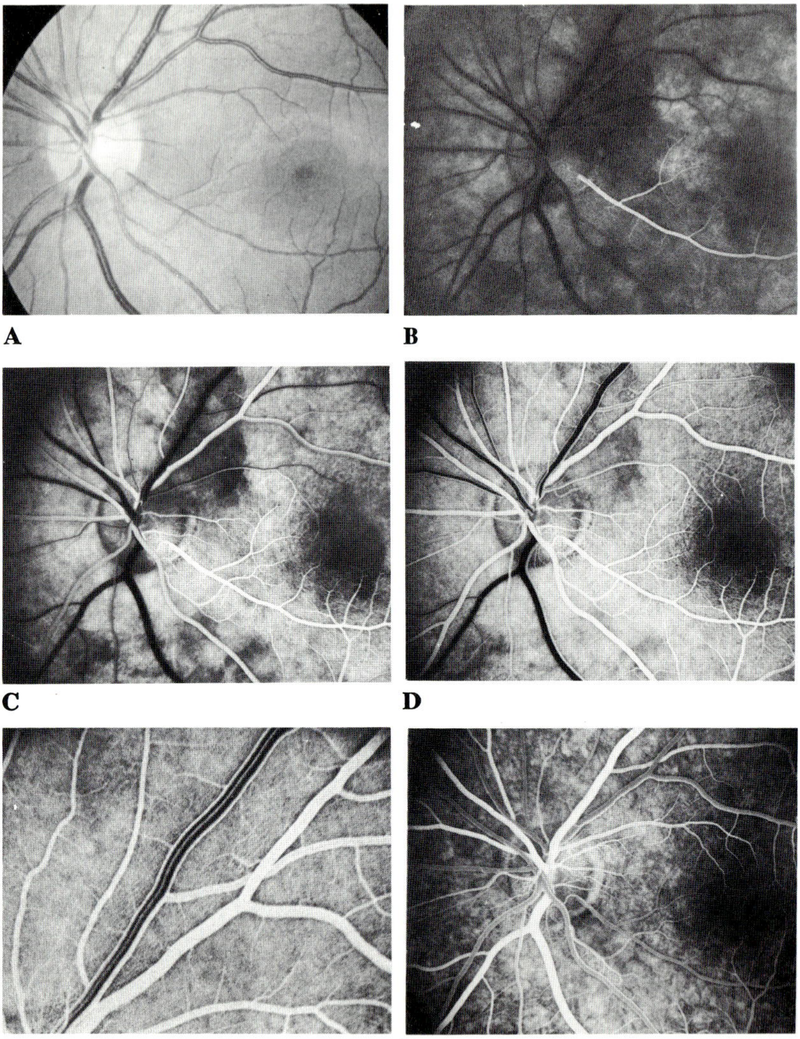

A B C D E F

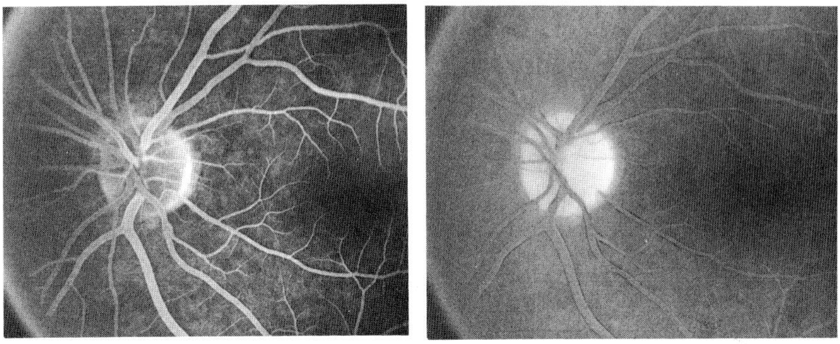

G H

Fig. 4-1. The normal angiogram. (A) *Red-free fundus photograph.* (B) *Cilioretinal artery filling before central retinal artery and simultaneously with the choroid (10 sec postinjection).* (C) *Perfusion of central retinal artery. Note normal patchy choroidal filling (11 sec).* (D) *Early laminar venous phase (13 sec).* (E) *Enlargement of later laminar venous phase demonstrating columns of dye (15 sec).* (F) *Uniform venous filling (23 sec).* (G) *Decrease in background fluorescence (206 sec).* (H) *Normal staining of the lamina cribrosa (15 min).*

dye normally leaks from the choriocapillaris, stains Bruch's membrane, and then diffuses into the extravascular spaces of the choroid, subsequently staining the sclera and the lamina cribrosa (Fig. 4-1H).

Basic Angiographic Interpretations

Hyperfluorescence

Hyperfluorescence can usually be classified as follows:

1. Leakage: pooling of fluorescein into an anatomic space such as a serous detachment of the retina (Fig. 4-2) or into cystoid spaces in the retina (see Fig. 4-5D).
2. Staining
   a. Leakage of fluorescein from the choroidal vessels will result in staining of large drusen (Fig. 4-3) and chorioretinal scars.
   b. Abnormal leakage of fluorescein from retinal vessels will result in perivascular staining as in venous occlusive diseases, (Fig. 4-4) and in inflammatory diseases affecting the retinal vessels.
3. Transmission (pigment epithelial window defect): Defects such as small drusen, atrophy, and absence of the retinal pigment epithelium will result in visualization of choroidal fluorescence through these defects (see Fig. 4-3).

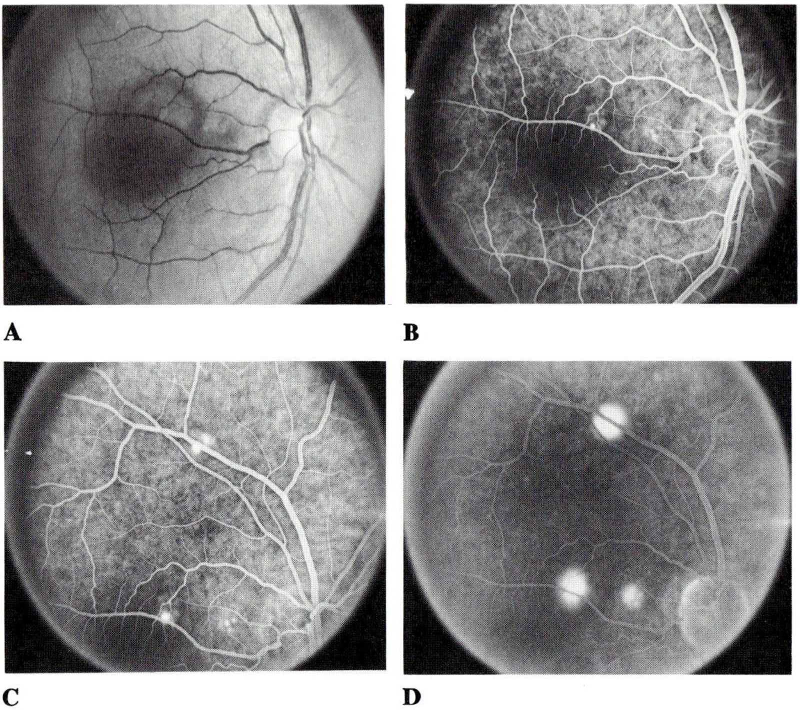

Fig. 4-2. Idiopathic central serous choroidopathy. (A) *Red-free fundus photograph.* (B) *Leakage sites* (*15 sec*). (C) *Additional active site* (*29 sec*). (D) *Late phase: pooling beneath sensory retina* (*15 min*).

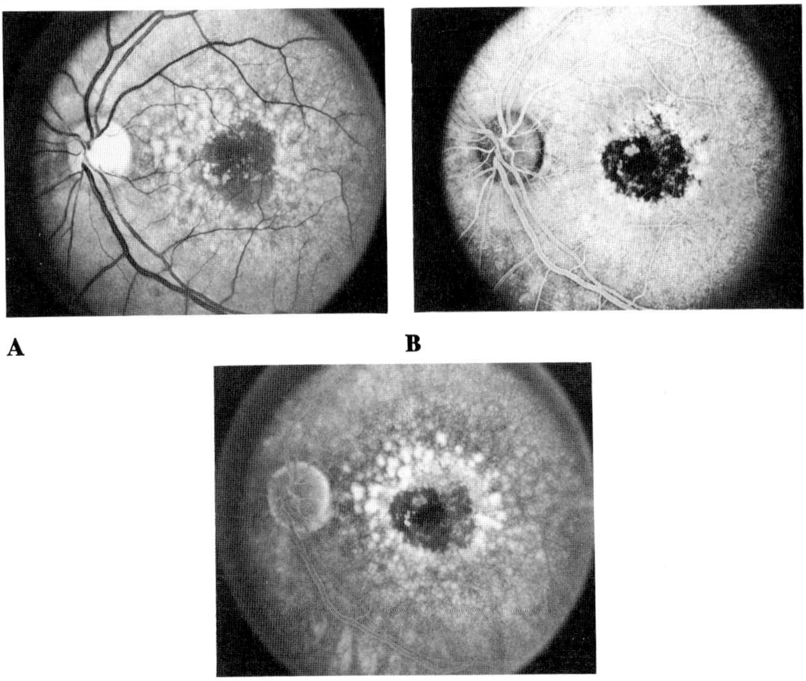

A B C

Fig. 4-3. Dominant drusen. (A) *Red-free fundus photograph.* (B) *Pigment epithelial window defect: small drusen and retinal pigment epithelium changes* (*20 sec*). (C) *Staining of large drusen* (*15 min*).

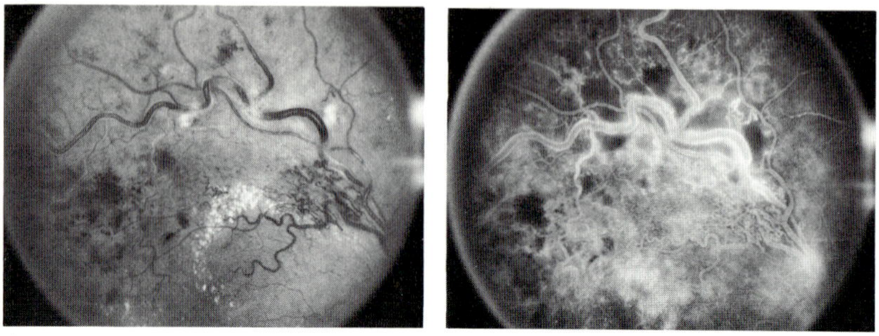

A B

Fig. 4-4. Branch vein occlusion. (A) *Red-free fundus photograph.* (B) *Perivascular staining caused by venous stasis* (*4 min*).

4. Abnormal vessels
    a. Retinal: Tortuosity, dilatation, neovascularization, macroaneurysms and microaneurysms, telangiectasis, shunts, and collaterals are dramatically demonstrated with angiography. Some of these abnormal vessels leak profusely; others do not (Figs. 4-5, 4-6).
    b. Subretinal: Neovascularization beneath the retina is very difficult to see ophthalmoscopically. Angiography is especially helpful in delineating these vessels (Fig. 4-7).
    c. Tumors: Ophthalmoscopically, retinal tumors such as angiomas and retinoblastomas are usually easily diagnosed; angiography is useful as a pretherapeutic and posttherapeutic test. Subretinal tumors such as hemangiomas, melanomas, and metastases are frequently difficult to diagnose accurately. Angiography is a helpful adjunct in a small percentage of subretinal tumors (Fig. 4-8). It is especially helpful in follow-up care, however.

Hypofluorescence

Hypofluorescence exists with any lesion that, by virtue of its relative nontransparency, blocks the blue (excitor) light from exciting fluorescence at the level of the retina and choroid; it also accompanies a filling defect caused by delay and occlusion.

1. Blockage of fluorescence: Pigments such as melanin, hemoglobin, xanthophyll, and lipofuscin are good examples. Hard and soft exudates, edema and transudates, and other abnormal material such as foreign bodies, as well as some diseases that affect the

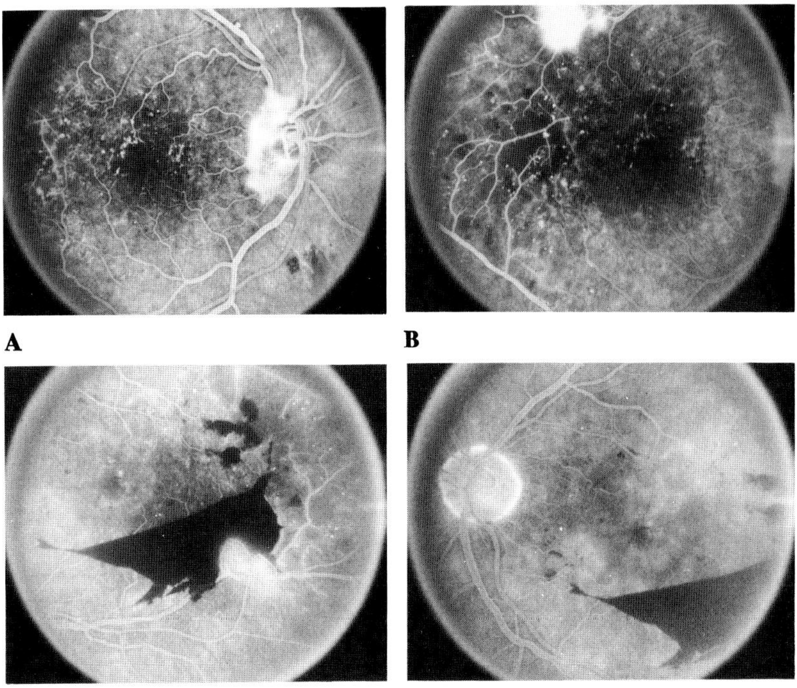

A B C D

Fig. 4-5. Diabetic retinopathy. (A) *Prepapillary proliferans* (*leakage*). (B) *Leakage from neovascularization. Note capillary avascularity and microaneurysms.* (C) *Blockage of exciting light by preretinal hemorrhage.* (D) *Cystoid macular edema* (*pooling*).

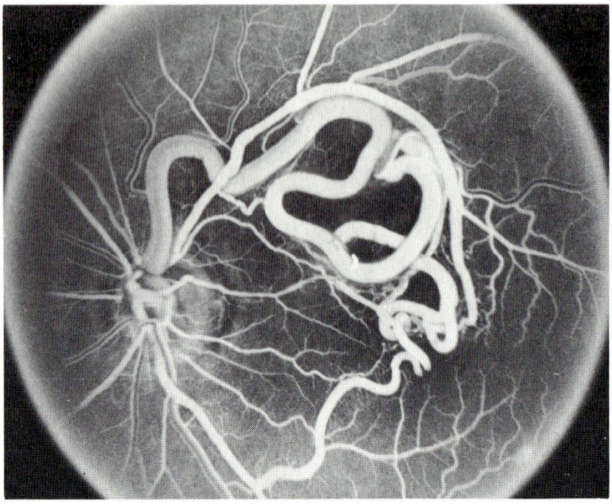

Fig. 4-6. Arteriovenous malformation (no leakage).

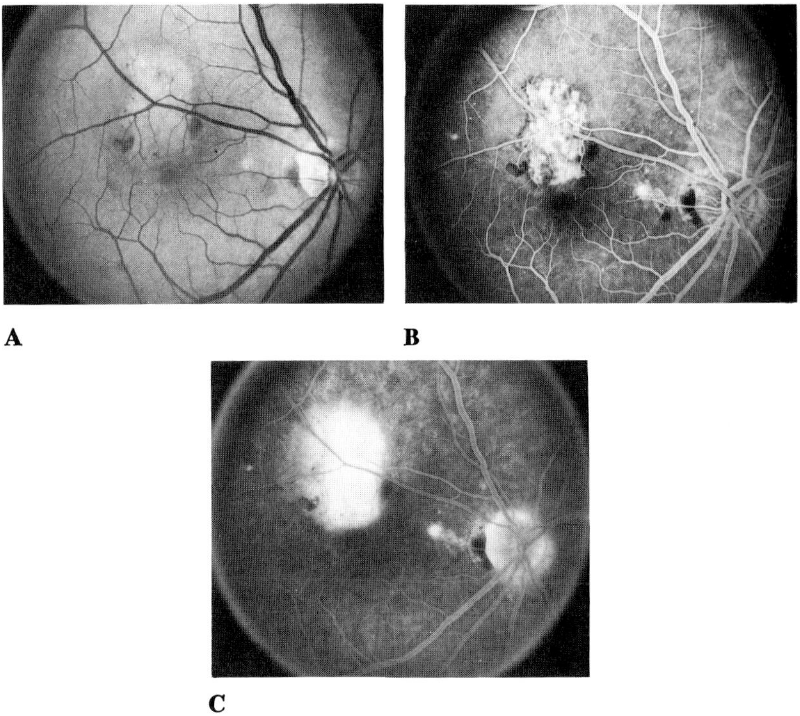

Fig. 4-7. Presumed ocular histoplasmosis. (A) *Red-free fundus photograph.* (B) *Subretinal neovascularization (leakage). Note "punched-out" lesions (window defect) and hemorrhage (blockage).* (C) *Pooling beneath the detachment.*

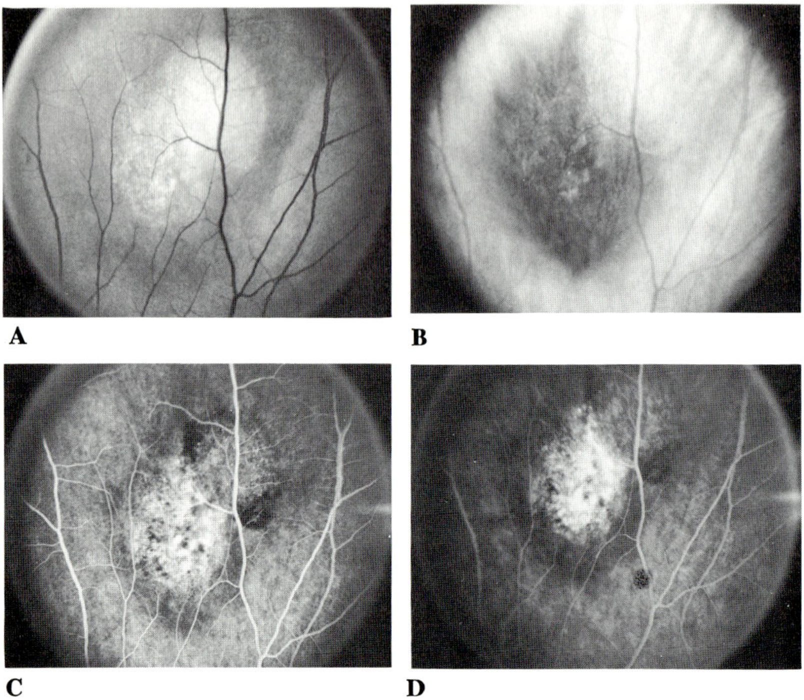

Fig. 4-8. Malignant melanoma of the choroid. (A) *Red-free fundus photograph.* (B) *Green-free fundus photograph.* (C) *Angiogram demonstrating a new area of recent growth. Note pinpoint leakage sites.* (D) *Pooling beneath the detachment.*

pigment epithelium are unusual conditions that can produce a hypofluorescent pattern (Fig. 4-9).

2. Filling defect: Occlusive diseases affecting the retinal vessels and capillaries frequently produce a hypofluorescent pattern due to nonperfusion (Fig. 4-10); diseases resulting in loss of tissue, such as dystrophies and degenerations, are other examples of hypofluorescence.

Pseudofluorescence

Pseudofluorescence is usually the result of an inefficient filter system and, with proper filters, can be kept to a minimum.

Autofluorescence

Autofluorescence occurs with some intraocular lesions. It is particularly notable and helpful in locating drusen of the optic nervehead, especially when the drusen are not obvious ophthalmoscopically (Fig. 4-11).

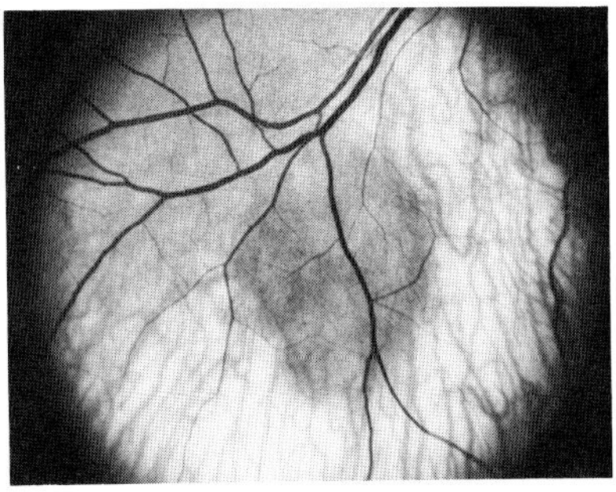

A

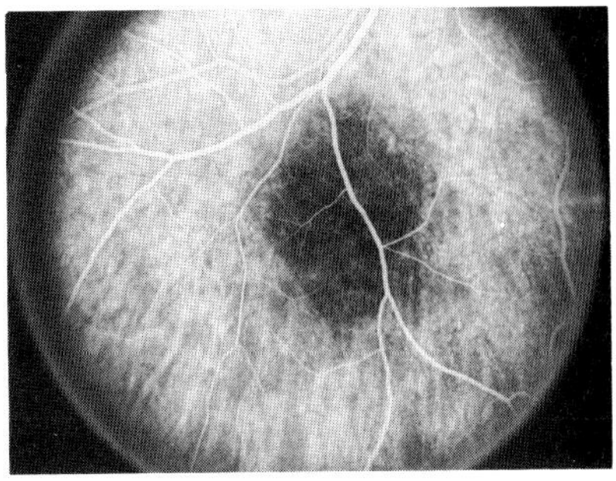

B

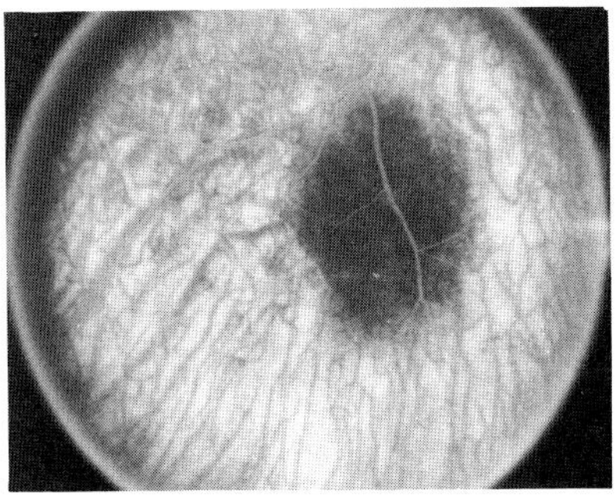

C

Fig. 4-9. Nevus of the choroid. (A) *Fundus photograph with an orange filter.* (B) *Blockage of choroidal fluorescence.* (C) *Blockage of scleral staining.*

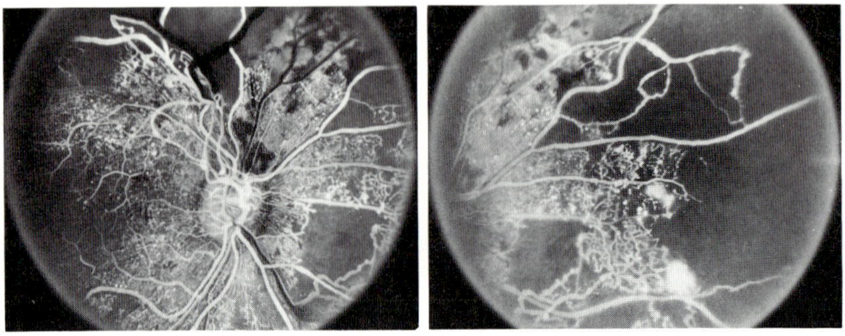

A B

Fig. 4-10. (A) *Diabetic retinopathy.* (B) *Capillary nonperfusion.*

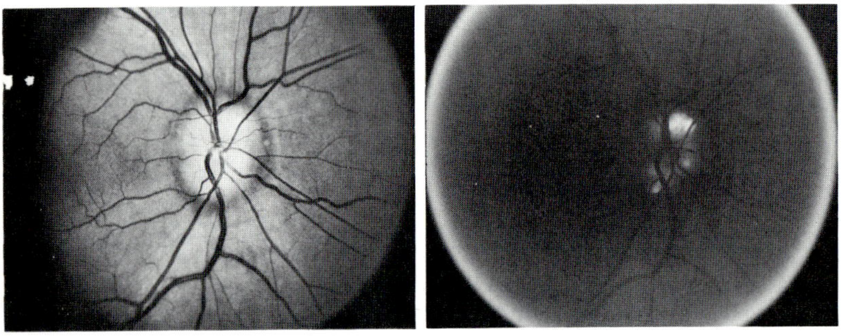

A B

Fig. 4-11. Pseudopapilledema with autofluorescent drusen. (A) *Red-free fundus photograph.* (B) *Autofluorescent drusen.*

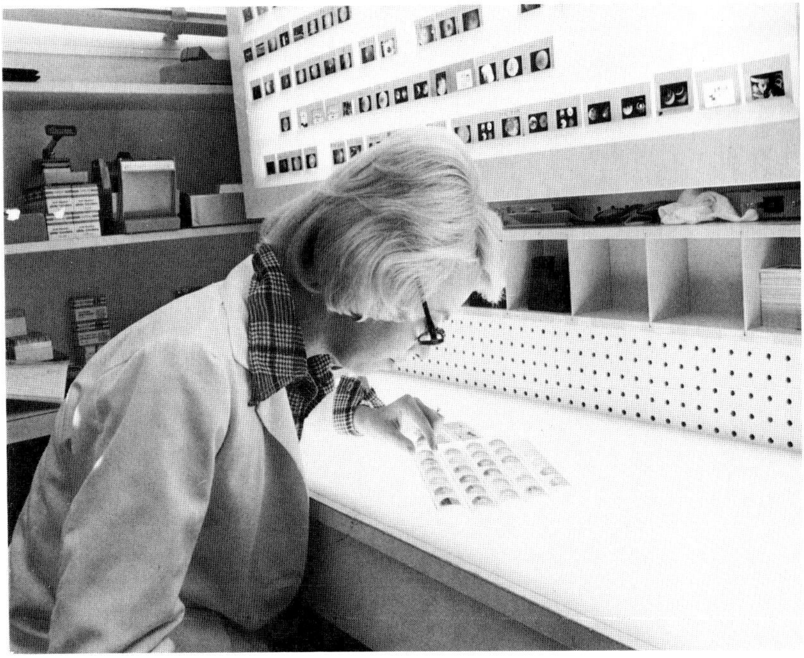

Fig. 4-12. Reviewing fluorescein angiography with special +15 stereo glasses.

Reading Fluorescein Angiograms

When preparing to dictate a report of a fluorescein study, the person interpreting the angiograms ideally should have: (1) a contact sheet of the entire study, (2) one or more enlargements of specific angiograms, (3) the entire set of negatives, (4) a view box, (5) special stereo glasses with plus lenses (Fig. 4-12), and (6) if available, stereo fundus photographs.

It is important to read the angiograms as negatives, since the positive angiograms simply do not have all the detail of the negatives. With practice, the transition from reading positives to reading negatives will result in more accurate interpretations.

Suggested Reading

Gass, J. D. M. *Macular Diseases*. St. Louis: Mosby, 1970.

Gass, J. D. M. *Differential Diagnosis of Intraocular Tumors*. St. Louis: Mosby, 1974.

Yannuzzi, L. A., Glitter, K. A., and Schatz, H. *The Macula*. Baltimore: Williams & Wilkins, 1978.

5

Introduction of the New Kowa Fundus Camera and Kowa Photo Slit Lamp

SADAO KANAGAMI

In this chapter I describe a new fundus camera (Fig. 5-1) and photo slit lamp (Fig. 5-2) that my experience as an ophthalmic photographer led me to design, after having for many years used various types of fundus cameras and photo slit lamps. Most of the cameras already in use were designed and developed by optical companies. My impression is that considerable training is necessary before beginners can take good photographs. There are also inconveniences in daily use of these cameras.

Because of this situation, I investigated the development of a simple, easily operated camera. I discussed my idea with several manufacturers, suggesting that they make prototypes based on my ideas, and KOWA, Co. agreed. I then introduced these models at the Ophthalmic Photographers' Society meeting held in 1980 in Chicago. Many members of the American Academy of Ophthalmology and the Ophthalmic Photographers' Society have shown keen interest in these new instruments. They have asked many detailed questions and requested that I introduce these cameras at the earliest convenience.

The Kowa RC-XV Fundus Camera

This new camera has the following features:

1. The overall length is about 2 inches shorter than the current model, which allows easier operation. The patient can maintain a comfortable position when raising the eyelid to take the photograph is necessary.
2. Two camera backs can be mounted simultaneously. At present, a 35-mm horizontal winding motor drive camera and a SX-70 Polaroid back are available; a 120/220 camera back and another type of 35-mm motor drive camera back are planned in the future.
3. The power unit has four buttons for automatic exposure and manual control. The optical pathway and proper exposure can be set automatically by simply pressing the appropriate button. When using 35-mm color film, the operator has only to set the dial for ASA sensitivity. When using special films or achieving special effects, the automatic program is released by pressing the manual-mode button; the operator can then freely adjust the flash

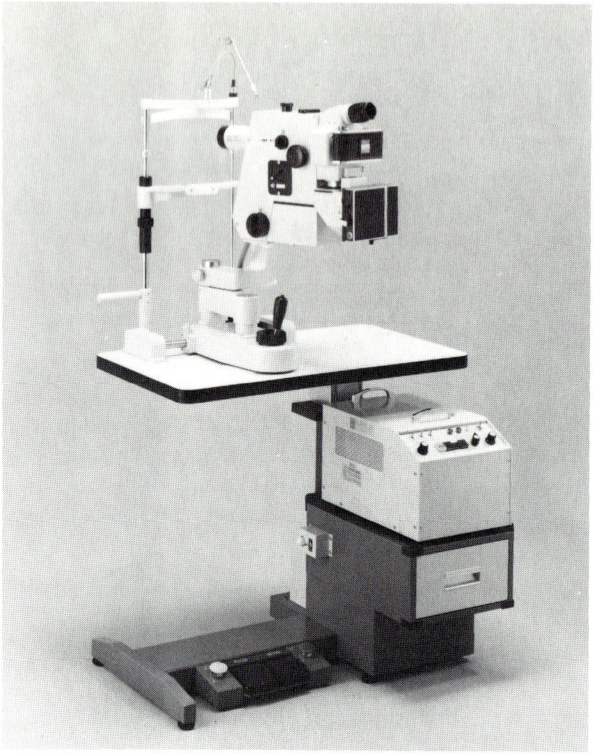

Fig. 5-1. The Kowa RC-XV fundus camera.

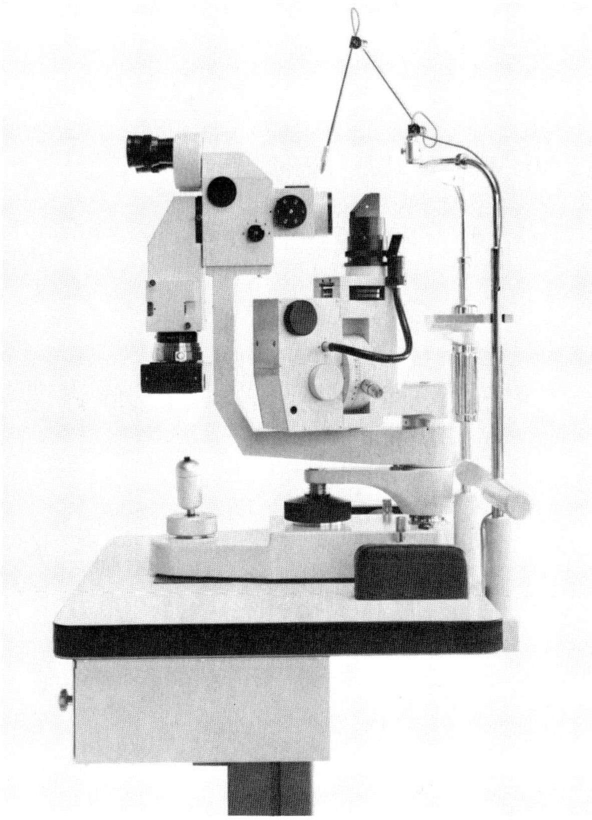

Fig. 5-2. The Kowa ASL-6 photo slit lamp.

intensity, set the illumination for data and counting, and select the optical pathway. For fluorescein angiography, the flash intensity is automatically adjusted for ASA 400 film by simply pressing the button. Inserting the excitor filter automatically sets the illumination at maximum. This function is released when the filter frame is turned upside down.

4. Every camera back has terminals that connect directly to the camera body. Because no cords are visible, accidental cord disconnection during photography is avoided. The operator has only to mount the camera back to the instrument. Also, the film counter can be illuminated for use in a darkened room.
5. The angular field of view can be easily selected from three, 45-, 30-, and 20-degree settings, by adjusting the lever on top of the instrument. With an angle change, illumination intensity auto-

matically adjusts to the proper exposure according to the angle selected.

6. For a Polaroid SX-70 back, the exposure can be properly adjusted for SX-70 film by pushing a button on the power unit. Two quick-return mirrors exchange the optical pathway to the Polaroid back, a newly designed mechanism. This back has automatic film feed linked to the shutter release; therefore, one need only remove the safety cover to take 66-mm diameter photos. A Polaroid back for stereoscopic photos is planned for this camera.
7. The data recording unit is interchangeable, and the data are displayed in the viewfinder on the left of the unit while one takes photos. The 4-digit space on the data unit is available for time recording in fluorescein angiography of identification number, with a space for the patient's name beside the number. The illumination control is linked with the power unit push button and automatically adjusts to the film sensitivity.
8. The halogen bulb is compact and very bright. The flashtube power is 300 watts per second at maximum, fully enough for every photographic purpose. This unit is located in an isolated and flocked compartment in the main body in order to prevent any serious heat effect on the other units in the body.
9. The excitor filter is a Delori type with the peak at 520 nm; the barrier filter has spectral characteristics that perfectly match this filter. On the barrier filter frame is a green filter for red-free photography, which is an interference filter (peak 570 nm) and is effective in photography of retinal blood vessels.
10. The internal fixation target can be inserted in the optical pathway by removing the cover.
11. Another feature of the Kowa RC-XV is that the camera combines with the table top. The alignment is almost that of the Goldmann cameras. The camera is simply connected to the power control unit (right side of instrument table) with single cabtive cord. Camera alignment is free of interference by heavy wiring. The support pole which moves the table up and down is electrically operated and located under the right side of the table. There are four foot pedals on the table base: The middle two pedals are foot switches to adjust the table height; the left pedal is a timer start button which is convenient for the photographer who performs the intravenous injection and takes the photographs; and the right pedal releases the shutter. The shutter can be operated by hand or by foot.

    There are many advantages in combining the camera and table. Placing the pole on the side rather than in the center is helpful for photographing a patient in a wheelchair and also provides leg room for patient and operator.

The Kowa ASL-6 Photo Slit Lamp

Simultaneous stereoscopic photos can be taken with this new photo slit lamp by easily moving a flip-flop lever from single to stereo mode. An automatic exposure control system will soon be incorporated since exposure control is one of the most difficult parameters of a photo slit lamp.

Figure 5-3A shows the illumination unit of this model. The lamp house (*1*) contains both a halogen bulb (*2*) for observing and an electronic flashtube (*3*). The mirror (*4*) changes the light pathway from these sources. A slit whose width and height can be adjusted to arbitrary openings and rotated by 90 degrees is controlled by a knob (*5*). A filter wheel (*6*) controls a diffusion glass plate, a blue filter for fluorescence observation, a green filter for red-free light, and a polarizing filter. Another wheel (*7*) above the filter wheel controls a diaphragm that adjusts the slit beam's depth of focus. Since, by rotating the wheel (*9*), a slit mirror (*8*) moves up and down, the slit beam can be inclined up to 15 degrees. A lever (*10*) swings the slit beam.

The microscope unit of the Kowa ASL-6 is shown in Figure 5-3B. After the rays from the patient's eye pass through the objective lens (*11*), they enter the magnification change unit (*12*), which presents five magnification choices: ×0.4, ×0.6, ×1.0, ×1.6, and ×2.5.

A 5-stage diaphragm ring controls the depth of focus (*13*). The rays reach the eyepieces (*15*) after being reflected by the mirror (*14*). One can see the exact image to be taken on film. Diopter scales are imprinted on both eyepieces. When the shutter is released, the mirror springs up to send the light to the camera and then returns quickly to its original position. One can select the optical axis for taking photographs or easily change the axis, by moving the lever near the camera back.

With most photo slit lamps, either the right or the left axis is used for taking photographs. Two camera backs should be prepared for stereoscopic photos; otherwise, one must use the adapter, and exchanging the camera or attaching the adapter is troublesome. For pictures of the anterior chamber angle or the vitreous humor, one can see the target area very well, but the camera axis does not always exactly encompass that area. In such a case, it is seen through the other axis (not used for photographing). The Kowa ASL-6 was developed to remedy these defects.

The light passes through the prism (*16*) and comes to the rotary lens unit (*17*). In the stereo mode, the light goes through two relay lenses (*18*) and makes a pair of simultaneous stereoscopic images on a full frame of 35-mm film. Each photograph is 24 by 17 mm in size. In the single mode, the light strikes the film after passing through paired mirrors (*19*) and relay lens (*20*). The rotary lens unit (*17*) can be rotated 90 degrees on either side to choose either axis.

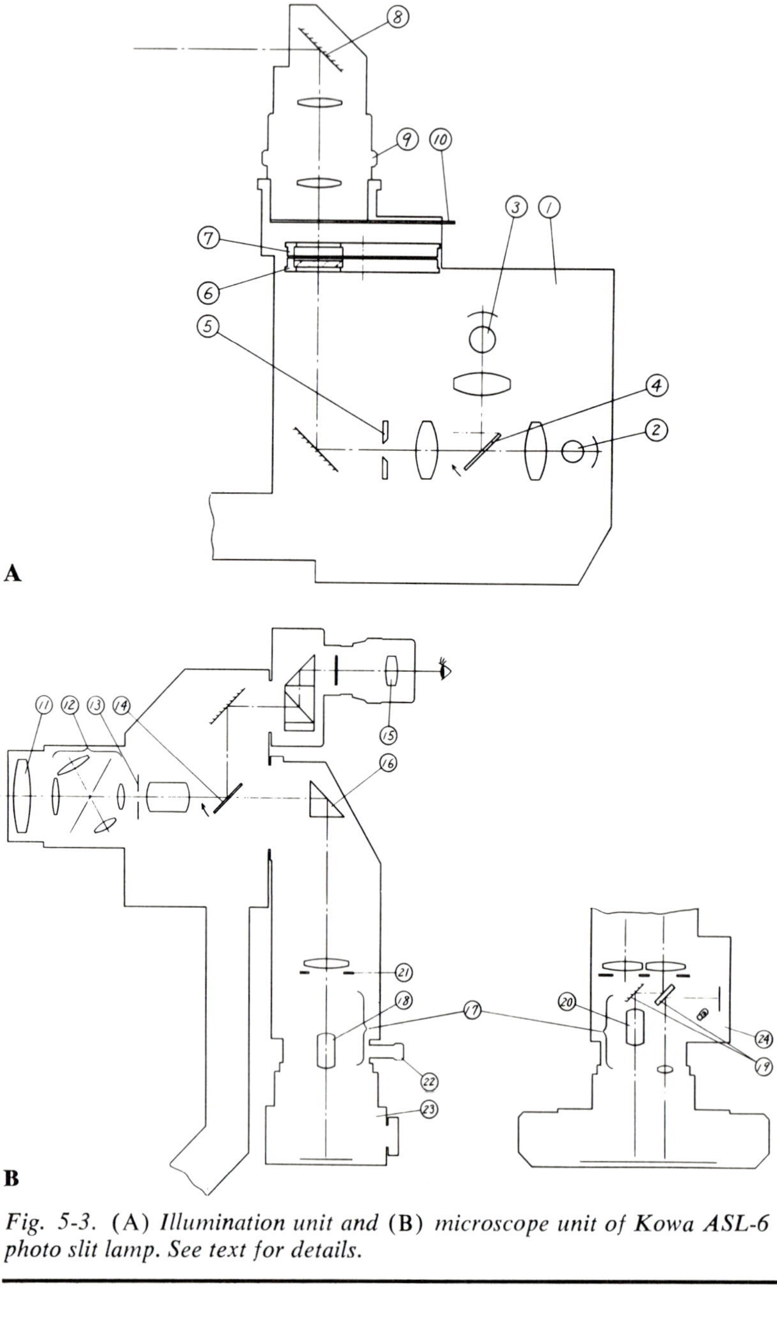

A

B

Fig. 5-3. (A) *Illumination unit and* (B) *microscope unit of Kowa ASL-6 photo slit lamp. See text for details.*

The identification recording unit (*24*) can be used only when the right axis is employed. The space occupied by this unit will soon be taken by the timer for anterior segment fluorescein angiography.

The automatic film-winding camera (*23*) can be used in the model RC-XV system. The circuit is connected to the main body circuit through built-in terminals. The film counter has internal illumination for use in a darkened room. The camera also has threads for an extra filter in front of the objective lens. The alignment is almost that of the Goldmann slit lamps; the shutter release button is on the top of the "joystick" mechanism.

One can use the RC-XV fundus camera system's table stand. Since the support pole is at the right of the stand, both operator and patient can be seated without any physical interference. The unit's location under the table means that no troublesome wiring will complicate alignment. The stand has pedals in the center of its base to adjust elevation, and the footswitch for shutter release is next to them.

Based on my experience as an ophthalmic photographer, I believe that these two new instruments will make it possible for the novice as well as the advanced ophthalmic photographer or ophthalmologist to obtain fundus and slit-lamp photographs of excellent quality.

6

Management of Adverse Reactions to Intravenous Fluorescein

STEPHEN N. SCHINDLER,
JOHNNY JUSTICE, JR., AND
RICHARD A. LEVACY

Although fluorescein angiography is regarded as a relatively safe diagnostic tool in ophthalmology, undesirable and potentially life-threatening side effects occasionally occur. The intent of this chapter is threefold: (1) to present to the practicing ophthalmologist the potential hazards of intravenous fluorescein, (2) to recommend safety precautions necessary in the office, and (3) to present a rational approach to the management of possible adverse reactions to intravenous fluorescein.

Adverse Reactions

Local Effects

EXTRAVASCULAR. Extravasation of fluorescein at the injection site results in intense local pain. The greater the amount of fluorescein extravasated, the more severe the pain [14]. Usually, extravasation is accompanied by a dull, aching pain in the injected arm. The discomfort lasts from 20 to 45 minutes. Sloughing of the skin [6, 9] and eczematous dermatitis [13] following extravasation of fluorescein have been reported. Kratz [6] reported a case of skin necrosis following extravasation of fluorescein that required later skin grafting.

INTRAVENOUS. Intravenous fluorescein may very rarely initiate a chemical thrombophlebitis with associated pain and tenderness along the course of the involved vein. The inflammatory reaction generally subsides in 1 to 2 weeks.

INTRAARTERIAL. Intraarterial fluorescein results in intense staining of the distal extremity and severe pain. The duration of discomfort is quite variable, ranging from 1 to 24 hours.

Systemic Effects

MILD. The most commonly encountered mild side effect of intravenous fluorescein is nausea. Various studies have shown an incidence of 2 to 15 percent of patients [1, 3, 10, 11, 14]. The incidence of nausea appears to be less when injection pressure is increased and when the patient is lying down rather than sitting [1]. Emesis occurs in about 2 percent of patients [1, 10, 11, 14].

Systemic effects of an allergic nature may include flushing of the skin, pruritis, urticaria, paresthesias of the lips and tongue, angioedema, wheezing, and pyrexia. *Urticaria* (hives or wheals) refers to localized patches of edema in the superficial layers of the skin that have erythematous margins and blanched centers. Patients with angioedema have localized dermal edema with an essentially normal epidermis.

SEVERE. Severe systemic effects associated with intravenous fluorescein have an incidence of 0.1 to 0.5 percent (1–5 reactions per 1000 angiographic studies) [1, 2, 7, 10, 11, 12]. These effects can include laryngeal edema, bronchospasm, pulmonary edema, respiratory arrest, hypotension, shock, syncope, cardiac arrhythmias, cardiac arrest, and myocardial infarction. In most instances, recovery is uneventful. Stein and Parker [10] reported one patient who sustained a myocardial infarction within a few hours following fluorescein angiography. The various presentations of adverse reactions to intravenous fluorescein are given in Table 6-1.

Two side effects of intravenous fluorescein administration are present in 100 percent of patients: skin staining, which is a yellow tinting of the skin and conjunctiva that lasts from 6 to 12 hours, and staining of the urine that can last from 2 to 3 days.

Fluorescein angiography is a valuable diagnostic tool that is being used with increasing frequency. The overall incidence of untoward reactions is quite low (1–5 reactions per 1000 procedures), but undoubtedly numerous severe reactions occur that remain unreported in the medical literature.

Table 6-1. Manifestations of Adverse Reactions to Intravenous Fluorescein (Can Occur in any Combination)

Mild Reactions	Severe Reactions
Nausea	Laryngeal edema
Emesis	Bronchospasm
Flushing of skin	Pulmonary edema
Pruritis	Respiratory arrest
Urticaria	Hypotension, shock
Paresthesias of lips, tongue	Syncope
Angioedema	Myocardial infarction
Wheezing	Cardiac arrhythmia, arrest
Pyrexia	Skin necrosis

Safety Precautions

The package insert of one of the commercially available fluorescein preparations* includes the following warning: *An emergency tray for appropriate treatment should be on hand.* With regard to total patient care and medicolegal responsibility, such an explicit warning cannot be ignored. The physician who performs fluorescein angiography must have available equipment, well-trained ancillary personnel, and a definite plan of action to meet a crisis should it occur. Such safety precautions warrant further discussion. The following are precautions taken in the photographic laboratory of the Cullen Eye Institute, Baylor College of Medicine. They require a minimal investment of time and expense; such an investment is greatly appreciated when the rare adverse reaction to intravenous fluorescein does occur.

History

The patient should be questioned about former allergic reactions (hay fever, asthma, fluorescein). A positive history of allergy should alert the physician to potential problems that could result from fluorescein injection. A negative history is no guarantee of impunity. Taking a careful history with specific emphasis on diabetes mellitus, hypertension, angina pectoris, or previous myocardial infarction is essential. A recent change in the pattern of angina pectoris or evidence of uncontrolled hypertension or cardiac arrhythmia are all good reasons to defer angiography until the problem or problems have been carefully investigated or corrected. Physicians who perform fluorescein angiography should also be aware of some important properties of fluorescein. Fluorescein:

1. Is nontoxic
2. Has molecular weight 332
3. Remains intravascularly in the retina
4. Is excreted unchanged in the urine within 24 to 36 hours
5. Emits green yellow light detectable visually and photographically
6. Does not cross-react with iodinated radiographic contrast dyes
7. Elimination prolonged by renal insufficiency
8. Does not cause teratogenicity or embryocidicity in mice and rabbits [8]

Trained Staff

The ancillary personnel in any office where fluorescein angiography is performed should be well trained and aware of their roles in the event of a severe reaction. They should be thoroughly familiar with the emergency equipment available and the location of such equipment.

* Fluorescite injection 5%, Alcon Laboratories, Inc., Fort Worth, TX 76134.

Table 6-2. Recommended Basic Emergency Equipment and Drugs

Item	Specific Description
Airway	Oral, endotracheal tube, Ambu bag
Oxygen	Portable cylinders, appropriate delivery tubing
Blood pressure cuff	
Parenteral fluids	IV stand, D_5W or saline, intravenous catheters, tubing, syringes, needles
Drugs	Epinephrine 1 : 1000 injectable
	Diphenhydramine (Benadryl) injectable
	Aminophylline parenteral
	Metaraminol bitartrate (Aramine) injectable
	Hydrocortisone sodium succinate (Solu-Cortef) injectable
	Promethazine (Phenergan) injectable

Medical Equipment and Drugs

Adequate medical equipment and emergency medications should be within immediate access in the event they are needed. The photographic laboratory shown in Figure 6-1 has emergency equipment readily available. The *minimum* in terms of an adequate emergency tray is presented in Table 6-2. We use the emergency kit illustrated (Fig. 6-2). The advantages of such a kit are that it (1) provides complete medical supplies, with the exception of oxygen and an Ambu bag; (2) is compact; and (3) is easily replenished if items are used.

Consent

One further medicolegal precaution we require is a signed consent form (Fig. 6-3). After obtaining an allergic history, we inform all patients of the potential adverse reactions, obtain the signed consent, and perform fluorescein angiography only when a physician is immediately available.

Practical Management of Adverse Reactions

In most instances of severe reactions to intravenous fluorescein, recovery is the rule. The following is intended as a practical approach to the management of these reactions, a guide for training ancillary personnel, and a brief review for physicians who have not treated such cases recently. The indications and dosages of all drugs mentioned have been recommended in the medical literature. The package insert for each drug should be consulted for use and dosage as approved by the FDA. Dosages given are for *adult* patients.

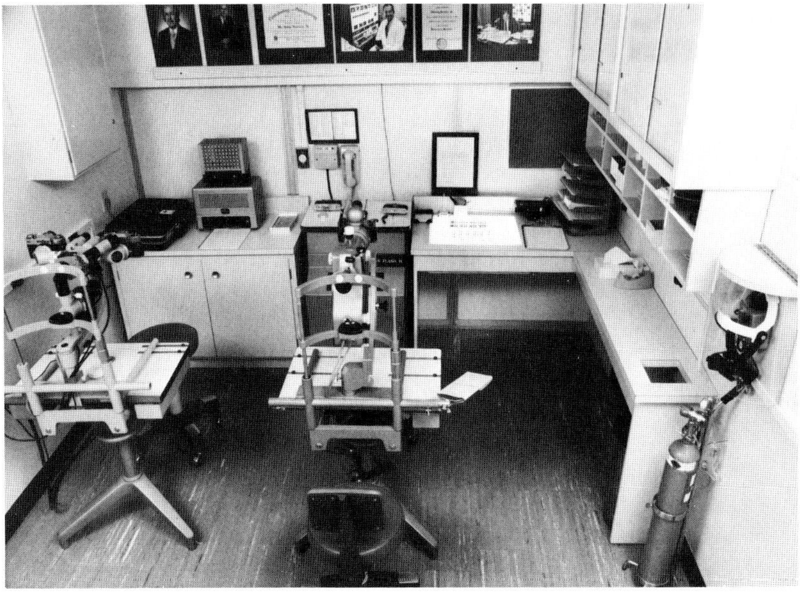

Fig. 6-1. Ophthalmic photographic laboratory, Department of Ophthalmology, Baylor College of Medicine, Houston, Texas. Note emergency kit at far left and oxygen at right.

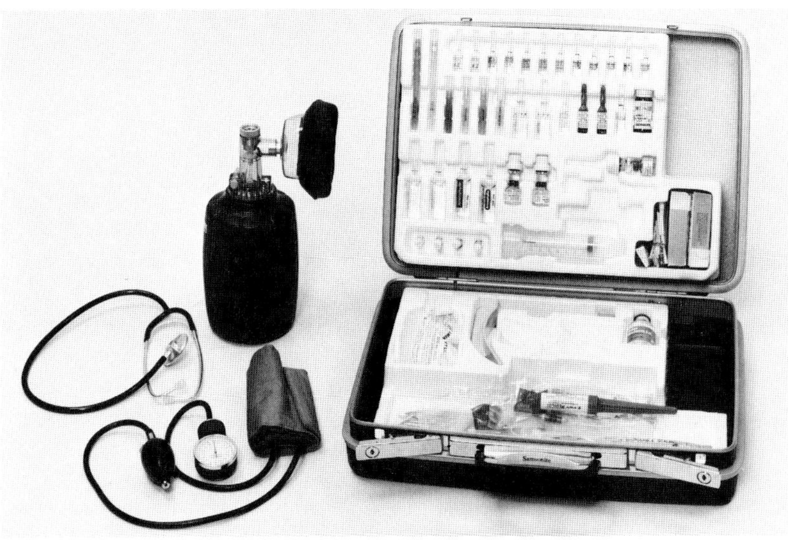

Fig. 6-2. Emergency-1 Kit. Manufactured by Banyan International Corporation, Abilene, Texas.

BAYLOR OPHTHALMOLOGY CONSULTANTS
Fluorescein Angiography Laboratory

CONSENT FOR FLUORESCEIN ANGIOGRAPHY

NAME OF PATIENT: ____________________________

1. I hereby authorize the ophthalmologist and/or the ophthalmic photographer in the Department of Ophthalmology at Baylor College of Medicine to administer intravenous fluorescein for the purpose of fluorescein angiography as requested by ________________, M.D.
2. This is a diagnostic study and I understand that no warranty or guarantee has been made as to the results or cure.
3. I authorize and direct the aforementioned physician and/or The Baylor Ophthalmology Associates and Assistants to provide such additional services as they deem reasonable and necessary.
4. *FOR WOMEN ONLY:* Although there is no scientific evidence of damage to unborn babies, intravenous fluorescein is not customarily administered to pregnant women. I clearly state that I am not pregnant.
5. Having received an explanation and given informed consent, I hereby agree to release The Baylor Ophthalmology Consultants, its employees, agents, and medical staff from further responsibility with regard to permission for this procedure.

I have read this form carefully before signing it and have been given an opportunity to question my physician about this procedure.

____________________	____________________
Patient's Signature	Witness (Must be an adult)
Date: ________________	Time: ________________ AM / PM

Fig. 6-3. Consent form for fluorescein angiography.

Local Irritation

The pain resulting from local extravasation of fluorescein or the dull ache in the injected arm after administration of the dye is self-limiting. Treatment consists of cold compresses and reassurance to the patient.

Nausea and Vomiting

Although approximately 10 percent of patients experience nausea, only 2 percent actually vomit. Usually this reaction is transient, requiring no therapy other than reassurance. In patients with a history of marked nausea or vomiting who require repeated fluorescein injections, premedication with promethazine hydrochloride (Phenergan) 25 mg intramuscularly 30 minutes before the fluorescein injection could be considered.

Urticaria, Pruritis, or Angioedema

Immediate allergic reactions occur generally within 1 hour and consist of pruritis, urticaria, or other manifestations of an anaphylactic reaction.

ANTIHISTAMINES. Given orally or parenterally, antihistamines, which are mediated through the release of histamine, inhibit urticaria, pruritis, hypotension, and bronchospasm. The physician should administer an antihistamine, diphenhydramine (Benadryl), 50 mg orally or intramuscularly, depending on the severity of the reaction.

EPINEPHRINE. With urticaria combined with angioedema, administration of epinephrine 1 : 1000 0.2 to 0.3 ml subcutaneously results in rapid resolution of wheals and edema. Continue antihistamines orally for an additional 24 hours.

Bronchospasm or Asthma

Sympathomimetics are the mainstay for an acute asthmatic attack.

EPINEPHRINE. Administer epinephrine 1 : 1000 0.2 to 0.4 ml subcutaneously (if no contraindication); this dose may be repeated as often as necessary.

AMINOPHYLLINE. Inject aminophylline 250 mg intravenously slowly over 5 minutes.

Hydrocortisone Sodium Succinate

For a prolonged reaction or severe bronchospasm, administer hydrocortisone sodium succinate (Solu-Cortef) 500 mg intravenously. The patient might require corticosteroids administered orally for a short period.

Anaphylactic Shock

Generally the rapid onset of symptoms signifies a more severe reaction.

EPINEPHRINE. Administer epinephrine 1 : 1000 0.3 to 0.5 ml subcutaneously and repeat every 15 to 30 minutes as needed. With *severe* shock, administer epinephrine 1 : 1000 0.5 ml in 10 ml D_5W or saline intravenously. If no response occurs, repeat the dose every 5 to 15 minutes.

INTRAVENOUS FLUIDS. Administer intravenous fluids to replenish intravascular volume. With prolonged shock, administer sodium bicarbonate 50 ml every 5 minutes to correct acidosis.

OXYGEN, AMINOPHYLLINE, SOLU-CORTEF. Maintain an adequate airway and administer oxygen as required. Bronchial and laryngeal edema are hazards. For bronchospasm, aminophylline 500 mg intravenously should be injected slowly over 10 minutes; for prolonged or severe bronchospasm, Solu-Cortef 500 mg intravenously should be administered.

ANTIHISTAMINES. Antihistamines block further histamine binding and can shorten the duration of the reaction. Administer Benadryl 10 to 20 mg intravenously.

METARMINOL BITARTRATE. Unless the blood pressure is raised excessively, metarminol bitartrate (Aramine) increases cardiac output. If it is used, attempt to bring the systolic blood pressure to only 90 to 100 mm Hg, using 25 to 100 mg in 500 ml D_5W or saline infusion as necessary to maintain blood pressure at that level.

TREATMENT SETTING. Transfer the patient to adequate medical facilities as rapidly as possible.

References

1. Chazan, B. I., Balodimos, M. C., and Koncz, L. Untoward effects of fluorescein retinal angiography in diabetic patients. *Ann. Ophthalmol.* 3 : 42, 1971.
2. Chung, E. K. Drug-associated EKG changes. *Fluor. Drug Ther.* 89 : 89, 1976.
3. Greene, G. G., et al. Adverse reactions to intravenous fluorescein: Evidence for sex difference. *Ann. Ophthalmol.* 8 : 533, 1976.
4. Hess, J. B., and Pacurariu, R. I. Acute pulmonary edema following intravenous fluorescein angiography. *Am. J. Ophthalmol.* 82 : 567, 1976.
5. Ingelstedt, S., and Iustam, B. Hypersensitivity to fluorescein. *Int. Arch. Allergy Appl. Immunol.* 1 : 157, 1950.

6. Kratz, R. P., Mazzocco, T. R., and Davidson, B. A case report of skin necrosis following infiltration with I.V. fluorescein. *Ann. Ophthalmol.* 12 : 654, 1980.
7. La Piana, F. G., and Penner, R. Anaphylactoid reaction to intravenously administered fluorescein. *Arch. Ophthalmol.* 79 : 161, 1968.
8. McEnerney, J. K., Wong, W. P., and Peyman, G. A. Evaluation of the tetratogenicity of fluorescein sodium. *Am. J. Ophthalmol.* 84 : 847, 1977.
9. Schatz, H. Sloughing of the skin following fluorescein extravasation. *Ann. Ophthalmol.* 10 : 625, 1978.
10. Stein, M. R., and Parker, C. W. Reactions following intravenous fluorescein. *Am. J. Ophthalmol.* 72 : 861, 1971.
11. Trimble, G. X. Low incidence of reactions during fluorescein angiography. *J. A. M. A.* 227 : 1448, 1974.
12. Wesley, R. E., Blount, W. C., and Arterberry, J. F. Acute myocardial infarction after fluorescein angiography. *Am. J. Ophthalmol.* 87 : 834, 1979.
13. Wing, G. L., and Weiter, J. J. Eczematous dermatitis following fluorescein extravasation. *Ann. Ophthalmol.* 12 : 825, 1980.
14. Yannuzzi, L. A., Justice, J., Jr., and Baldwin, H. A. Effective differences in the formulation of intravenous fluorescein and related side effects. *Am. J. Ophthalmol.* 78 : 217, 1974.

7

Use of the Astigmatism Correction Device on the Zeiss Fundus Camera for Peripheral Retinal Photography

BRUCE J. BUSSE AND
DAVID MITTELMAN

The ability to photograph lesions accurately in the peripheral regions of the fundus of the eye is extremely important in ophthalmology. Such peripheral lesions include sea fans in sickle cell retinopathy, angiomas in von Hippel-Lindau disease, and peripherally located malignant melanomas. Our earlier attempts to obtain good photographs were extremely disappointing (Fig. 7-1); however, through trial and error, we were able to improve their quality as well as that of fluorescein angiograms (Fig. 7-2). This great improvement was possible primarily through better understanding of the use of the astigmatism correction device incorporated into the Zeiss fundus camera. Unfortunately, the Zeiss fundus camera operating manual [2] does not contain information concerning this device, nor is it available in any other source. The purpose of this chapter is to present a brief and simple explanation of astigmatism and the use of the astigmatism correction device in achieving high-quality peripheral fundus photographs.

Types of Astigmatism

The two types of astigmatism that we wish to discuss are paraxial (refractive) astigmatism and astigmatism of oblique incidence, with particular emphasis on the latter [1]. Paraxial astigmatism is a difference in the refracting power of the eye in two planes or meridians caused by one or more of the refractive surfaces (cornea, anterior or posterior surfaces of the lens). In a simple spherical lens (Fig. 7-3), all meridians of the lens surface have the same degree of curvature, allowing parallel rays of light entering the lens to be refracted to a sharp point focus. When all the meridians do not have the same curvature, this sharp point focus is not possible, and such a lens is called astigmatic. When a ray of light strikes an astigmatic lens (Fig. 7-4), it is not refracted to a fine point; instead, astigmatic line imagery is formed. This astigmatism results from the fact that the front lens surface has two radii of curvature and therefore two refracting powers. Thus, two line foci are formed at right angles to each other separated by a vari-

This study was supported in part by contract NIH 72 2956B and grant IP HL 15168-03 from the National Heart and Lung Institute.

The authors thank Rosalind Stephens and Jane Lantz for their help in preparing this chapter.

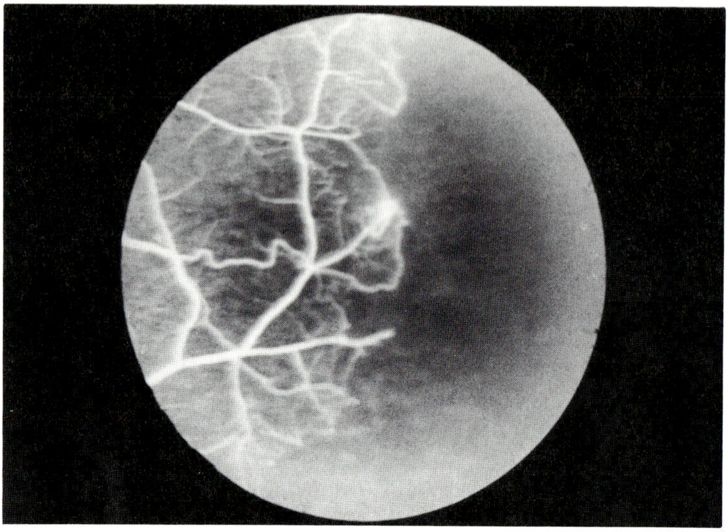

Fig. 7-1. Peripheral sickle cell avascular zone photographed without the astigmatism correction device.

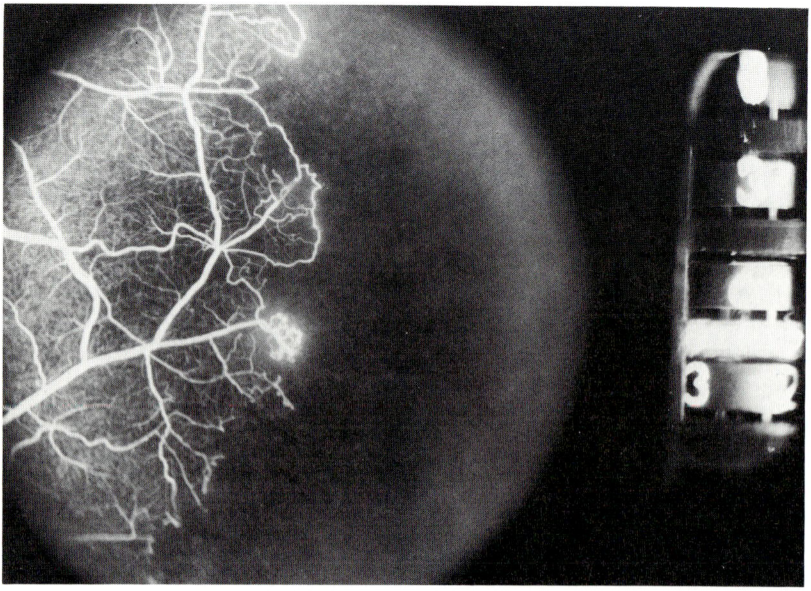

Fig. 7-2. Same peripheral sickle cell avascular zone as Fig. 7-1, 3 months later, with astigmatism correction device.

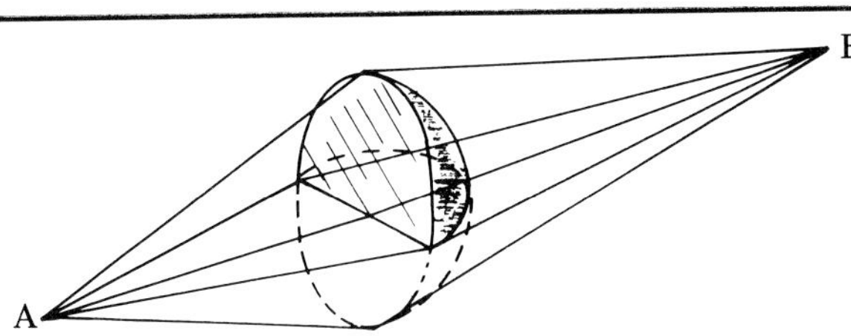

Fig. 7-3. Spherical lens with ray of light (A) *being refracted to focused point* (B).

able distance (Sturm's interval), which includes a circle of least confusion.

Parallel rays of light striking a spherical lens at an oblique angle also cause astigmatism. The rays do not come to a sharp point focus; instead, line imagery similar to that produced by a toric (astigmatic) lens is formed. This type of astigmatism is caused by rays of light passing obliquely through the refracting surfaces of the eye in a manner similar to that which occurs when one attempts to visualize the retinal periphery (Fig. 7-5).

Astigmatic Correction

The cylinder is a type of astigmatic lens that also may be used to correct astigmatism. Some simple diagrams are shown that explain the principle of the cylinder, how it corrects for astigmatism, and its relation to the line imagery formed. A cylindrical lens is not symmetric about its optical axis. Light that strikes such a lens in a plane parallel to the axis of the cylinder (Fig. 7-6) passes through in a straight line. These rays meet a linear surface and are not refracted in any way. Therefore, one can say that there is no curvature in the meridian parallel to the axis of the cylinder. A plane at a right angle to the axis of a cylinder (Fig. 7-7) intersects the cylinder in the arc of a circle and is refracted in the same manner as in a spherical lens. A point light source, when passed through a cylindrical lens, will bring all rays to a line focus parallel to the axis of the cylindrical lens; Figure 7-8 shows that rays emitting from point *A* and passing parallel to the axis are not refracted at all, and rays passing perpendicular to the axis are refracted and form the focused line *B*.

Figure 7-9, which is a combination of Figures 7-5 and 7-8, illustrates how astigmatism correction works. Light reflecting off the retina strikes the optical surfaces of the eye at an oblique angle and causes astigmatism. The proximal rays are brought to focus along a plane at point *H*. The difference in refraction of the distal rays causes these rays to focus along a plane at point *V*. Insertion of a plug cylinder of a given power between the eye and the focused plane at point *H* with

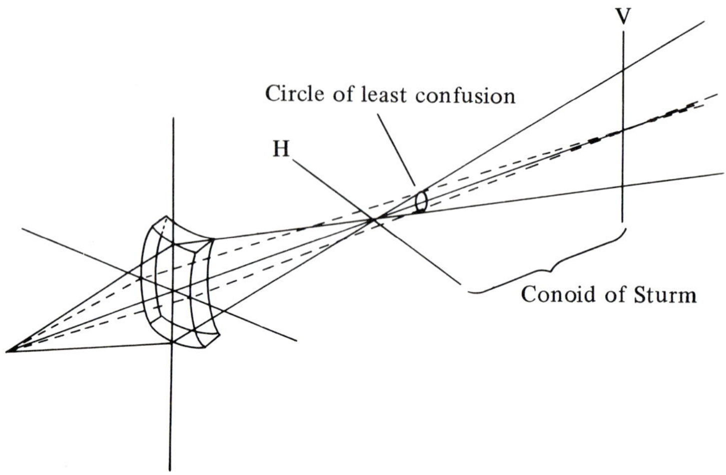

Fig. 7-4. Astigmatic lens with ray of light being refracted to form line foci (H and V). *Foci form right angle. They are separated by Sturm's conoid, which contains a circle of least confusion.*

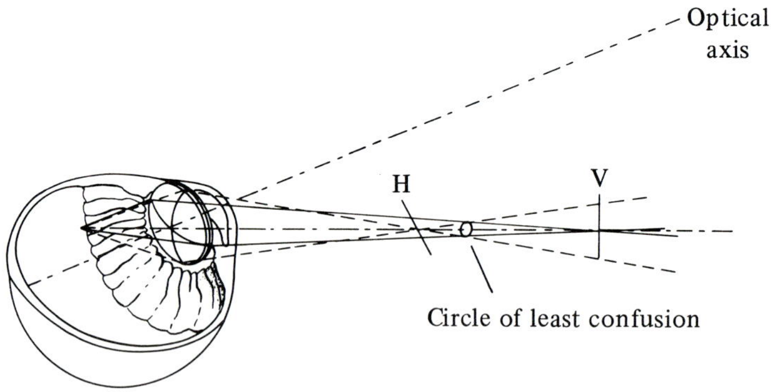

Fig. 7-5. Astigmatic line imagery formed when viewing peripheral fundus through lens at oblique angle (e.g., when photographing the periphery).

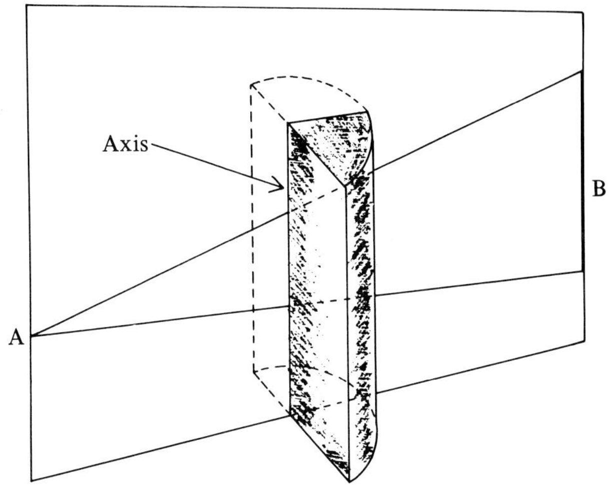

Fig. 7-6. Cylindrical lens, with ray of light (A) *in plane parallel to the cylindrical axis.* A *is unrefracted and forms focused line* (B).

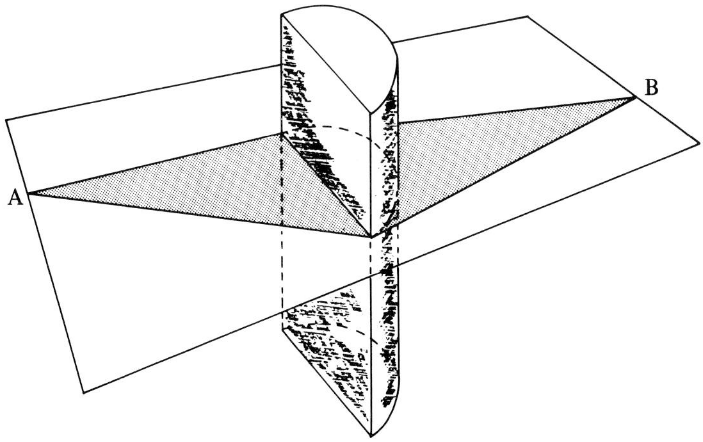

Fig. 7-7. Cylindrical lens, with ray of light (A) *in plane perpendicular to cylindrical axis.* A *is being refracted and forms the focused point* (B).

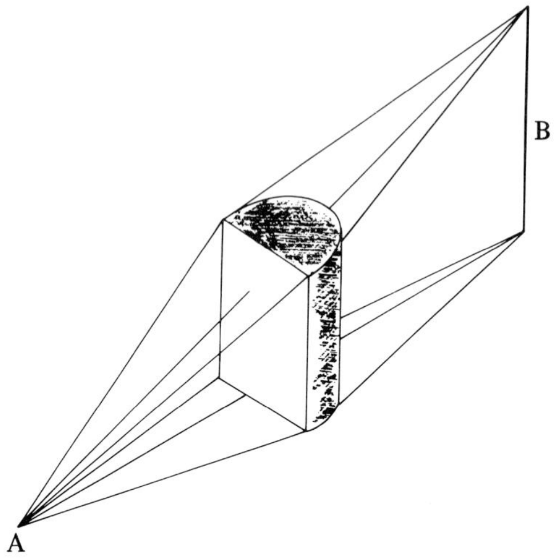

Fig. 7-8. Combination of Figs. 7-6 and 7-7: astigmatic line imagery formed when ray of light (A) *is refracted to form image line* (B).

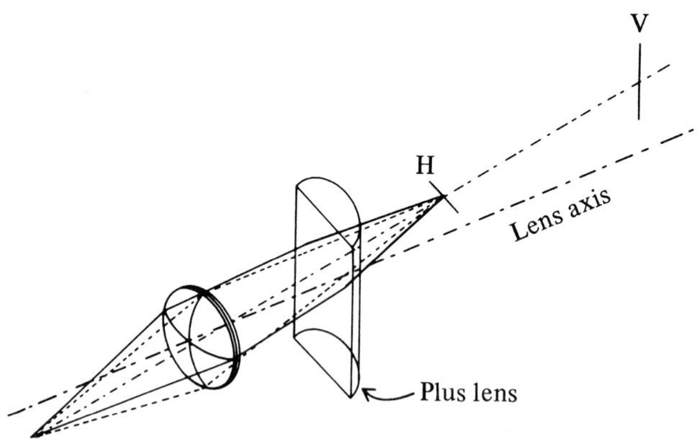

Fig. 7-9. Plus cylinder, perpendicular to optical axis of spherical lens, when viewed obliquely refracts distal rays (V) *to same point of focus as proximal rays* (H).

the cylindrical axis perpendicular to the axis of the eye will refocus the distal rays to the same point at which the proximal rays are focused. The proximal rays are unaffected by the vertical placement of the cylinder as they pass through its linear surface. This placement of the cylindrical lens corrects any astigmatism and gives a sharp image over the entire field.

Astigmatic Correction Device

To neutralize the astigmatism induced when peripheral pictures are taken, a variable cylindrical lens system is used within the Zeiss fundus camera to give a ± cylinder in the range of 0 to 10 D or 3 to 20 D, depending on the camera model (Fig. 7-10). The degree of astigmatism produced by peripheral retinal photography varies with the square of the tangent of the angle of oblique incidence. Thus, light striking the refractive surfaces of the eye at an angle of 30 degrees will produce 10 to 15 D of astigmatism. Neutralization of this induced astigmatism along with collapse of Sturm's conoid is crucial in achieving the sharpest possible focal imagery when photographing the peripheral retina.

Limitation of movement of the astigmatism correction device (110°) often prevents placement of a plus cylinder perpendicular to the axis of the eye, in which case a minus cylinder of a given power should be placed parallel to the axis between the eye and the focused plane at point *H* (Fig. 7-11). The distal rays will be unaffected by the horizontal placement of the cylinder and will not be refracted: These rays will focus at plane *V*. The proximal rays will be diverged by the minus cylinder to refocus at the same point at which the horizontal rays are focused. Again, this should correct for the induced astigmatism and give sharp imagery over the entire field.

Positioning the astigmatism correction device in relation to the eye in the different positions of gaze is shown in Figure 7-12. Position A illustrates a gaze up and to the left. The astigmatism correction device is placed perpendicular to the axis of the eye, and plus diopters of cylinder are dialed into the instrument. Position B illustrates a gaze down and to the right. Again, the astigmatism correction device is set perpendicular to the axis of the eye, and plus diopters of cylinder are dialed into the instrument to correct for the induced astigmatism.

As mentioned previously, limitation of movement often requires positioning the astigmatism device parallel to the axis of the lens and dialing minus diopters of cylinder into the instrument. Position C illustrates a gaze down and to the left with the astigmatism correction device set parallel to the axis and minus diopters of cylinder dialed into the instrument. Position D illustrates a gaze up and to the right, with the astigmatism correction device set parallel to the axis of the eye and minus diopters of cylinder dialed into the instrument.

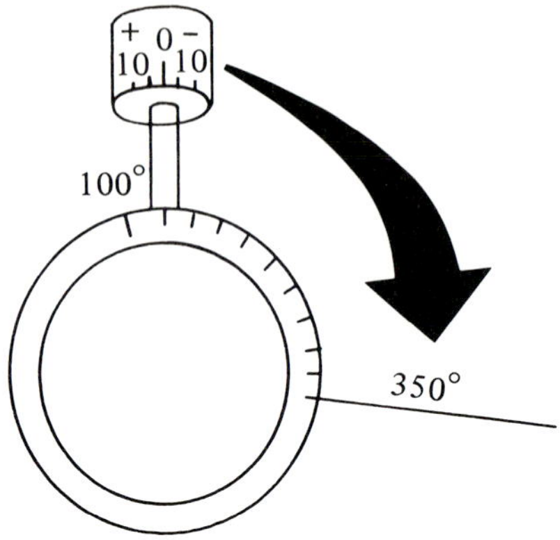

Fig. 7-10. Astigmatic correction device on Zeiss fundus camera. Arrow *indicates limitation of movement.*

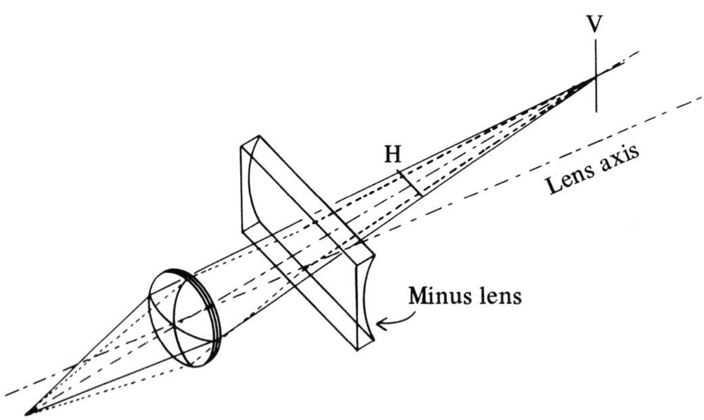

Fig. 7-11. Minus cylinder, parallel to optical axis of spherical lens, when viewed obliquely refracts proximal rays (H) *to same point as distal rays* (V).

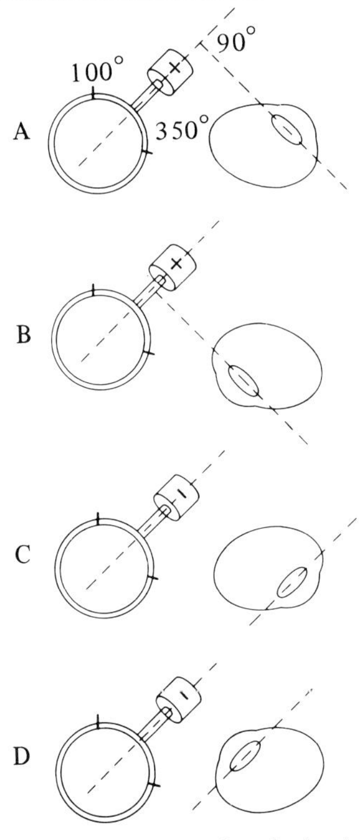

Fig. 7-12. Position of astigmatism correction device in relation to patient's gaze (explained fully in text).

Because of the many variables existing in the eye (differing degrees of rotation, variations in the surface of the cornea, and the possibility of refractive astigmatism), the exact amount of power needed can be determined only by viewing the fundus through the camera and adjusting the astigmatism correction device until the entire field is brought into focus.

Figure 7-13 shows the difference in detail of the peripheral retina obtained with and without the astigmatism correction device.

When taking photographs of the posterior pole, one can also use the astigmatism correction device to correct for refractive astigmatism. The device works in the same manner except for the amount of cylindrical power needed to make corrections. Figure 7-14 shows the fine capillary network in the macula which can be recorded after fine tuning the focus with the astigmatism correction device.

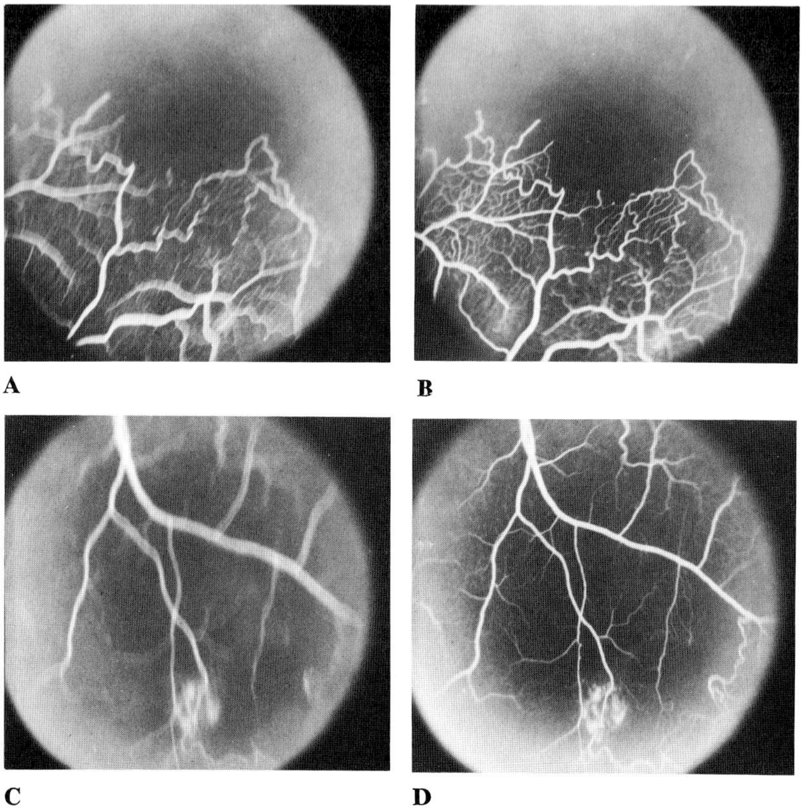

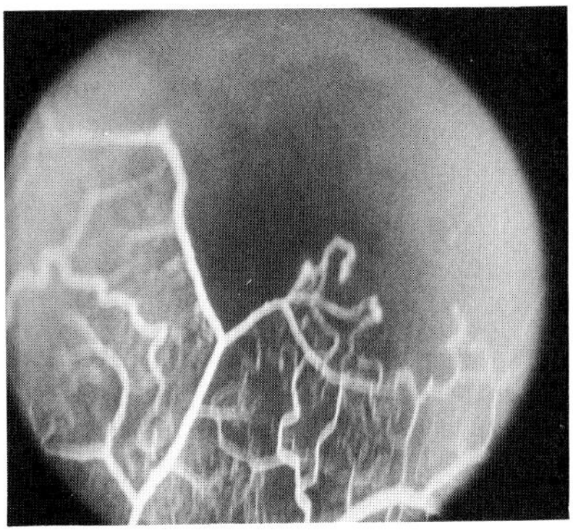

E

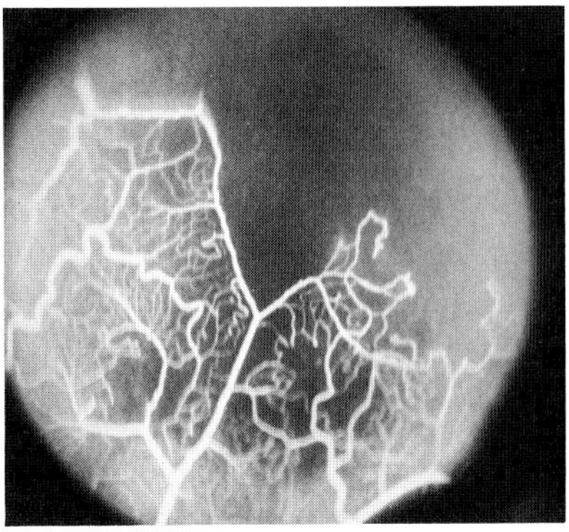

F

Fig. 7-13. Peripheral fundus photographs of sickle cell retinopathy. A, C, and E show areas photographed without use of astigmatism correction device; B, D, and F show same areas photographed using the device.

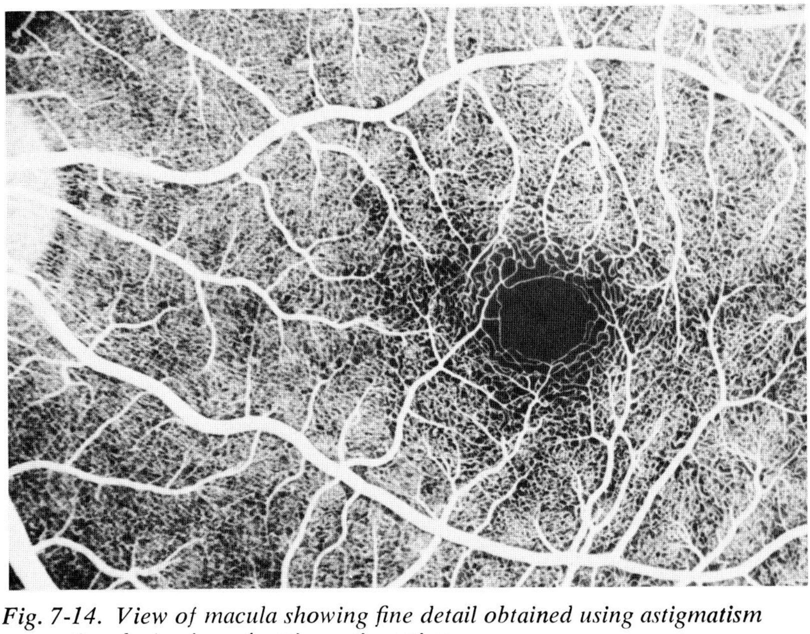

Fig. 7-14. View of macula showing fine detail obtained using astigmatism correction device for refractive astigmatism.

Conclusion

High-quality photographs of the peripheral retina are made possible by the proper positioning of the astigmatism correction device on the Zeiss fundus camera. Using a plus cylinder, axis perpendicular or a minus cylinder, axis parallel to that around which the eye is rotated will eliminate the astigmatism induced by viewing the retina obliquely through the optical surfaces of the eye, resulting in a sharply focused image at the film plane. Proper use of this instrument can be helpful in evaluating and diagnosing retinal lesions that occur in the peripheral fundus.

References

1. Davson, H. *The Physiology of the Eye.* Boston: Little, Brown, 1963. P. 423.
2. Zeiss, C. *Description and Instruction Manual for Fundus Flash 3.* 1974.

8

Film, Developing, and Printing Techniques for Fluorescein Angiography

ARTHUR SMIALOWSKI

Film Used in Black-and-White Fluorescein Angiography

In black-and-white fluorescein fundus angiography two types of film are used, that employed for routine photographs and that used for special purposes. During the last 15 years, Kodak Tri-X film (ASA 400) has been found to produce good results regardless of any difficulties the photographer may experience in taking fundus angiograms. This type of film has a wide latitude of exposure and will produce adequate photographic images in patients with minimal pupillary dilatation or cloudy media as well as in peripheral views. To increase the exposure latitude, sensitivity, and contrast even further, this film should be overdeveloped by doubling the speed. Tri-X film is panchromatic and has good sensitivity in red, green, and blue spectrums. The combination of speed, balance, and color sensitivity ideally suits it for fundus fluorescein angiograms. In addition, Kodak Tri-X gives excellent gradation and brilliant highlights, which provide good tonal separation between blood vessels and surrounding pathologic changes. This medium–fine-grain film of medium resolving power produces negatives of good quality even when it is not precisely exposed or developed.

Special Purpose Black-and-White Film

When maximum sharpness, contrast, and resolving power are required, Kodak Plus-X panchromatic film (ASA 125) is an excellent choice. This film has a fine grain and medium speed, which permit maximal reproduction of fine details for special studies. Because of the film's narrower exposure latitude and speed, patients must be cooperative and have clear media and widely dilated pupils. Usually it is necessary to increase the flash intensity to compensate for the lower speed of the film. Plus-X film is used extensively when photographing the fundus with red-free light and in ordinary black-and-white fundus photography of the eye. However, for routine fluorescein fundus angiography, Tri-X film is preferable.

Roll Film Capacity

For black and white fluorescein fundus photography, standard 35-mm roll film with 36 frames is of adequate length to record the sequential

For help with this manuscript, I would like to thank Ann Smialowski, Linda A. Huett, William N. Milan, Jr., Dr. Dwain G. Fuller, and Dr. Richard A. Lewis.

fluorescein events. A second roll can be quickly loaded if additional exposures are needed, which is often the case in recording late stages of fluorescence. For extended, uninterrupted high-speed photography, such as that required for research purposes, Tri-X and Plus-X films are available in large rolls suitable for motor-driven, large capacity cameras. In routine photography, bulk capacity cartridges are cumbersome to handle, and the entire film must be processed if immediate access to a single angiogram is necessary.

Film Storage

With time, film becomes subject to deterioration which is accelerated by high temperature and humidity. Film should be stored in a cool, dry place away from chemicals, vapors, and radiation. It should not be stored longer than 6 months without proper refrigeration. Exposed film should be processed as soon as possible (within 1 or 2 days) to avoid deterioration of the latent image. Film that has been refrigerated should stand at room temperature for 3 to 5 hours in the original package to prevent moisture condensation on the film emulsion. Modern film will take a reasonable amount of abuse, but careful handling and application of basic knowledge are necessary to ensure consistently good results.

Film Developing

Fluorescein fundus angiograms exposed on black-and-white Tri-X panchromatic film require a developer of high energy to increase film speed and contrast within a reasonable time with low film fog. Kodak D-11 developer has proved satisfactory for this purpose if used at full strength for 6 minutes at 68°F (20°C). Both D-11 and D-76 are clean-working developers with good latitude and produce low fog on forced development.

Other developers are used for special purposes. The ultrafine-grain developers usually are not recommended because of their relatively low contrast with loss of effective film speed. It is best to use just one or two developers because, with constant use, the photographer learns their characteristics and capabilities.

Commercially Prepared Chemicals

The photographer has little time to spend mixing complicated formulas de novo. The prepared chemicals that require only dissolving or dilution in water are convenient and assure a solution of the proper strength and chemical properties. Prepared photographic chemicals have a long shelf life, are of uniformly high quality, and can be readily mixed into working solutions.

Preparing Developing Solutions
For photographers who prefer to mix their own developing solutions, the following are two examples from standard Kodak formulas of developers for black-and-white Tri-X panchromatic film used for fluorescein fundus angiograms.

KODAK D-11 DEVELOPER
Water, about 50°C (125°F): 500.0 ml
Elon developing agent: 1.0 gm
Sodium sulfite (anhydrous): 75.0 gm
Hydroquinone: 9.0 gm
Sodium carbonate (monohydrated): 30.0 gm
Potassium bromide (anhydrous): 5.0 gm
Cold water to make 1.0 liter

Use this developer full strength at 68°F for 6 minutes with intermittent agitation.

KODAK D-76 DEVELOPER
Water, about 50°C (125°F): 750.0 ml
Elon developing agent: 2.0 gm
Sodium sulfite (anhydrous): 100.0 gm
Hydroquinone: 5.0 gm
Borax (granular): 2.0 gm
Water to make 1.0 liter

Use this developer full strength at 68°F for 8 minutes with Tri-X panchromatic film. When developing Plus-X panchromatic film, dilute this agent with equal parts of water (1 : 1). Develop at 68°F for 10 minutes.

Paper and Graphic Film Developer
Kodak Dektol developer has a high capacity, uniform rate of development, and high energy. These qualities are suited for developing photographic paper and graphic films in trays when making positive contact slides of angiograms.

DEKTOL DEVELOPER
Water, about 50°C (125°F): 500.0 ml
Elon developing agent: 3.0 gm
Sodium sulfite (anhydrous): 45.0 gm
Hydroquinone: 12.0 gm
Sodium carbonate (monohydrated): 80.0 gm
Potassium bromide (anhydrous): 2.0 gm
Water to make 1.0 liter

Dilute one part of stock solution with two parts water to make a working solution. Average developing time in a tray with continuous agitation at 68°F is 2 to 3 minutes.

Stop Bath and Fixing Solution for Film and Paper

KODAK SB-5 STOP BATH
Water: 500.0 ml
28% acetic acid: 32.0 ml*
Sodium sulfate (anhydrous): 45.0 gm†
Water to make 1.0 liter

Bathe the films or plates for about 30 seconds, with agitation, at 18° to 21°C (65°–70°F) between developing and fixing. This bath should be replaced after approximately 13 rolls of film per liter (quart) have been processed.

KODAK F-5 FIXING BATH
Water, about 50°C (125°F): 600.0 ml
Sodium thiosulfate (pentahydrated): 240.0 gm
Sodium sulfate (anhydrous): 15.0 gm
28% acetic acid: 48.0 ml
Boric acid, crystals: 7.5 gm‡
Potassium alum, fine granular (dodecahydrated): 15.0 gm
Cold water to make 1.0 liter

Films or plates should be fixed for 5 to 10 minutes in a freshly prepared bath. The bath need not be discarded until fixing time exceeds 10 minutes. Kodak F-5 fixing bath is recommended for general use.

Containers for Film Developing
Thirty-six–exposure lengths of 35-mm film are processed in spiral reels, either singly or in groups. Automatic processing machines are commonly used for developing large numbers of film rolls or when quick developing is necessary. For small quantities of roll film, use Kinderman or Honeywell-Nikor stainless steel tanks and spiral reels. For large quantities of roll film, use hard rubber or stainless steel 3½ gallon tanks 8 by 10 inches in dimension (Fig. 8-1).

To save time, labor, and working space in processing bulk quantities of 35-mm film, an automatic processor can be used, although its

* To make approximately 28% acetic acid from glacial acetic acid, dilute 3 parts glacial acetic acid with 8 parts water.
† If crystalline sodium sulfate is preferred to the anhydrous form, use 2¼ times the quantity listed.
‡ Crystalline boric acid should be used as specified, since powdered boric acid dissolves with great difficulty.

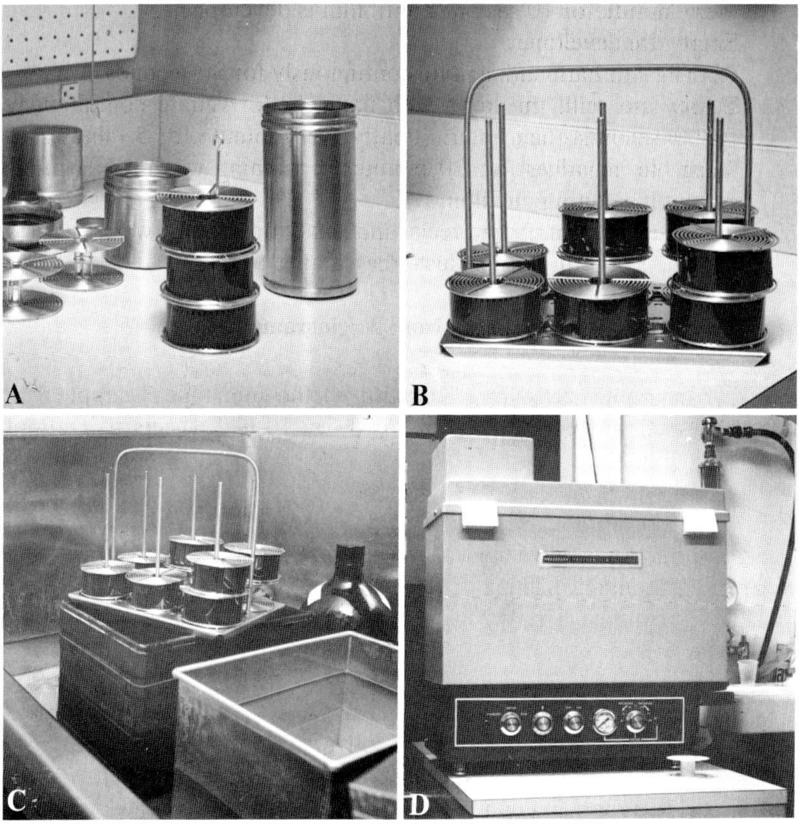

Fig. 8-1. Angiograms are usually processed on spiral reels in tanks. (A) *Suitable method for developing one to four rolls of film.* (B and C) *One to twenty rolls of film can be developed easily by using spiral reels in a basket with deep tanks.* (D) *For large volume of film, automatic processor is recommended.*

initial cost is high. The Kodak Recordak Prostar DVR model will process negatives in minutes. In my experience, however, manual developing is a requisite for the highest quality.

Steps in Processing Film in Small Tanks

1. Fill the tank with developing solution at 68°F; turn room lights off.
2. Load the film on spiral reels.
3. Immerse the loader film in the tank containing the developer.
4. Start the timer.

5. Agitate the film for 10 seconds. Continue intermittent agitation every minute for 10 seconds until film is developed.
6. Empty the developer.
7. Pour in stop bath and agitate continuously for 30 seconds.
8. Empty and refill the tank with fixing bath. Agitate continuously for 30 seconds, then intermittently every minute for 5 minutes.
9. Wash the negatives for 20 minutes in running water while intermittently agitating the film.
10. Remove the film from reels and soak up excess water with a sponge. Hang in warm, dust-free cabinet to dry.

Making Positive Transparencies from Angiograms

Material

Use Kodak graphic arts film, Kodalith, Ortho film type 3 supplied in 10- by 12-inch sheets, 50 per box, or 8- by 10-inch sheets of DuPont Cronar A (Fig. 8-2).

Printing

Contact print the sandwiched negative film and Kodalith, emulsion to emulsion, in contact printer or frame. Develop in Dektol diluted 1 : 3 for 2 to 3 minutes. Fix, wash, dry, and mount for positive transparency (Fig. 8-3).

Contact Prints

Contact positive prints of an entire roll of film, cut into six exposure strips, are often made for records and reports. The negatives and photographic paper are contact printed using a procedure similar to that employed in making positive transparencies. Glossy surface, single weight paper is best suited for contact prints because it gives maximum detail and contrast. Both Kodabromide and Kodak Polycontrast rapid RC paper F are good for this purpose.

Enlarging the Angiogram

Selected enlarged frames of the angiograms are used for records, referrals, publication, and diagnostic purposes (Fig. 8-4). A standard 35-mm negative carrier can be used. To achieve a crisp, round outline, a custom-made round negative carrier should be used; a selection of round openings of varying diameters is useful. A selection of photographic papers should be available for trial. Glossy finish paper is preferable for obtaining maximum detail and contrast and is required by most publishers (Fig. 8-5). A popular paper for making positive enlargements is Kodak Polycontrast rapid RC paper F, available in 5- by 7-inch and 8- by 10-inch sizes. This modern photographic paper provides good exposure latitude, detail, and contrast, and a glossy surface obtained without ferrotyping; in addition, it has a short processing,

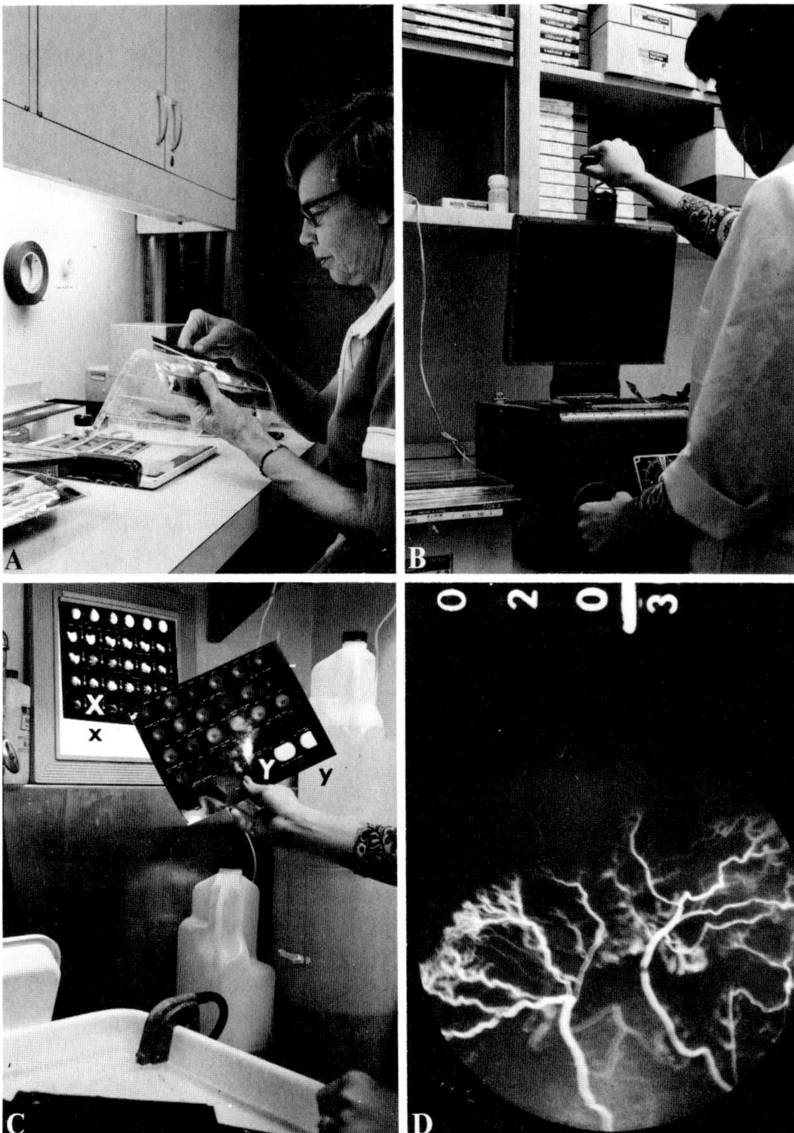

Fig. 8-2. Developed negatives are cut into strips and placed in a protective envelope. (A) *36-exposure film cut into strips of 6 frames and placed in plastic envelope for easy handling and viewing.* (B) *For making positive film or prints, contact printer or frame is used.* (C) *Developed positive transparency* (X) *is inspected. To make 2- by 2-inch slides, the frames are cut out and mounted.* (D) *Typical angiogram transparency.*

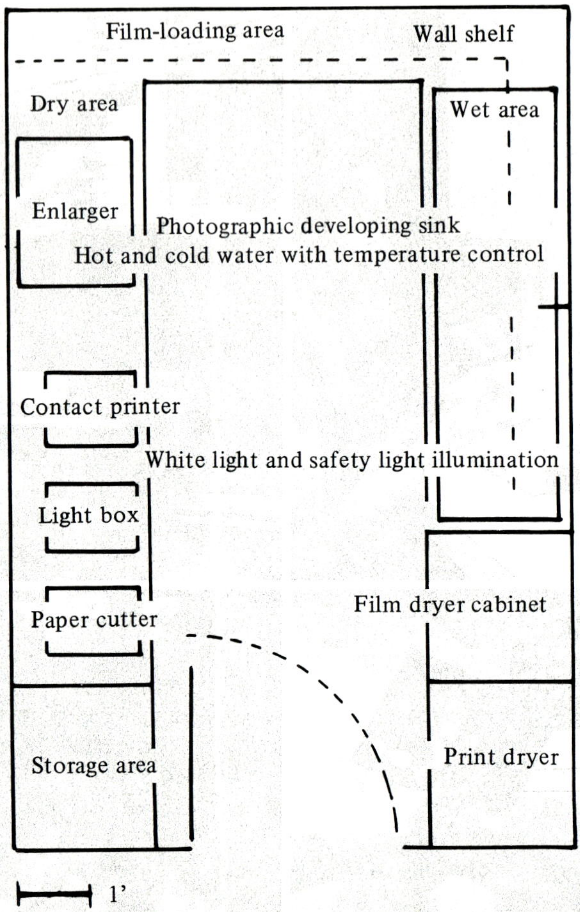

Fig. 8-3. Darkroom suitable for developing, printing, and finishing fluorescein angiograms.

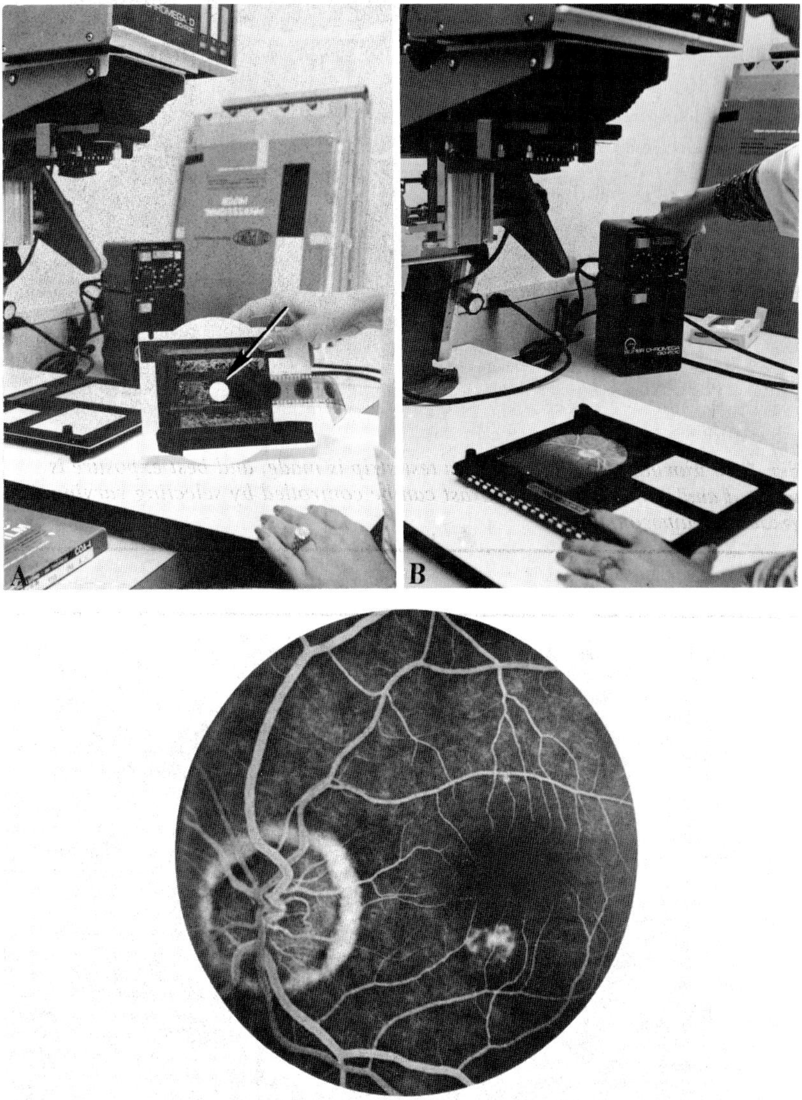

C

Fig. 8-4. Making enlargements of angiograms for records and publication. (A) Negative carrier with appropriate mask gives sharp, round outline. (B) Proper framing and focusing is important to bring out details. (C) Sample of finished print.

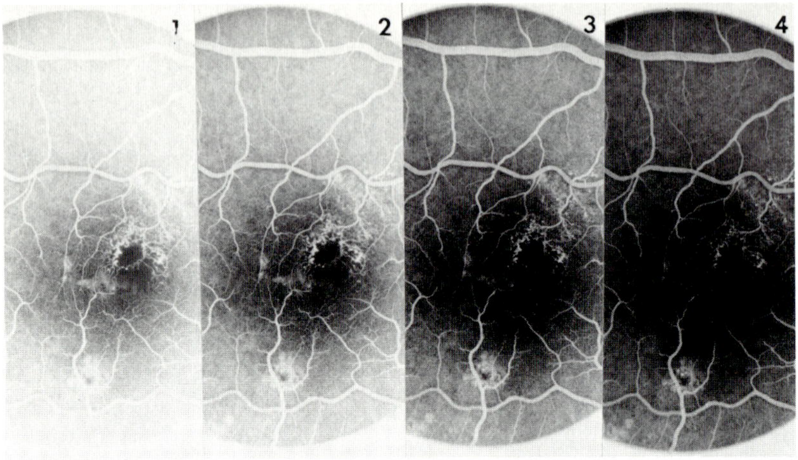

Fig. 8-5. For high-quality prints, a test strip is made, and best exposure is selected and printed. Print contrast can be controlled by selecting varying grades of paper or filter.

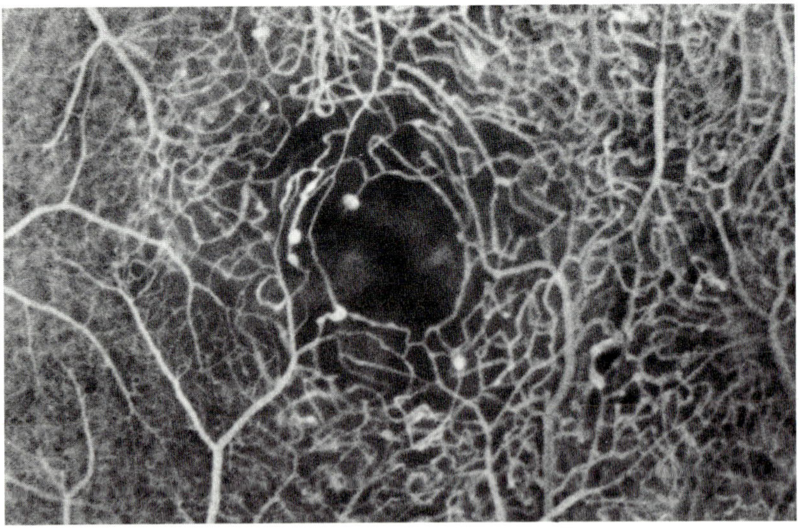

Fig. 8-6. Tri-X film properly exposed, developed, and printed yields good contrast and resolving power. This portion of negative was enlarged ×15 and still retains good detail. It shows the left macular area of a 22-year-old man with Coats syndrome. Fine retinal capillary network surrounding the foveal avascular zone has been brought out by antecubital injection of sodium fluorescein. The capillaries are slightly dilated and considerable disruption of the geometric vascular network is evident. Multiple short capillary segments are either nonperfused or missing, a number of microaneurysms are present, and the caliber of the lumen of some vessels varies pathologically.

washing, and drying time. By using polycontrast filters, one can easily adjust the contrast of the final print (Fig. 8-6).

Processing Procedure

Kodak Polycontrast rapid RC paper should be developed in Dektol solution diluted 1 : 2 for 2 to 3 minutes and continuously agitated. The paper should be fixed for 3 minutes, washed for 5 minutes, and dried at room temperature for 15 minutes. For exhibits, a matte surface on double weight paper is preferable.

Fundus fluorescein angiography is a specialized field; therefore, commercial developing and printing techniques do not give adequate results. Conscientious photographers will do their own developing and printing.

9

The Clinical Application of Televised Fluorescein Angiography

W. A. J. VAN HEUVEN AND
MICHEL MEHU

Television systems for recording the fluorescein angiogram have been used clinically since 1969 [3], and a commercial television attachment for the Zeiss fundus camera has been available since 1972 [5]. Still, television has not replaced photographic methods. There are several reasons for this seeming lack of popularity: First, the resolution of any television system cannot match that of the sensitive, fine-grain films available today. Thus, when one compares a single television frame with any photograph of the same fundus, the latter will inevitably be clearer and have more detail. Of course, this comparison may not be valid, because a single television frame records every 1/60 of a second while most film systems record, at best, each 1/4 of a second.

Second, for clinical purposes, there is as yet no proven need for more rapid sequential imaging than that provided by most film methods. In the present state of the art, most fundus conditions can be adequately diagnosed and evaluated for treatment with recording rates of one frame per second. Although at times multiple fluorescein injections are required, even procedures such as finding the feeder vessel in a diabetic neovascular frond can be done successfully with relatively slow sequential imaging.

Third, a television tape does not permit side-by-side still frame comparisons of different phases of the angiogram, which are customarily done with still photographs. Also, the careful study of a single image of good quality is not possible without stopping the videotape, which leads to decreased resolution, or else photographing on Polaroid film several sequential images directly from the television monitor, which integrates out the random noise while reinforcing the repeating vascular image. The later method, however, sacrifices the rapidity of sequential imaging.

Stereo viewing also is not easily done using television. At present, the only stereo television systems for fluorescein angiography [1, 4] utilize sequential rather than simultaneous images. Thus the stereoscopic image is lost when the tape is slowed down for slow motion or stop-frame viewing. Adaptation of a television recording system to a simultaneous stereo camera will largely obviate this drawback.

This work was supported by Research Grant 1 RO 1 EY 00791-04 from the National Eye Institute.

Another disadvantage of television is that many classrooms and auditoriums are still inadequately equipped to show videotapes. Because ceiling-mounted monitors are small compared to film screens, audiences prefer the magnification and resultant ease in detail viewing of film. Transposing videotapes to film for large audiences is expensive because of problems with synchrony. Videotape is recorded at 60 fields per second, while film is recorded at 24 fields per second; therefore, special equipment, not available everywhere, is required for transposition. Hopefully, the more recent development of large screen television projection systems will become standard in most auditoriums.

Furthermore, if publication of a particular patient's angiogram is contemplated, photography must be used instead of television. Enough detail is already lost in most printing for publication so that the best possible original is required, which only high-quality photographs can provide.

Finally, there is an undercurrent of uninterest by photographers in using other than photographic means for recording. Their attitude is hardly surprising, since most of them are artistically inclined and trained in the art of photography rather than in the engineering of electronic systems. Film developing and printing, which represent an important part of the photographer's art, are eliminated. Thus, it is difficult to generate enthusiasm for televised recording in any clinical unit where photographic systems are also available.

The Present Television System

Since the development of the original prototype television system for recording the fluorescein angiogram [3], the hardware has continued to change as improved electronic components have become available. The details of our system's development have already been described [2] (Fig. 9-1). Presently, our equipment consists of a high-sensitivity vidicon camera coupled to a three-stage image intensifier; these are attached to the Zeiss fundus camera in place of the eyepiece.* A sliding mirror is installed in front of the glass beam-splitter of the Zeiss unit to make full use of the observation lamp. A special-effects generator is used to include frame counting in the video signal, which is then fed through a 1/2-inch videotape recorder (VTR) to a television monitor. A wide-band, delayed-sweep cathode ray oscilloscope can be connected between the VTR and the monitor for line-selection photometry.

Advantages

The question of whether televised angiography is better than photo-

* More detail can be obtained by writing the authors.

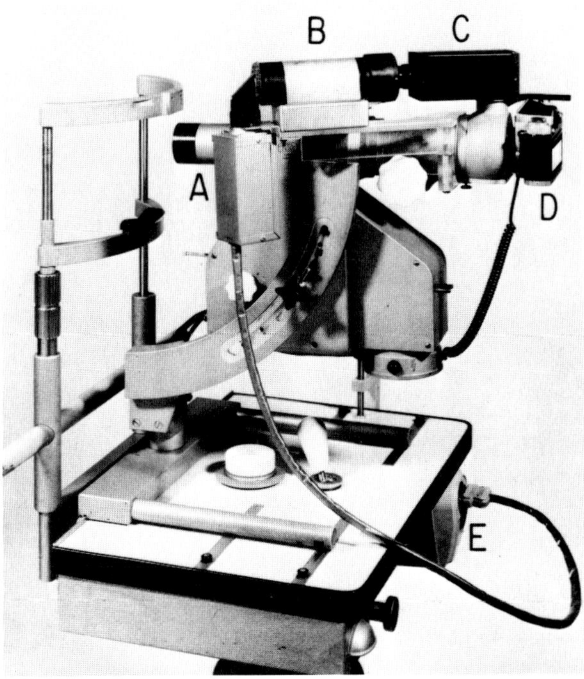

Fig. 9-1. (A) *Television camera;* (B) *image intensifier;* (C) *coupling optics;* (D) *still camera;* (E) *television control unit. Miniaturized television camera coupled to the intensifier is attached to the Zeiss fundus camera in place of the eyepiece. Optical connection has been folded for compactness. A film camera remains attached to permit film photography whenever desired.*

graphic angiography can be answered only when the needs of a particular clinical setting are known.

If instant results are required, television is superior. The angiogram is immediately available; it can be studied in time lapse, real time, slow motion, or stop frame; it can be photographed from the monitor on Polaroid; and it can be broadcast instantly to monitors in other hospital areas for teaching, consultation, or treatment purposes. Such instant results have been important in our own study of vascular occlusions, when an immediate decision had to be made concerning treatment with streptokinase or heparin, depending on the clinical angiogram. Instant results are also valuable when, for the convenience or peace of mind of patient or physician, immediate treatment is desirable. Thus the patient who lives at a distance is often saved much time and money otherwise spent on hotels or travel. The positive public-relations aspects of this fast service are not without reward.

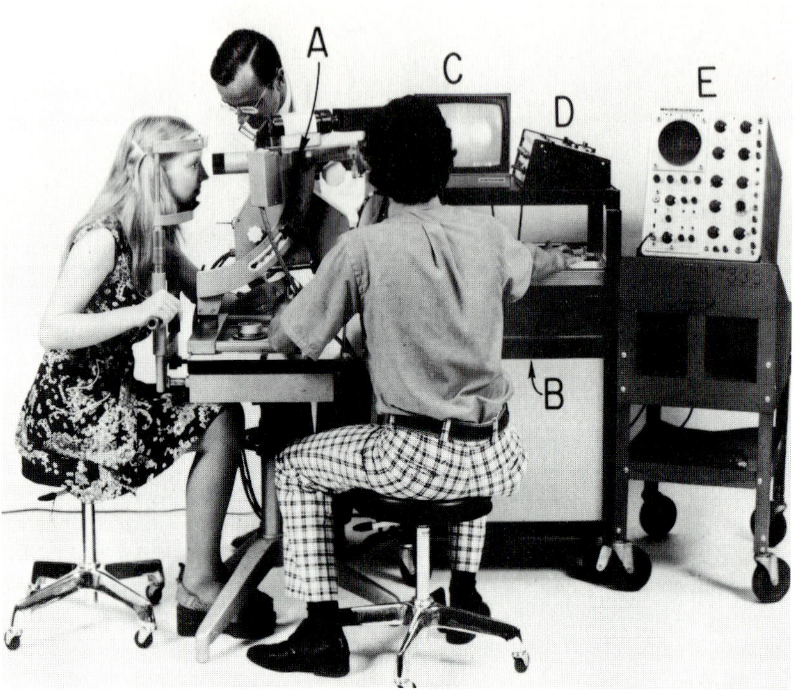

Fig. 9-2. (A) *Television camera system;* (B) *videotape recorder;* (C) *television monitor;* (D) *special effects generator;* (E) *oscilloscope. Photographer focuses by viewing the monitor. Oscilloscope is used for photometric quantification after record is made.*

Furthermore, the quality of the angiogram is virtually assured because the technician views the monitor (not the patient) while recording, permitting continuous adjustment of light levels, centering, and focusing (Fig. 9-2). Repeated fluorescein injections and patient visits, because "the pictures didn't come out" or because a certain flow phase was missed, are obviated.

In the study of rapidly occurring events, such as those of the first 2 seconds of chorioretinal fluorescence, television provides an essentially continuous record at 60 frames per second. In our own search for the feeder vessel in a frond of diabetic neovascularization, we have confidence that televised recording after a single fluorescein injection can give us the information we need. In previous years, multiple injections were often required to find the feeder vessel when recording photographically.

If patient expense is an important factor, television is also preferable. The basic television equipment is less expensive than a fundus flash system, particularly when one considers that darkroom facilities and personnel for film processing are not needed. The expense of a television angiogram is about one-tenth that of a photographic angiogram, and those portions of the videotape that contain no significant information can be erased and reused for other patients.

For teaching purposes, television has one important attribute: It is kinetic. As a result, fluorescein angioscopy, namely, the observation through an ophthalmoscope (with blue filter) of the dye passing through the fundus, can be taught. In the usual setting of clinical teaching at a medical center, where a fluorescein angiography laboratory is available, assistants and residents order fluorescein angiograms on patients as an alternative rather than an adjunct to clinical examination. This procedure is similar to ordering a chest x-ray without having used a stethoscope. Much money and time could be saved if angiograms were not recorded until angioscopy had revealed an abnormality worthy of recording, as well as its approximate location. Photographers could then improve their results by concentrating on different areas at certain specific times, giving the clinician more diagnostic information. The teaching of the concept that clinical angioscopy precedes angiography and should be part of a complete eye examination in selected patients, just like visual fields, gonioscopy, and indirect ophthalmoscopy, hopefully will lead to a new generation of ophthalmologists who stock fluorescein in their offices.

In addition to these presently known advantages of televised fluorescein angiography, it is hoped that investigations currently underway will make this recording system a quantitative and reproducible method for measuring blood volume flow. This achievement will not only elevate the system into the realm of a research tool, but it may also produce clinical data presently not available from photography that could increase the diagnostic perception of and change our therapeutic approaches toward a variety of fundus disorders.

References

1. Heuven, W. A. J. van, and Schaffer, C. Televised Fluorescein Angiography. In K. Shimizu (Ed.), *Fluorescein Angiography*. Tokyo: Igako Shoin, 1974. Pp. 10–14.
2. Heuven, W. A. J. van, and Schaffer, C. Electronic imaging systems for fluorescein angiography. *Int. Ophthalmol. Clin.* 14(3) : 31, 1974.
3. Heuven, W. A. J. van, Schaffer, C., and Mehu, M. The use of low light level television in fundus imaging. *Mod. Probl. Ophthalmol.* 9 : 6, 1971.
4. Heuven, W. A. J. van, Schaffer, C., and Mehu, M. The Evolution of Electronic Recording Systems for Fluorescein Angiography. Presented at the 25th Anniversary Congress, Retina Service, Boston, Massachusetts, September, 1972.
5. Yuhasz, Z., Akashi, R. H., Urban, J. C., and Mueller, M. M. H. A new apparatus for videotape recording of fluorescein angiograms. *Arch. Ophthalmol.* 90 : 481, 1973.

10

Spectral Reflectance Photography

THOMAS BEHRENDT AND
EILEEN SLIPAKOFF

Monochromatic light photography became a practical reality after the development of the modern electronic xenon flash fundus camera, the availability of fast, high-contrast, low-granularity films, and advances in interference filter technology. Before these developments, various attempts had been made to observe the fundus in monochromatic light. The work of Vogt led to the classic examination of the fundus with red-free light, which is now incorporated in almost all modern direct ophthalmoscopes. However, such attempts had to be made through visual observation alone, as none of the above technical prerequisites were available. The use of the human eye, however, was a poor system of direct observation, not only because of the lack of good documentation, but also because of the lack of sensitivity and resolution at the extremes of the visual spectrum—mainly in the blue range. The early experiments were, however, successful enough to warrant continued interest in the concept once adequate technology was available.

Direct examination of the fundus with monochromatic light presented several problems. Mainly, the quantity of light available was not sufficient when rather close monochromatic observation was desired. Line sources of light (monochromatic) were not nearly intense enough. Monochromatic filters were totally inadequate for selection of narrow bands of light from polychromatic sources.

Techniques

With the development of the xenon flashtube, a ready source of high-intensity light of short-duration pulses became available for fundus photography. Interference filter technology advanced to such a point that filters with band widths of 10 to 20 nm (at half width) with better than 50 percent peak transmission became available. Thus it is now possible to illuminate the eye with nearly pure monochromatic light derived from the xenon flashtubes and passed through narrow band filters. The amount of light is adequate to expose modern films such as Tri-X properly with some forced development. The technique per se requires only the introduction of the filters in some convenient position in the light path of the fundus camera, a procedure easily accomplished in the Zeiss camera system. Placement of the monochromatic filters in the combined illumination and flash path ensures proper filtration of all the light reaching the subject's eye, but it creates some difficulty in visualization for the photographer. To avoid such a problem, place the filter in the path of the flash light in a position prior to the beam-splitter, thereby combining the flash illumination with the observation light. This placement permits excellent observation in the white light while delivering monochromatic light to the eye during photography, with only a small amount of impurity present which does not usually modify the picture to an appreciable degree. The effect of this impure light can be easily judged by trying to obtain photographs without the flash light operating. It will be found that only the extreme bright settings of the observation light will result in even slight exposure of the film.

The selection of the characteristic values (peak transmission wavelength) of the filters currently used is rather arbitrary, spanning the spectrum in band passes of approximately 20-nm half widths. The extremes were selected based on the sensitivity of Tri-X film and on the scattering properties of the lens in the human eye. At present, our selection consists of a series of 7 filters, ranging from 431 to 640 nm.

Tri-X film is handled basically in the same way as film for fluorescein, except that a developer with somewhat less contrast is used. This is desirable because unlike fluorescein, significant information may be obtained from the gray scale (optic density) values of the recorded image.

Clinical Use

Although the analysis of the results of spectral reflectance photography is still in its early stages, some basic observations can be made.

Red Wavelengths

Red wavelengths tend to penetrate all fundus structures except accumulations of melanin and are reflected heavily by the sclera. In most cases they are able to penetrate the retinal pigment epithelium, thus making it possible to evaluate the melanin-containing structures in the choroid. This property, however, does not open up as large possibilities for the study of the choroidal vessels as might be expected, since these vessels as well as most other structures of the fundus interact poorly with the long wavelengths, making them next to invisible. However, this system does allow for a meticulous documentation of melanin distribution in the choroidal space (Fig. 10-1).

Green Wavelengths

Green wavelengths do not penetrate the retinal pigment epithelium-Bruch's-choriocapillaris complex. A rather effective barrier to these and shorter wavelengths is present somewhere at the level of these structures. It is thus possible, for example, to differentiate between melanin pigment accumulations on either side of an intact retinal pig-

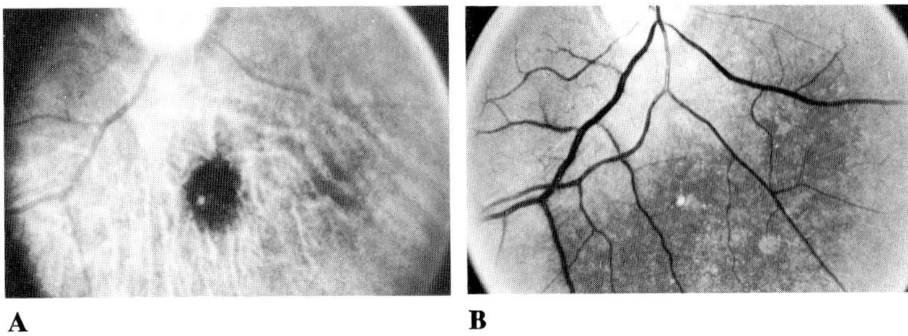

Fig. 10-1. *Choroidal nevus seen* (A) *in monochromatic red light and* (B) *in monochromatic green light. The very well-defined pigmented structure seen in red disappears in green. Drusen known to be superficial to the inner limiting membrane are visible in green and red (difficult to see in red because of low contrast).*

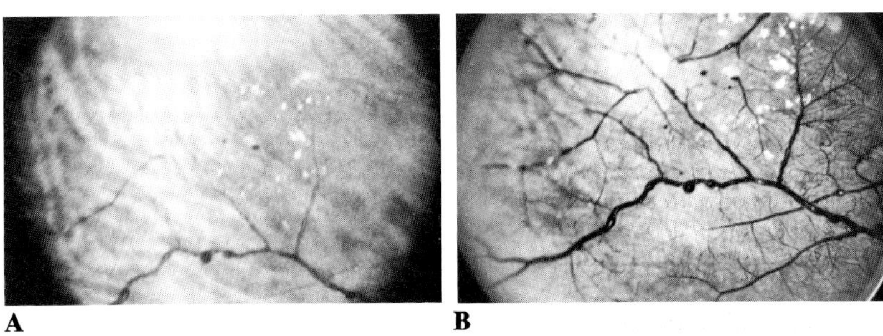

Fig. 10-2. *Angiomatosis of retina seen* (A) *in monochromatic red and* (B) *in monochromatic green. Observe the extreme vascular detail appreciable in green. White patches are visible in both red and green, as is blood in stagnant areas.*

ment epithelium-Bruch's-choriocapillaris complex. Furthermore, these wavelengths allow an extreme contrast between blood in the retinal vessels and in the surrounding background structures of the retina; thus they form an excellent medium for recording vessels, either normal or abnormal, and hemorrhages. The difference between the background and the majority of the so-called white lesions (e.g., hard exudates, myelin, cotton wool patches) is the same as with color film (Fig. 10-2).

Blue Wavelengths

Blue wavelengths penetrate poorly even into the matrix of the retina; the waves seem to interact significantly with the nerve fibers. One consequence of this interaction is that the high optical density of the image

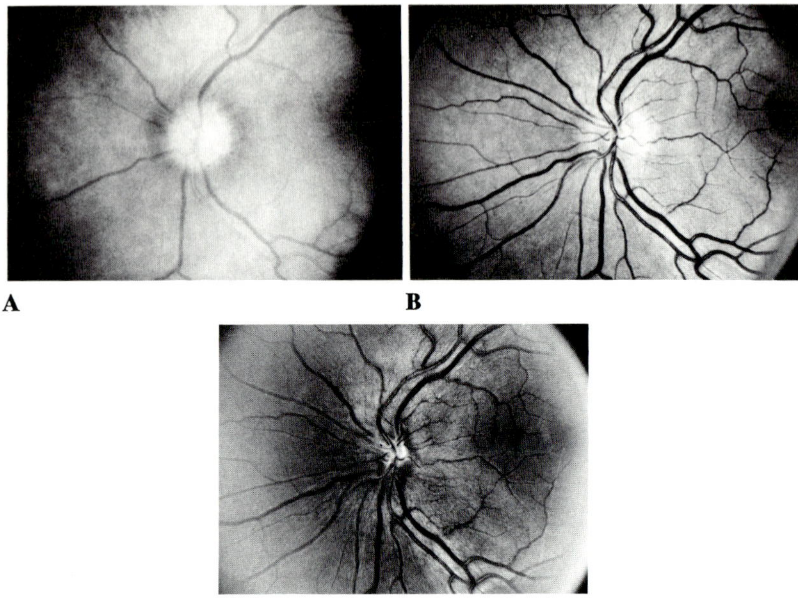

Fig. 10-3. Normal fundus seen (A) *in red,* (B) *in green, and* (C) *in blue. Observe details of choroidal pigmentation in red, vascular pattern in green, and nerve fiber pattern in blue. Note difference in density of normal disc: very pale in red, becomes darker than surrounding area in blue.*

of the normal optic disc is often significantly darker than the peripapillary area. This property is lost in modifications of the nerve fibers that are closely related to clinically demonstrable atrophy. The marked contrast between the reflectance of the papillary tissue and that of the vessels crossing the nervehead results in excellent visibility of even the smallest superficial vessels in the disc itself. Photography of the disc in blue light may thus be a useful additional tool in studying optic atrophy (Fig. 10-3).

Conclusion

It can be seen that the technique of using properly selected filters to provide rigidly defined monochromatic bands with which to observe the fundus presents interesting and challenging information that is as yet mainly untapped. The applications quoted present only a small part of the areas that can be investigated. The technique is basically standard, but advances can still be made in optimizing filters. The question of what band width to use for a given application is by no means solved and presents a challenging avenue of inquiry.

It should be pointed out that the use of color film with interference filters offers no advantage. The only dimension being recorded at each point in the film is reflectivity of the structure at the wavelength of the filter being used. Documenting the color of this wavelength by the use of color film is a fruitless exercise.

References

1. Behrendt, T., and Duane, T. D. Investigation of fundus oculi with spectral reflectance photography. *Arch. Ophthalmol.* 75 : 375, 1966.
2. Behrendt, T., and Wilson, L. A. Spectral reflectance photography of the retina. *Am. J. Ophthalmol.* 59 : 1079, 1965.

A Lens System for Wide-Angle Fundus Photography

OLEG POMERANTZEFF

In any conventional fundus camera, the lens that faces the patient's eye can be considered an objective lens. The field of view of the fundus that can be photographed by this camera depends on the numeric aperture of this lens. The illumination of the fundus is also transmitted through the same lens. Each of its surfaces, acting as a mirror, forms an image of the light source. These images are superimposed on the image of the fundus. Therefore, to avoid multiple reflections, this lens is usually of the single-element variety. Even when an aspheric surface is used, the aperture of such a lens can hardly be larger than f/1, corresponding to an angular field of 45 degrees. To increase the field of view beyond this limit, the objective lens must be in contact with the patient's cornea.

With a normally constricted pupil of 1 to 2 mm, the angular visual field extends temporally beyond 90 degrees. Therefore, rays incident upon the cornea at a 90-degree angle enter such a pupil and reach the retina. Conversely, rays originating at the peripheral retina and entering this small pupil emerge from the eye at an angle of approximately 90 degrees. Thus the entire retina can be seen through a very small pupil, which can be considered the entrance pupil of the observation system. However, the image (for an emmetropic eye) is formed at infinity in a solid angle of 180 degrees.

If a contact lens is constructed using a glass with a high refractive index and is placed on the cornea, the solid angle containing the image of the fundus is reduced accordingly, and an additional lens can be designed to accept the reduced solid angle and focus it in the observer's eye or on a photographic film [1].

Illumination of the Fundus

Illumination of the fundus can be achieved by placing a ring-shaped bundle of optical fibers in contact with the cornea. The central part of the cornea covered by the contact lens must be kept free of any obstruction in order that the image of the fundus may be observed.

From the Department of Retina Research of the Eye Research Institute of Retina Foundation, Boston, Massachusetts. This work was supported by Public Health Service Research Grant EY-00227 from the National Eye Institute, National Institutes of Health, by United States Army Grant DADA 17-73-c-1344, and by the Massachusetts Lions Eye Research Fund, Inc.

I wish to express my gratitude to Miss Julianne Schneider for her technical assistance and particularly for her volunteering as a subject throughout this study.

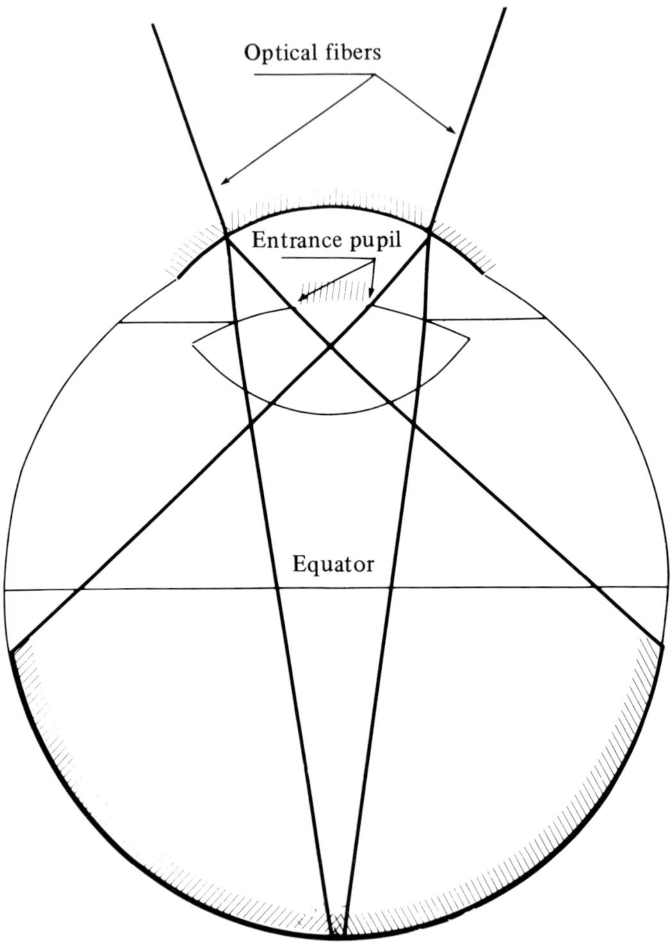

Fig. 11-1. Single-ring illumination.

Only the periphery of the cornea can be used for illumination [1].

In Figure 11-1, the ring of fibers has an inside diameter of 8 mm. The pupil of the patient's eye should be widely dilated (7–8 mm). As is shown, the beam of light from the right side of the illuminating ring is limited by the ray that touches the edge of the iris and is incident upon the retina before intersection with the longitudinal axis of the eye. If the pupil is smaller than 7 to 8 mm, this ray intersects the axis

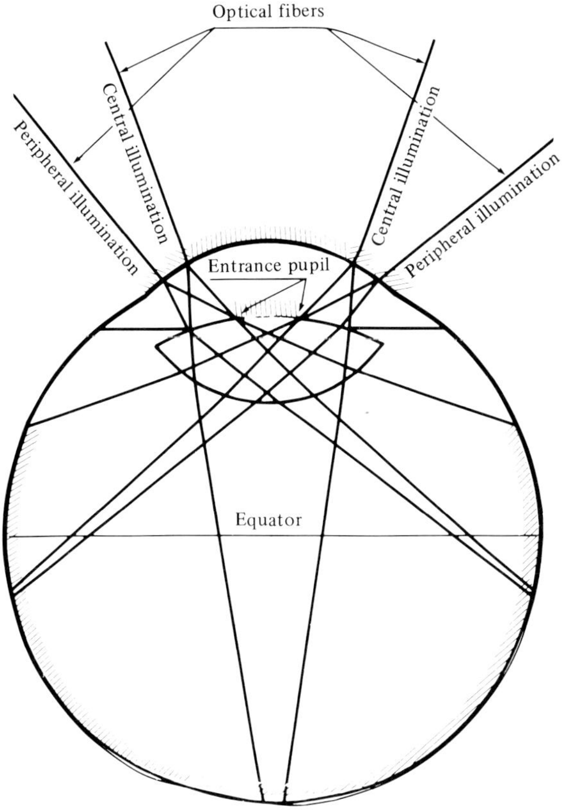

Fig. 11-2. Double-ring illumination.

before reaching the retina, and the area around the posterior pole is not illuminated. Therefore, illumination of the posterior pole is dependent on maximum pupillary dilatation.

To avoid reflection from the crystalline lens, no direct light should be incident upon the entrance pupil of the observation system. As a result, only a small field in the retina can be illuminated by this ring of light fibers (Fig. 11-1). To illuminate the peripheral retina, another ring of fibers must be placed more peripherally on the cornea with a corresponding increase in the inclination of the fibers (Fig. 11-2). This method, termed *direct illumination,* provides sufficient illumination if the patient's pupil can be adequately dilated [2].

In some ophthalmic pathology, the pupil cannot be dilated more than 4 to 6 mm. In such cases, illumination of the fundus can be achieved by using a separate optical fiber bundle placed against the sclera at the pars plana (approximately 4 mm posterior to the limbus). This method is termed *transillumination.* Transillumination is recom-

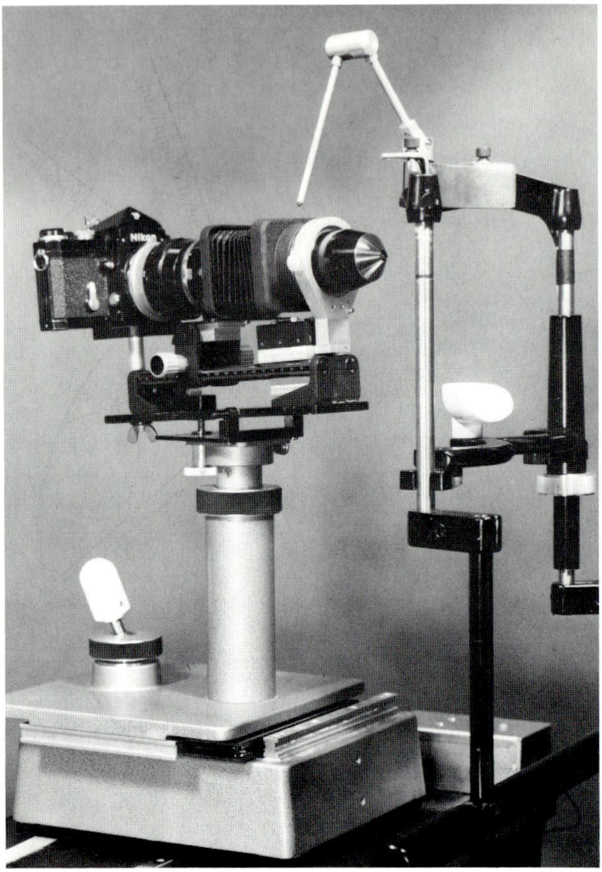

Fig. 11-3. Equator-Plus lens mounted on a simple 35-mm camera.

mended in all cases when the pupil cannot be dilated or when the media of the eye are not clear. This method is being investigated further for its applicability in patients with heavily pigmented fundi and also in fluorescein angiography.

The contact lens cone, equipped with either direct illumination or transillumination, can be attached either to an optical focusing system to provide a hand-held ophthalmoscope or to a camera, as in the following description.

Operation of the Camera Using the Equator-Plus Lens with Direct Illumination

The cone containing the contact lens and the focusing optical system (Fig. 11-3) is supported by a high-precision, ball-bearing slide mechanism preloaded with a constant-force spring. The spring is calibrated in such a way that the maximum pressure applied to the eye by the contact lens cannot exceed 20 to 30 mm Hg (30–50 gm of force). A microswitch activates a buzzer to warn the operator when this pressure has been attained.

The slide mechanism is attached to a camera body equipped with a close-up lens. A bellows joins the contact lens cone to the close-up lens. Focusing of the camera lens is performed in the usual manner; the bellows permits movement of the lens during focusing. The viewfinder is equipped with a transparent screen with a reticle and an eyepiece magnifier. The operator must focus the eyepiece magnifier sharply on the reticle in the following manner:

1. Rotate the ocular to its maximum clockwise position (maximum negative power).
2. Slowly rotate the ocular counterclockwise (toward maximum positive power) until the focus becomes sharp.
3. If the sharp focus point is passed, repeat the entire procedure in order that the sharp focus point is always approached by a counterclockwise rotation.

By following this sequence, the operator is forced to relax his accommodation when adjusting the focus on the reticle. When photographing, one must see both the reticle and the fundus in sharp focus.

When the reticle is sharply in focus, the operator must then focus the camera lens on a distant object, such as the wall of a room. This will give an approximate focus of the fundus of an emmetropic eye. Thus, when contact between the lens and the cornea is established, the operator will immediately perceive some fundus details.

While looking through the viewfinder, the operator slowly approaches the patient's eye using the "joystick" of the camera mount. One will initially see an entire view of the exterior of the eye and a small, circular reflection (corresponding to the illuminating ring) in the patient's cornea. While moving the camera forward, the operator must center this reflection in the patient's pupil using either the joystick or the vertical vernier. As the contact lens cone approaches the eye, the circular reflection expands peripherally. It is imperative that this reflection remain centered within the pupil.

When the contact lens, which is filled with a contact and moistening solution (methyl cellulose), touches the cornea, the operator will see this liquid spread across the field of view, expelling the air bubble that forms between the contact lens and the cornea. The interface between the cornea that is in proper contact with the lens and that which is still separated from the lens appears as a curved line moving toward the periphery of the field. Contact in the separated area may then be

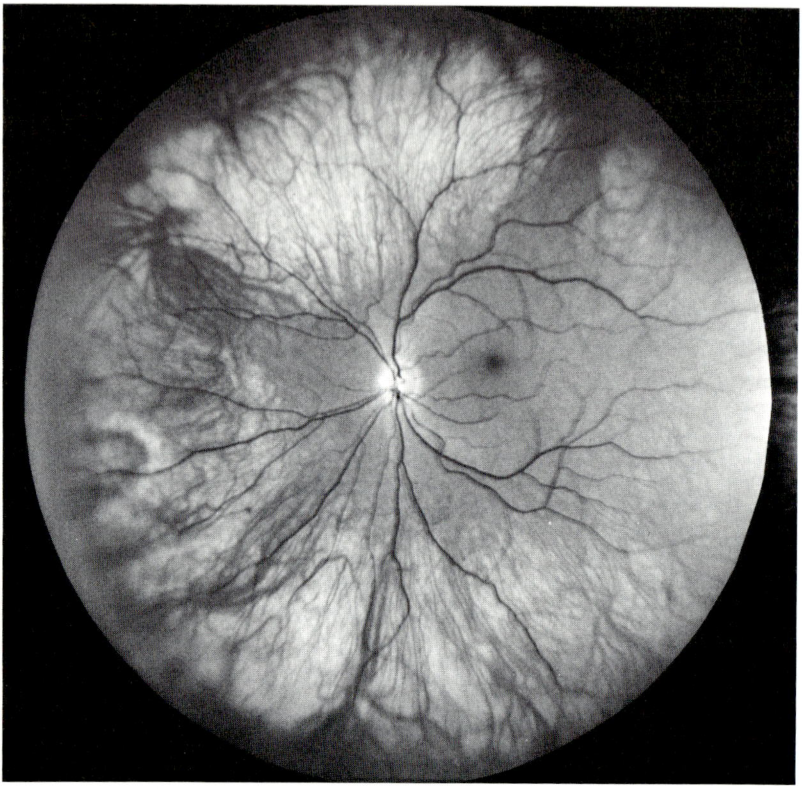

Fig. 11-4. Fundus photograph taken with the Equator-Plus lens mounted on a simple 35-mm camera.

improved using the joystick or the vertical vernier. If contact remains unimproved, the lens may be moved forward carefully to provide a slightly increased pressure on the cornea and thus better contact.

When proper contact has been achieved throughout the visual field, the operator should lock the joystick, focus the camera lens, and trigger the shutter. The results of such careful work are shown in Figure 11-4.

References

1. Pomerantzeff, O. Equator-Plus camera. *Invest. Ophthalmol.* 14 : 401, 1975.
2. Pomerantzeff, O., and Govignon, J. Design of a wide-angle ophthalmoscope. *Arch. Ophthalmol.* 86 : 420, 1971.

12

Stereophotographic Systems

DAVID D. DONALDSON

It is obvious that the primary objective of photography in the medical field is to reproduce actual visualization as exactly as possible. Stereography not only gives a stronger impression of reality than two-dimensional photography but also often illustrates features that cannot otherwise be shown photographically. Furthermore, the loss of detail caused by physical limitations of film and equipment is reduced appreciably in the stereoscopic presentation, because two pictures are being presented to the visual system simultaneously.

Various factors have been regarded as important in the development of stereophotographic systems and have been incorporated in them whenever possible:

1. Magnification, exposure, and stereoscopic effect are exactly reproducible.
2. An electronic flash, a short-duration variable-intensity light source, is utilized.
3. Lens apertures of relatively small size are used to obtain maximum depth of field.
4. The design of the camera is such that stereopsis is obtained by a parallel rather than a convergent optical system, thus minimizing distortion.
5. The operation of the camera is as simple as possible, thereby permitting persons untrained in photography to obtain consistently good pictures.

Stereophotography as applied to ophthalmology generally falls into three main categories: anterior segment photography (diffuse illumination), fundus or retinal photography, and slit-lamp photography.

Anterior Segment Photography

The anterior segment of the eye comprises the cornea, anterior chamber angle, iris, and lens, each of which offers special problems in recording it photographically.

The patient who has a photophobic eye (as in iritis) or a constant nystagmus requires photographic apparatus designed to function adequately under these adverse conditions. Such a system incorporates a camera, composed of two separate optical systems, and a power supply, which acts as a base or stand for the camera (Fig. 12-1). The

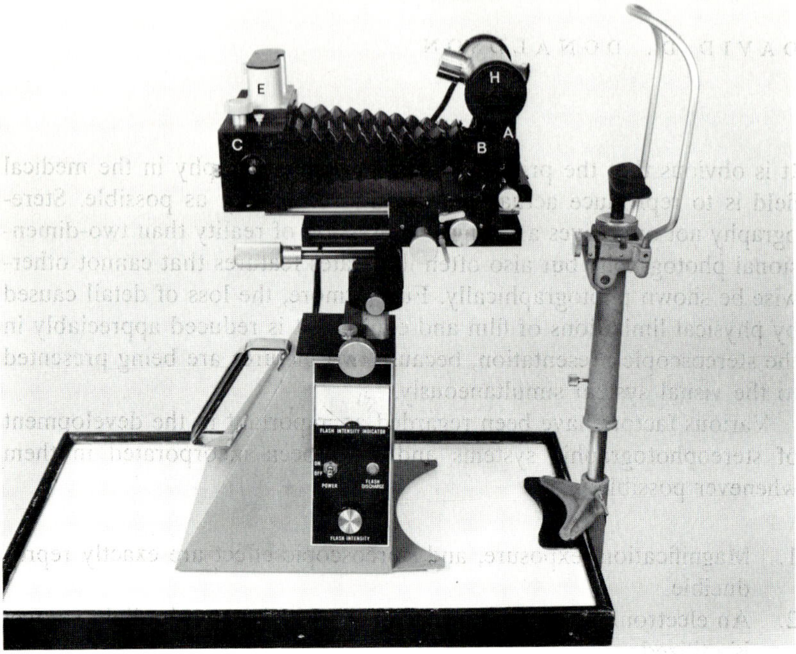

Fig. 12-1. Anterior segment stereocamera with power supply built into the base and chin rest as used for eye photography. A = *rhomboid prisms;* B = *lenses;* C = *reflex housing and film back;* E = *housing for focusing lights; H = electronic flash lamp housing.*

camera is utilized on a small table and requires a head and chin rest for the patient when it is used at higher magnifications.

The camera has nine different magnifications, each using a different inter-lens separation in order to obtain a natural appearance or equivalent depth effect. This requirement is important, whether the final photograph is to be used in the stereoscopic viewer or the stereoscopic projector. Correction for parallax is accomplished by linear movement of the lenses rather than convergence or "toe-in," which has been used commonly in the past. The latter method produces the well-known wedge-shaped distortion, which is particularly undesirable because it is opposite in the two images.

The optical portion of the camera involves two separate optical systems; each produces an image on a standard 35-mm film (Figs. 12-2 through 12-4). The use of the rhomboid prisms accomplishes two things. In the first place, the distance between the upper reflecting surfaces of the rhomboid prisms will determine the effective inter-lens separation and thus the depth effect. The separation of the two lower

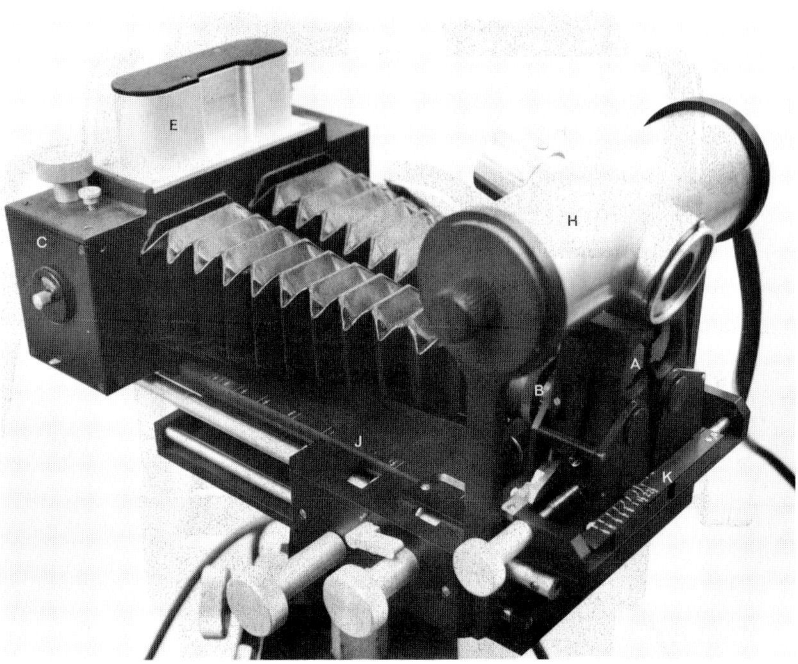

Fig. 12-2. Anterior segment stereocamera. A, B, C, E, H *as in Fig. 12-1;* J = *bellows extension scale;* K = *inner lens distance scale.*

surfaces will determine the horizontal positioning of the images at the film plane. Thus, separation of the lower two surfaces makes possible accurate correction for parallax by translation rather than convergence, which results in photographs without wedge-shaped distortion. The second advantage is the inward tilt (Fig. 12-3) of the rhomboid prisms and the fact that the faces of the prisms need only be large enough to cover the lens itself—the lens together with the mount is more than twice the diameter of the actual lens. Thus, with the magnification of ×2.5 on the film, the prisms are touching, and the effective inter-lens distance is 10 mm. The rhomboid prism system allows a magnification in the stereoviewer of ×13, whereas, if the lenses themselves determined the inter-lens separation, a viewer magnification of only ×3 would be possible. Lenses used in this camera are of the macro type (80 mm f/4.5 Leitz Microsummar*).

In focusing, the optical system is used in reverse (Fig. 12-4). Incorporated in the roof of the double-reflex housing are two incandescent ribbon filament lamps having filaments that produce vertical im-

* E. Leitz, Inc., Rockleigh, NJ 07647.

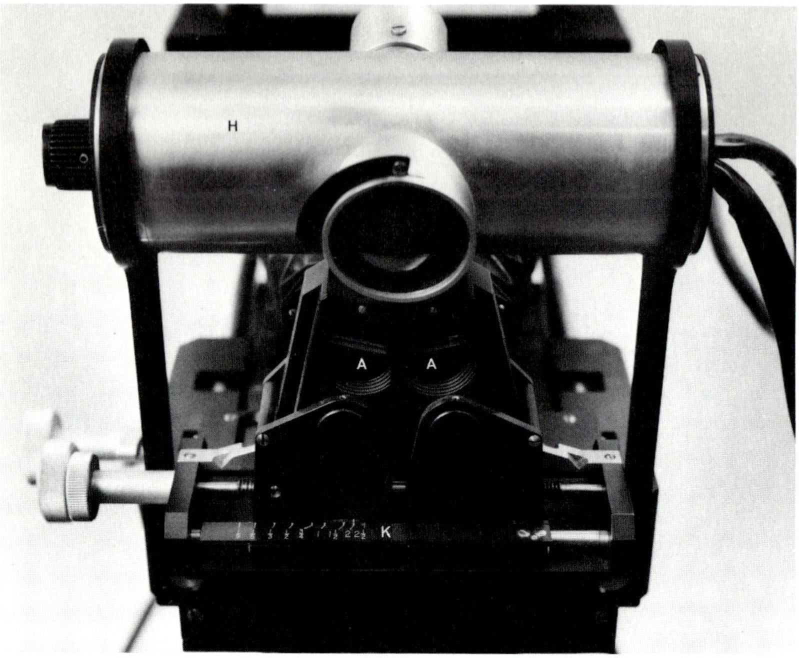

Fig. 12-3. Anterior segment stereocamera. Note relationships of rhomboid prisms with the camera set at ×2 magnification on the film. A = *rhomboid prisms;* H = *electronic flash lamp housing;* K = *inner lens distance scale.*

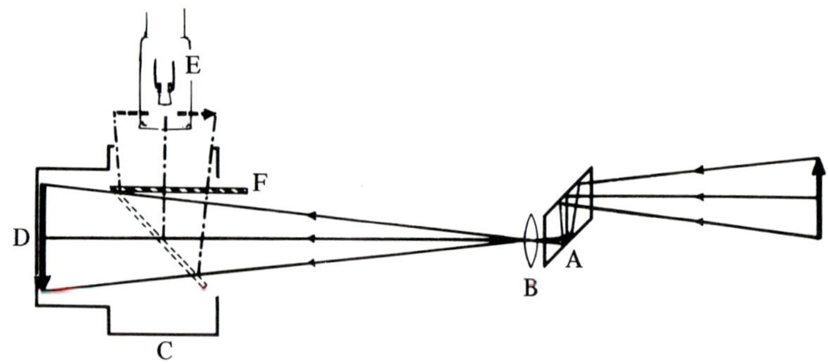

Fig. 12-4. Object image pathways and focusing system. D = *image at film plane;* E = *ribbon filament focusing light;* F = *reflex mirror in up position.*

ages. The position of these filaments is equated to the film plane. When the reflex mirror is down, the images of these filaments are projected onto the object being photographed. The camera is aligned and calibrated so that when the vertical filament images are aligned end-to-end (Fig. 12-5), the image will be in focus at the film plane. Not only does this method produce remarkably accurate focusing, but it also assures automatic parallax correction, because the vertical filament images aligned on the object are effectively in the centers of the two film planes, and thus duplicating areas must result. In addition to the projection of these filament images, there are eight small images that delineate the extent of the field (Fig. 12-5). These images are formed by eight small, concave reflectors that surround one of the bulbs in the roof of the reflex housing.

This method of focusing has a number of advantages:

1. It places a minimum of light onto the eye and thus can be tolerated easily by the subject being photographed.
2. Because the alignment of the filaments is even more accurate with a small aperture (f/18 is generally used), the picture can be taken immediately at the end of the focusing procedure without using automatic diaphragms.
3. Moreover, because the images of the filaments are similar to a slit-lamp beam, they can be visualized and aligned in an apparently clear cornea or lens; thus, even though the pathology in these various portions of the eye is not grossly visible, accurate focusing can still be accomplished.
4. It should be pointed out that in patients who are uncooperative, such as some children, if the filaments are seen to be aligned even momentarily on the portion of the eye to be photographed, it is possible to take the picture immediately. To do so would be very difficult, if not impossible, if the standard single-lens-reflex viewing device were being utilized.
5. It is also possible to align the filaments on portions of the eye, such as the cornea and lens, in which the opacities or abnormalities are not grossly visible, so that, in photographing an early cataract, the images of the filaments have an appearance similar to the slit-lamp beam and can be aligned in any portion of the lens desired. Thus, the multiple advantages of this method permit consistently excellent photographs of difficult subjects (Figs. 12-6 to 12-8).

The light source for taking the picture is an electronic flash unit that consists of a flash lamp (General Electric FT218*) mounted in front of a concave reflector. The voltage on this lamp can be varied up to

* General Electric Lamp Division, Nela Park, Cleveland, OH 44112.

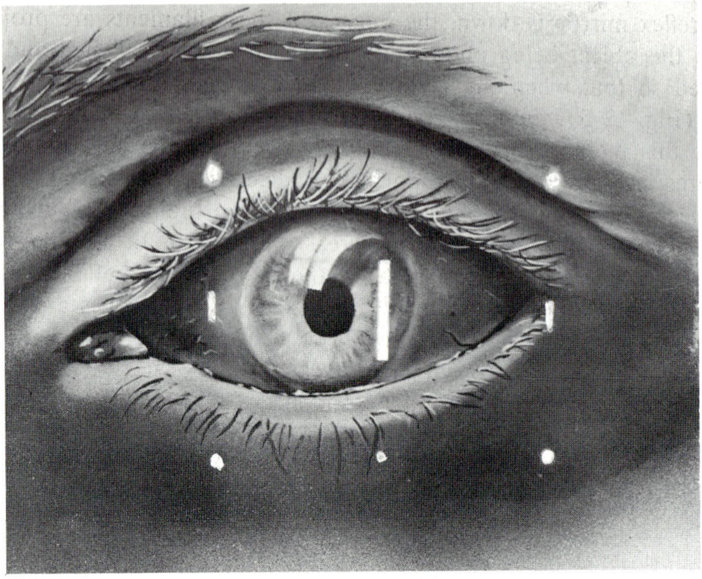

Fig. 12-5. Appearance of focusing light images on an eye and the eight field lights. The two focusing light images are aligned on the iris, giving the appearance of only one bright line.

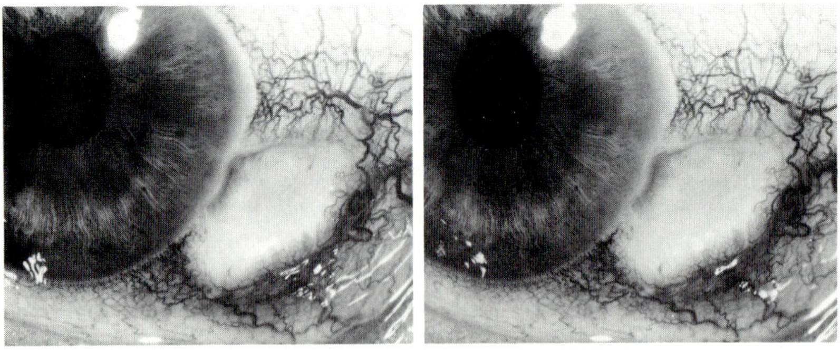

Fig. 12-6. Area of marked thinning of the sclera in a patient with scleromalacia perforans. Without the stereoscopic effect, it is impossible to determine whether there is elevation or depression of the lesion.

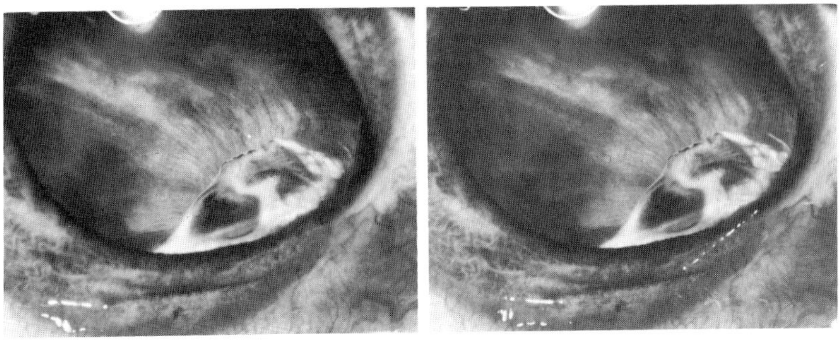

Fig. 12-7. A foreign body indenting a clear crystalline lens and retrolenticular vitreous membrane. The picture is almost meaningless without the three-dimensional effect.

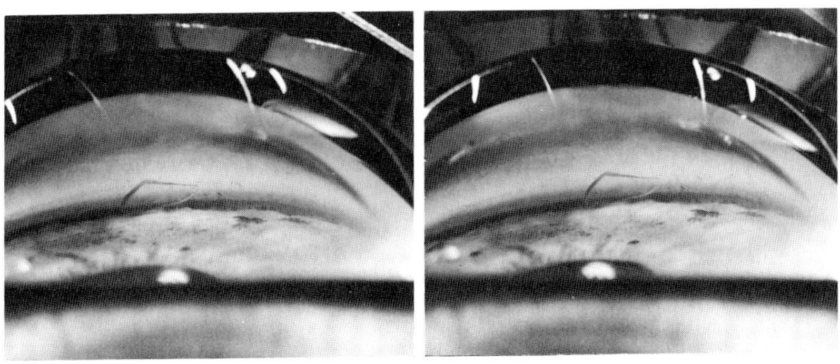

Fig. 12-8. A splinter of glass lying in the inferior angle as seen through a three-mirror Goldmann gonioprism. Depth relationships of the anterior chamber angle are far more meaningful when seen stereoscopically.

a maximum of 200 watt-seconds (joules). The amount of light required for any given magnification is determined by a voltmeter on the power supply, on which the various magnifications are indicated. The voltage is adjusted by means of a knob at the bottom of the power supply, and appropriate adjustments can be made at any given magnification for eyes that are unusually dark or light. Of course, this is accomplished simply by adjusting the voltage slightly higher or lower, depending on the light requirement. The aperture is kept constantly at f/18, which produces excellent depth of field, a particularly important factor in stereoscopic photography.

The camera has three calibrated scales, each with the various film magnifications indicated on it. The scale for bellows extension is along the side of the camera, while the scale for inter-lens separation (actually inter-aperture separation) is along the front of the camera. The third scale is on the power supply, on the face of the meter, and indicates flash intensity. Inasmuch as each scale is engraved with a similar set of numbers indicating the magnification on the film, setting of the camera before photographing the patient is relatively simple. As mentioned previously, nine reproducible magnifications are available, ranging from ×2.5 film magnification (×13 in the viewer) to a magnification low enough to take in the entire face.

Simultaneous Stereoscopic Fundus Photography

Stereoscopic fundus photographs in which both stereoscopic pictures of the pair are taken at the same time is referred to as the technique of *simultaneous* or *absolute stereoscopic fundus photography*. The relatively simple alternative to the simultaneous stereoscopic fundus camera is the technique of changing the position of the camera between successive exposures to obtain a slightly different viewpoint of the fundus, which can result in a pair of stereoscopic photographs. Another approach is use of the Allen separator, which also requires successive photographs. In both instances, a constant depth effect in the final result is not assured.

In recent years, the importance of depth relationships within the fundus has become increasingly evident, largely as a result of more extensive use of the indirect ophthalmoscope and the obvious advantages of this method of observation. The depth aspects of the excavation of the disc in determining the progress of glaucoma, particularly on continuing examinations, appear to be of considerable importance. More subtle depth relationships in lesions of the macula or choroid, or even in location of the vessels, may be overlooked or not readily appreciated in the standard two-dimensional stereoscopic fundus photograph. Repeated photographs of tumors in the fundus or lesions of the optic nerve head, such as papilledema, require stereoscopic photographs for definitive determination of the possible changes in such lesions.

The fundus camera that will be described involves the indirect ophthalmoscopic principle. It is a modification of the original Zeiss Nordensen camera developed more than 50 years ago to make single fundus photographs. The present camera utilizes optical components from the Olympus fundus camera, with modifications to adapt them for stereoscopic use. The stereoscopic fundus camera is mounted on a standard table utilizing a joystick for alignment. It allows binocular focusing of the fundus immediately before taking the picture (Fig. 12-9). A portion of the optical system (Fig. 12-10) is doubled so that the aerial image formed by the ophthalmoscope lens is photographed from two

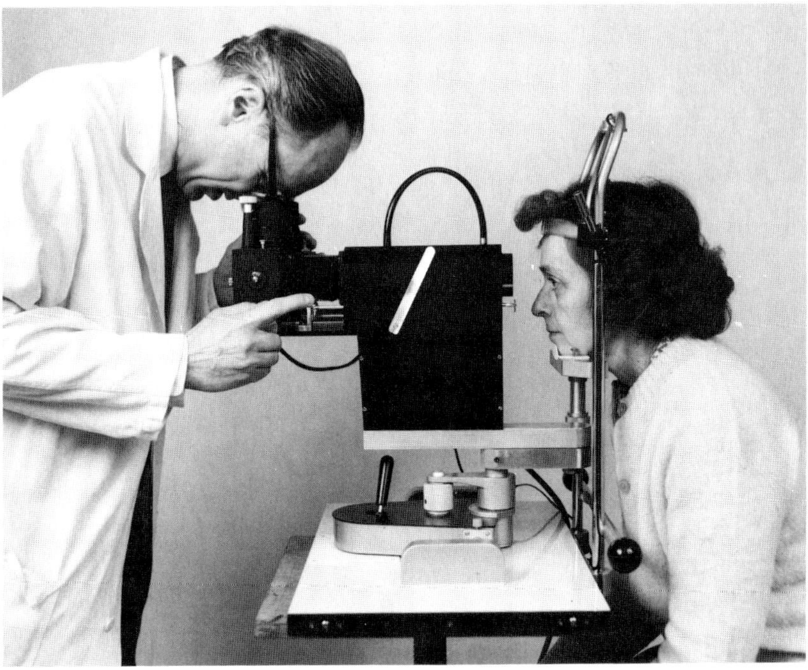

Fig. 12-9. Simultaneous stereoscopic fundus camera: patient and operator in position. Camera mounted on a table is aligned by using the joystick while focusing is performed with the operator's right hand.

slightly different vantage points. These are determined by the images in the dilated pupil of the eye (at the 3 and 9 o'clock positions) of two apertures immediately in front of the two rhomboid prisms. The size and separation of the points of view in the pupil are determined by the diameter and separation of the two apertures. Thus, an inverted image of the fundus is formed by the refracting system of the eye and the aspheric ophthalmoscope lens. Through the use of a matched pair of rhomboid prisms, the inverted aerial image is viewed from two points of view, and the light rays are carried into a pair of camera lenses. Depending on whether a higher or lower magnification is desired, a pair of Barlow lenses can be placed in the system. Focusing the image is accomplished by means of a double-reflex mirror system in which the mirror is in the down position during focusing; at the time of the exposure, it is automatically brought to the horizontal position so that the image is focused at the film plane. Focusing the image is accomplished by moving the entire reflex housing (including the Barlow lenses) backward and forward. The image is viewed through a pair of oculars (×8) that have a wide field and allow visualization of the entire fundus image.

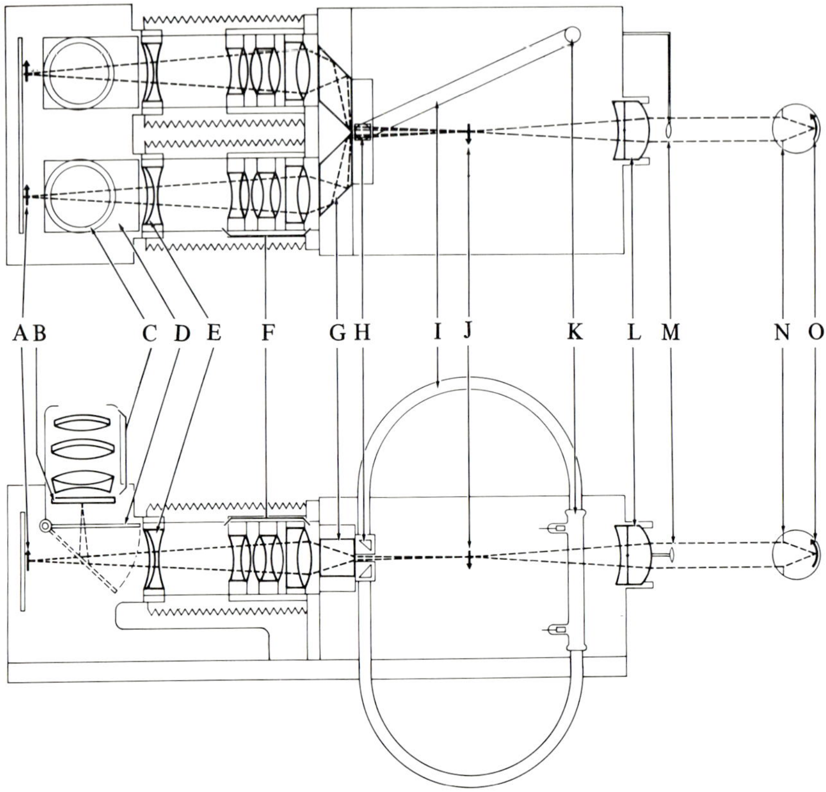

Fig. 12-10. Optical system of the simultaneous stereoscopic fundus camera. A = *image of fundus at film plane;* B = *reticle in focusing eyepieces;* C = *focusing eyepieces;* D = *reflex mirror;* E = *Barlow lens (negative achromat);* F = *camera lens;* G = *rhomboid prisms;* H = *small right-angle prisms;* I = *fiberoptic bundle;* J = *inverted aerial image of fundus;* K = *electronic flash tube (end-on type);* L = *aspheric ophthalmoscope lens;* M = *small plus spherical lens;* N = *pupil;* O = *fundus.*

A conventional reticle avoids errors in focusing caused by accommodation of the person taking the photographs.

The lighting system (Figs. 12-11 through 12-13) utilizes an end-on type of electronic flashtube, which has two tapered fiberoptic bundles in contact with each end of the tube. These fiberoptic bundles carry the light into a pair of apertures facing into the rhomboid prisms. Light emitted from these small right-angle prisms is transmitted through the ophthalmoscope lens and refocused at the iris plane as two small lights at the 6 and 12 o'clock positions near the pupillary margin in the same plane as the viewing apertures. In this way, one of the primary considerations for high-resolution fundus photography is met: The illumi-

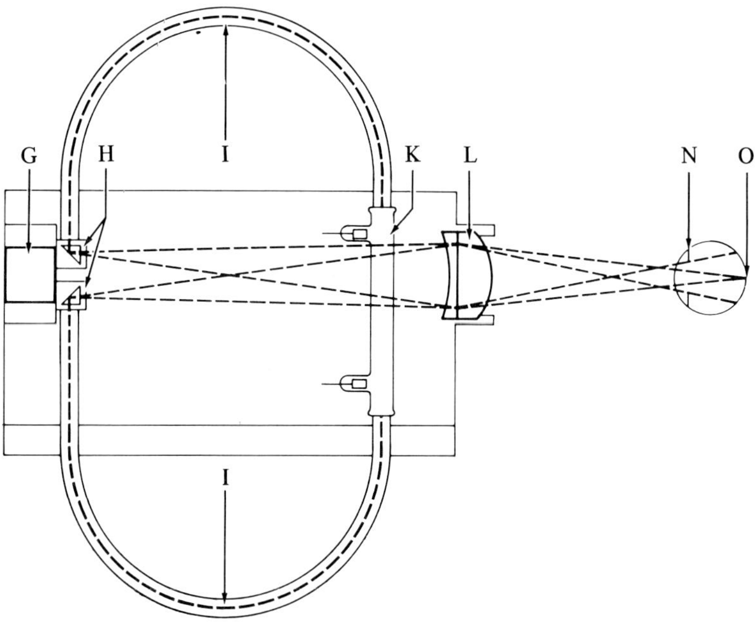

Fig. 12-11. Lighting system for the simultaneous stereoscopic fundus camera (G–I, K, L, N, O *as in Fig. 12-10.*)

nating light does not pass through the same portion of the pupil (and thus the crystalline lens) as that used in the imaging system. For focusing purposes, the electronic flash lamp is flashed at a rate of 60 flashes per second with a relatively low energy. When the picture is to be taken with the reflex mirror in the up position, a single flash is obtained at a power input of up to 300 joules. Thus, the light being used for focusing is from the same source as the light used for taking the picture. The two small prisms can be moved symmetrically toward or away from each other to allow adjustment for the separation of the lights as they pass through the pupillary aperture; therefore, they can be adjusted to fit into an 8-mm pupil or brought sufficiently close to each other to pass through a 4-mm pupil. On the power supply panel is a control, a meter that indicates the voltage on the tube, and a voltage control knob that allows variation in flash intensity for different magnifications and for different fundus reflectivities, magnifications, and apertures.

Four different magnifications are possible, depending on the combination of two variables. The first variable is whether or not the Barlow lenses (Fig. 12-10*E*) are used in the system. The second variable

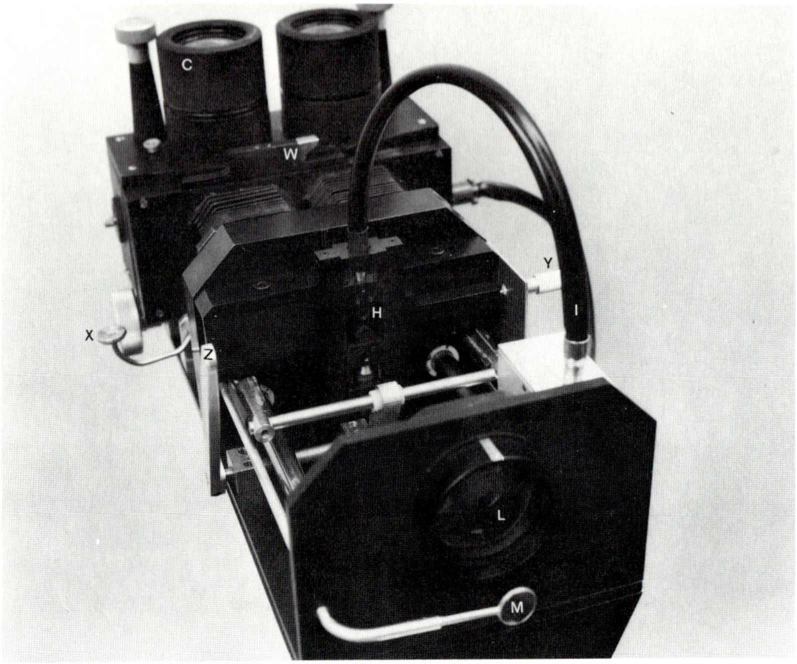

Fig. 12-12. Simultaneous stereoscopic fundus camera. Note location of fiberoptic bundle and housings for small right-angle prisms. C = *focusing eyepieces;* H = *housing for small right-angle prism;* I = *fiberoptic bundle;* L = *aspheric ophthalmoscope lens;* M = *small plus lens for alignment (see Fig. 12-11); W = release button incorporating Barlow lenses into optical system;* X = *push button for operation of* M; Y = *adjustment knob for changing separation of* H; Z = *knob for changing position of camera lenses.*

is the position of the camera lenses, which is accomplished by means of a lever (Fig. 12-12*Z*) that can be adjusted to a forward or backward position. When the camera lens is in the high-power position and the Barlow lens is adjusted into the optical pathway, a magnification is obtained that is about twice that of the lowest magnification, which includes about 30 degrees of the fundus. At this highest magnification, the diameter of a normal disc is close to 1 cm on the film, which is about 6 times the actual size of the disc. Another variable feature of the camera involves the use of interchangeable aperture plates that can be placed in front of the rhomboid prisms, allowing variation of the stereoscopic effect as well as the depth of field by varying the center-to-center distance and the diameter of the apertures utilized. Some loss of detail results if the separation of the apertures is too large, while the stereo effect is minimized if it is too small. In most

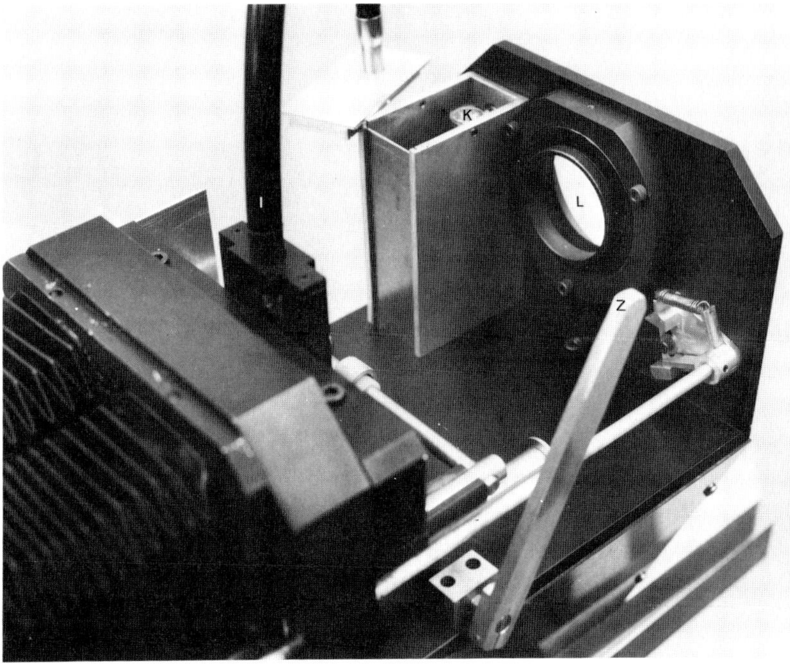

Fig. 12-13. Simultaneous stereoscopic fundus camera. Note electronic flash tube housing with cover removed. I = *fiberoptic bundle;* K = *upper end of electronic flash tube;* L = *aspheric ophthalmoscope lens;* Z = *knob for changing position of camera lenses.*

cases, the optimal separation is 5 mm and the optimal diameter is 4.5 mm.

The operation of the camera is simplified in that, during the focusing procedure, a small biconvex lens (Figs. 12-10, 12-12) can be moved in front of the ophthalmoscope lens by means of a lever. This lens allows a view of the pupillary aperture and the two small light sources as they pass through into the lens of the eye. Accurate positioning and focusing of these lights in the pupillary aperture make it possible to obtain pictures with maximum saturation (contrast) because backscatter of light is minimized. (The position of the lens during the alignment procedure is shown in Fig. 12-14.) The meter on the power supply is then adjusted to the proper setting for both the magnification being used and any variation in the lightness or darkness of the fundus. Following positioning of the two illuminating lights in the pupil, final critical focusing is accomplished by means of the focusing knob. A footswitch is then depressed, which turns off the rapid flashing of the electronic flashtube and produces one high-intensity flash at the mo-

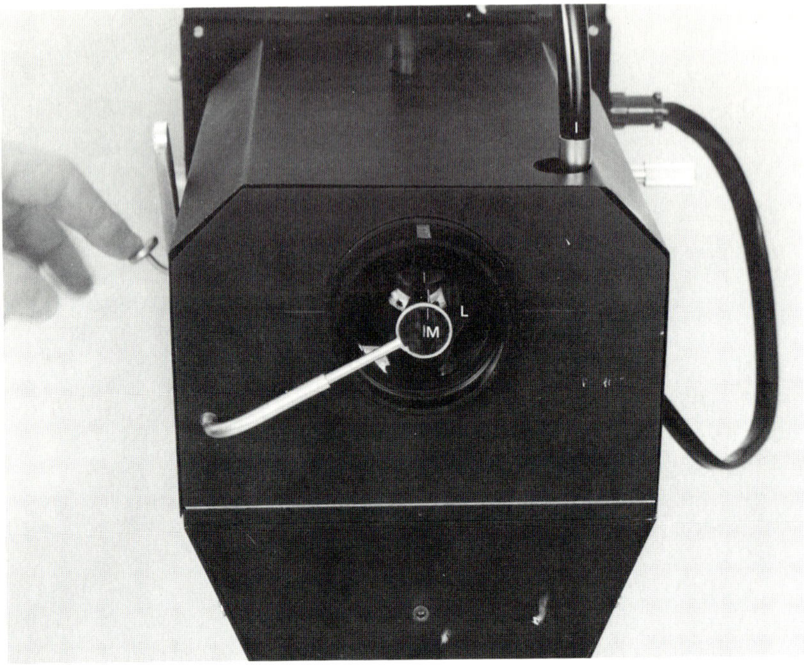

Fig. 12-14. Simultaneous stereoscopic fundus camera. Note position of small plus lens when used in the alignment procedure (see text). I = *fiberoptic bundle;* L = *aspheric ophthalmoscope lens;* M = *small plus lens.*

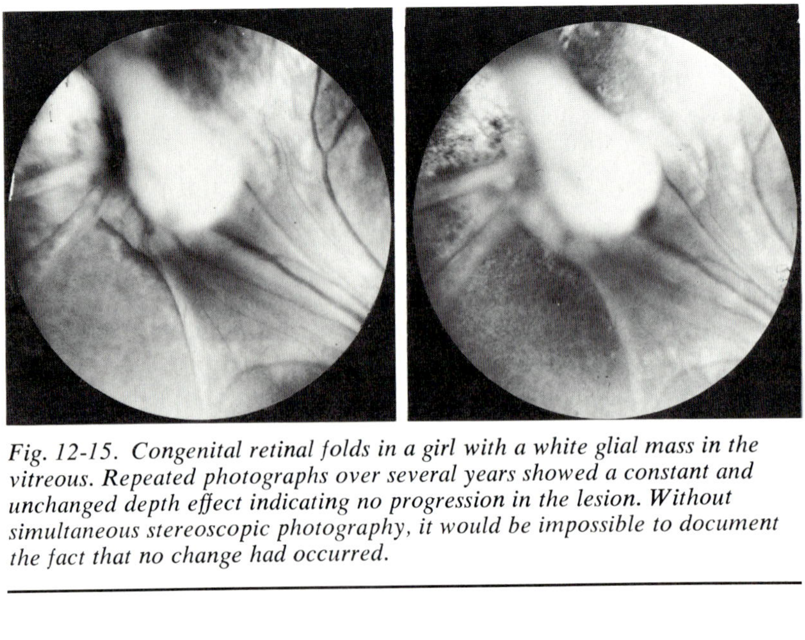

Fig. 12-15. Congenital retinal folds in a girl with a white glial mass in the vitreous. Repeated photographs over several years showed a constant and unchanged depth effect indicating no progression in the lesion. Without simultaneous stereoscopic photography, it would be impossible to document the fact that no change had occurred.

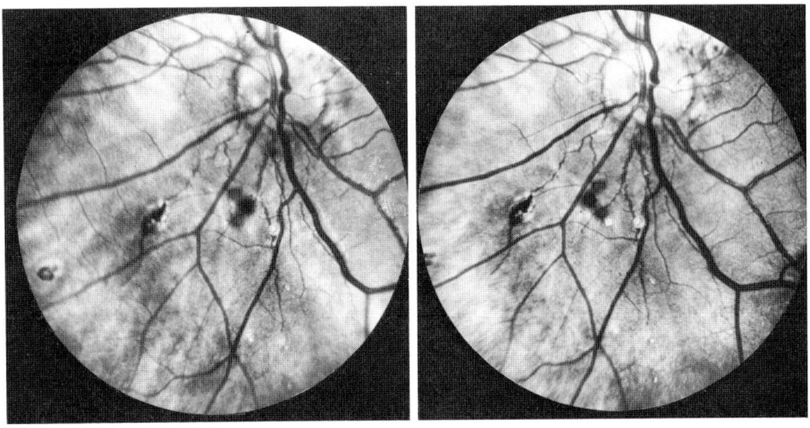

Fig. 12-16. Irregular streaks in the fundus with appearance of vessels in a patient with pseudoxanthoma elasticum and angioid streaks. The streaks are easily visualized stereoscopically to be deep to the vessels.

ment the reflex mirror is in the horizontal position. Not only are the resulting photographs valuable for recording small changes in subsequent pictures (Fig. 12-15) but subtle depth relationships are also evident (Fig. 12-16).

Stereoscopic Slit-Lamp Photography

The ability to record the appearance of the slit-lamp beam traversing the various portions of the eye is an important adjunct to ophthalmic photography. It appears that the Zeiss slit-lamp camera is at present the most satisfactory equipment for this purpose. However, the arrangement that makes it possible to take stereoscopic photographs leaves much to be desired. The two separate camera housings that must be utilized, along with the loss of light inherent in the system, are undesirable features. Because the slit-lamp beam traverses various portions of the eye that represent considerable depth, it would obviously be desirable to be able to use various apertures and, under certain circumstances, be able to take pictures with an increased depth of field.

As far as the light source is concerned, the camera (Fig. 12-17) remains essentially the same as the standard Zeiss slit-lamp camera. A major change, however, concerns the camera portion, which has been redesigned so that the stereopairs are recorded on one film. It has a fixed magnification of approximately ×3 on the film, and viewing of the stereoscopic image is obtained through a pair of high-power oculars, the same as those used in the stereo fundus camera. The lenses utilized are a matched pair of f/6.3 Zeiss Microtars, which are mounted

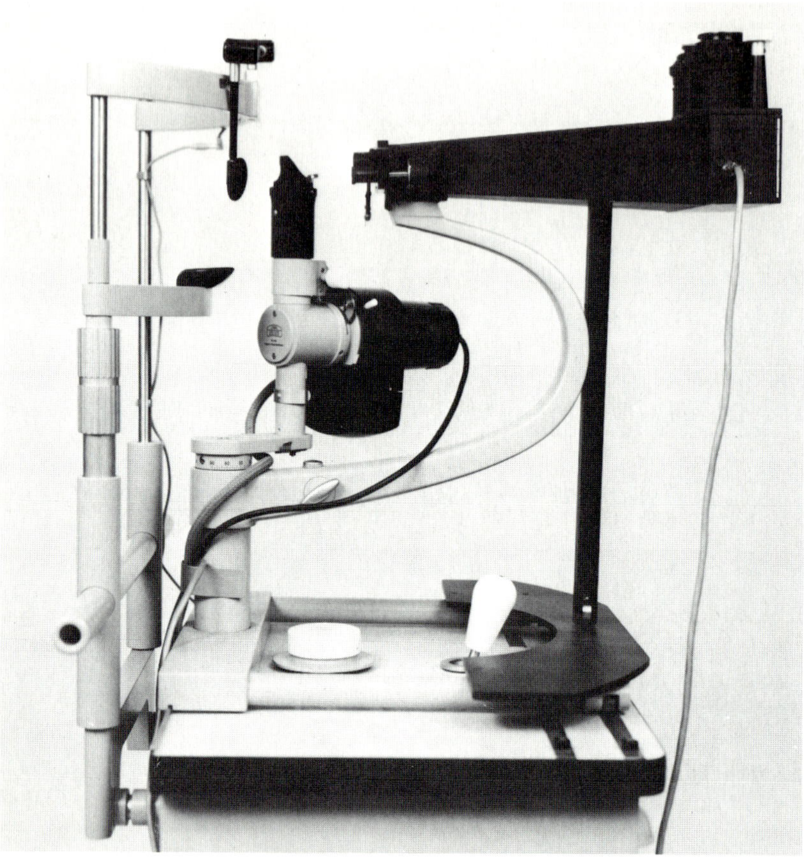

Fig. 12-17. Stereoscopic slit-lamp camera (modified from Zeiss slit-lamp camera). Here, single camera is producing a ×3 film magnification.

side by side and have the appropriate separation to give a good stereoscopic depth effect and to produce the proper separation of the images at the film plane.

Another important feature of the camera is an automatic diaphragm arrangement that allows one to focus with the apertures wide open but automatically reduces the aperture size at the time the pictures are taken. When photographing a cataract, for example, it is possible to obtain a depth of field great enough to bring into sharp focus almost the entire thickness of the normal lens. This is accomplished by a double pair of apertures mounted on a bar (Fig. 12-18). This bar can be rotated so that either pair of apertures can be used to stop down the lenses. During the focusing procedure, the apertures are in the

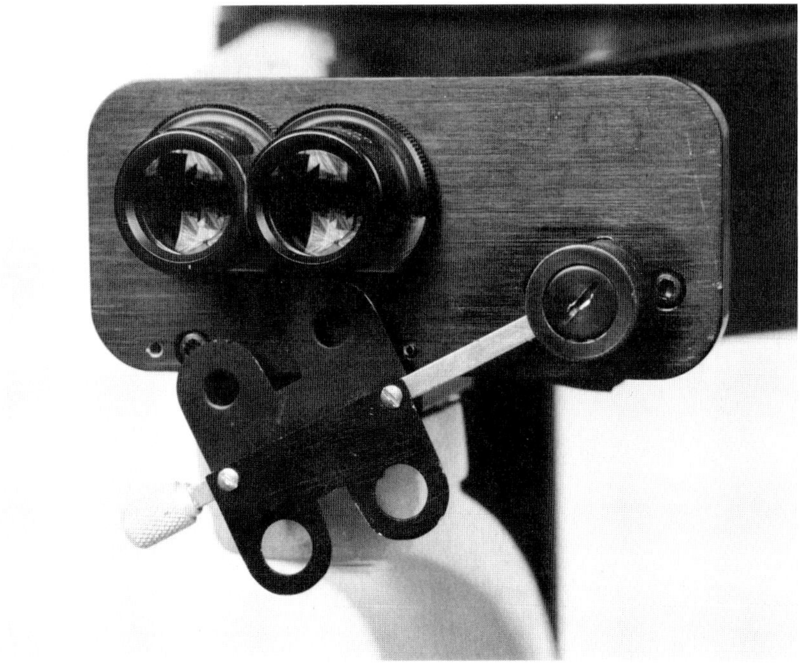

Fig. 12-18. Stereoscopic slit-lamp camera. Note paired lenses and aperture bar in the focusing position.

down position, but when the picture is to be taken and the footswitch is depressed, the apertures swing into a slot in the lens and are positioned to act as the apertures of the lens (Fig. 12-19). The lever then activates the reflex mirror and electronic flash to take the picture. The larger of the two sets of apertures closes the lenses down 2 stops (approximately f/12.5), and the smaller closes the apertures down 3½ stops (approximately f/22). Although the enhanced depth of field is more dramatic when seen stereoscopically, it can be appreciated two-dimensionally (Figs. 12-20, 12-21).

Iris Transillumination

The translucency of the iris is dependent almost entirely on the integrity of the pigment epithelium of the iris. The technique of transillumination depends on observation of the red reflex from the fundus as it is transmitted through various defects in the pigment epithelium. In the normal young person's eye, the iris does not show translucency, and in older individuals (over 45 years), translucency is sometimes found in the pupillary zone. Some of the more common conditions in-

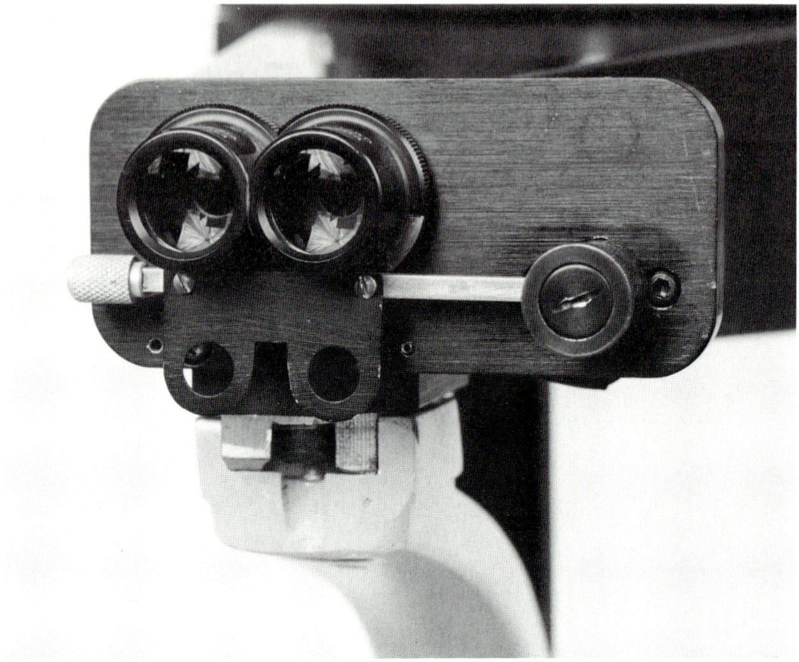

Fig. 12-19. Stereoscopic slit-lamp camera. Note smaller set of apertures swung up into the lens for taking the picture.

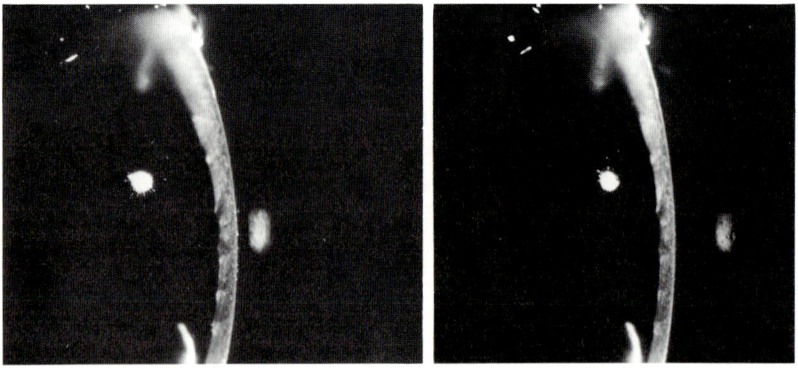

Fig. 12-20. Narrow slit-lamp beam passing through the cornea in a patient with corneal edema and folds in Descemet's membrane (striate keratopathy). Despite the curvature of the cornea, the entire extent of the beam is in focus due to the smaller aperture used in the slit-lamp camera.

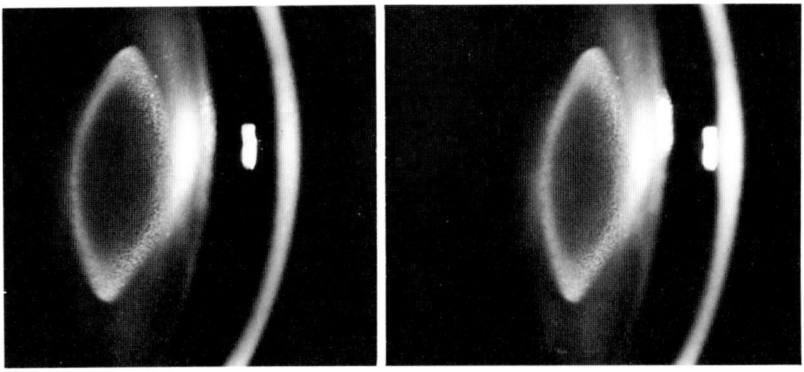

Fig. 12-21. Slit-lamp beam passing through the cornea and lens in a patient with a punctate cataract involving the adult nucleus. There is also a small anterior subcapsular opacity. Note that the beam as it passes through the cornea is only slightly out of focus.

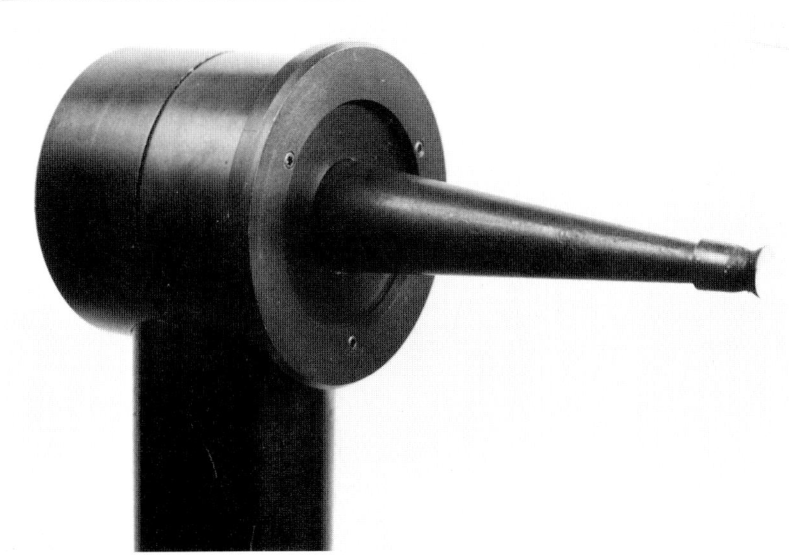

Fig. 12-22. Light pipe and electronic flash unit for iris transillumination photography (see text).

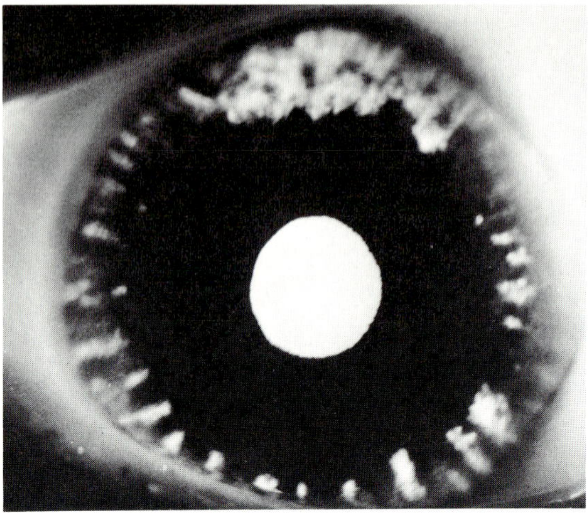

Fig. 12-23. The transilluminated iris of an elderly man with pigmentary dispersion syndrome. The iris periphery, as well as the pupil, shows the bright red reflex of the fundus and reveals the abnormal radial pattern of iris translucency.

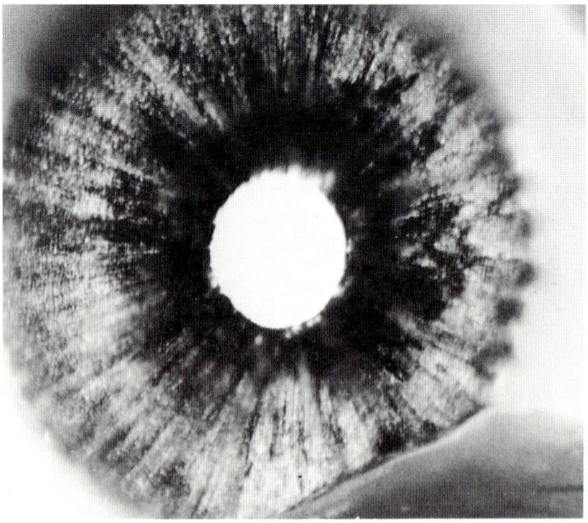

Fig. 12-24. Iris transillumination in a patient with chronic glaucoma with an irregular translucency of the entire iris due to generalized loss of pigment epithelium.

volving iris translucency are albinism, diabetes mellitus, pigmentary glaucoma, pseudoexfoliation, chronic glaucoma, and uveitis.

A satisfactory method for photographing iris translucency is use of a light pipe made of Pyrex glass. This solid pipe is 4 inches long and has a diameter of 1 inch at one end, tapering to 1/8 inch at the other (Fig. 12-22). The large end of this pipe comes in direct contact with a 600-joule electronic flash lamp. The small end is fitted with a rubber tip to avoid leakage of the light around the edge of the pipe. This end is placed in contact with the sclera temporally. Light from the end of the pipe is transmitted through the sclera onto the fundus, the red reflection of which is seen through the iris defects as well as through the pupil. Areas of abnormality are seen as red patches surrounded by the dark iris, which does not transmit light (Fig. 12-23, 12-24).

Before the procedure is carried out, a topical anesthetic is placed in the eye, so the patient experiences little or no discomfort except for the momentary brightness of the flash. The translucency of the iris is recorded on color film (Kodachrome II) at ×2 film magnification. The stereoscopic anterior segment camera appears to be a satisfactory unit for this procedure, but the apertures of the lenses must be opened to f/6.3.

Suggested Reading

Donaldson, D. D. A new camera for medical stereophotography with special reference to the eye. *Arch. Ophthalmol.* 52 : 564, 1954.

Donaldson, D. D. A stereocamera for medical photography. *Med. Biol. Illus.* 5(4) : 209, 1955.

Donaldson, D. D. A new camera for stereoscopic fundus photography. *Trans. Am. Ophthalmol. Soc.* 62 : 429, 1964.

Donaldson, D. D. A new camera for stereoscopic fundus photography. *Arch. Ophthalmol.* 73 : 253, 1965.

Donaldson, D. D. Transillumination of the iris. *Trans. Am. Ophthalmol. Soc.* 72 : 89, 1974.

Donaldson, D. D., Prescott, R., and Kennedy, S. Simultaneous stereoscopic fundus camera incorporating a single optical axis. *Invest. Ophthalmol. Vis. Sci.* 19(3) : 289–297, 1980.

External Eye Photography: Equipment and Technique

KENNETH W. CHRISTOPHERSON

External eye photography can easily be achieved with a single-lens reflex camera system throughout a wide range of magnifications, making focusing possible from infinity to extremely close up. There are a variety of accessories and lenses designed for the single-lens reflex camera, which make it a versatile and practical system.

The image seen in the viewfinder of the single-lens reflex camera is exactly the image captured by the film because the image is viewed through the same lens that takes the picture. At the instant the shutter release is pressed, the mirror that reflects the image onto the viewing screen moves out of the image path and the shutter is opened to allow the film to be exposed. This mechanism provides an accurate means of photography at increasingly higher magnifications and eliminates many of the problems encountered with systems that do not permit accurate viewing through the lens that takes the picture.

Equipment Selection: The Camera

There are 35-mm film format and roll film format single-lens reflex cameras. The 35-mm single-lens reflex cameras are smaller, far less expensive to equip, and more easily utilized than roll film cameras. The cameras and lenses discussed and illustrated throughout this chapter pertain to the 35-mm film format, but the principles apply to all film formats.

Deciding on a camera should be a mixture of personal preference, cost, and feasibility. The only features a camera must have are: (1) interchangeable lenses; (2) a suitable close-up system which can be attached to the camera; (3) the ability to operate completely manually (the f/stop and the shutter speed can each be selected independently); and (4) electronic flash synchronization. Some additional features to consider are interchangeable viewing screens and auto-winders.

Optics Selection

The Normal Lens

The normal focal length lens for the 35-mm film format is 50 mm. Designed for general photography, this is the lens normally purchased with a camera: It usually focuses only as close as 1½ or 2 feet, which will allow a magnification of about 1/10 lifesize. The range of magnification necessary for external eye photography is from about 1/10 to 3

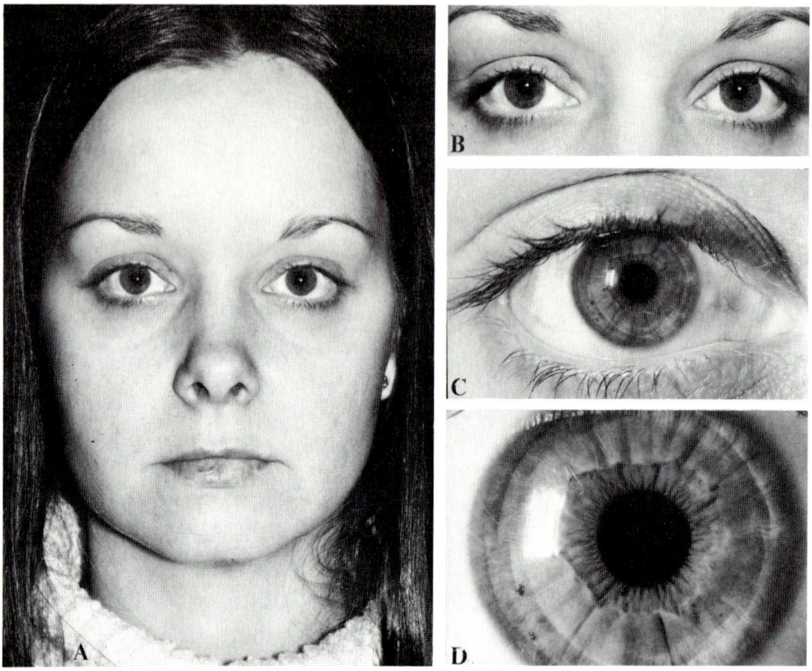

Fig. 13-1. Range of magnifications most often required in ophthalmology. (A) ×*1 : 8.* (B) ×*1 : 3.* (C) ×*1 : 1.* (D) ×*3 : 1. Photographs* A–C *were taken with the Canon 50-mm macro lens used with the Canon FD2X-B Telextender. Photograph* D *was taken with the Canon 50-mm macro lens reversed on a bellows. The illustrations are enlargements of the negatives and are used to show what a typical picture would include on a slide.*

times lifesize (3 : 1) (Fig. 13-1). Focus and magnification are directly related to the distance between the lens and the film plane. When a lens is focused at infinity, it is at its closest relationship to the film plane. Greater magnification and closer focusing are achieved by extending the lens away from the film plane and closer to the object.

Bellows and Extension Rings to Increase Magnification

Magnification can be increased by the use of extension rings or a bellows unit between the lens and camera body. Extension rings are fixed millimeters of extension which couple between the lens and the camera body. They can be added one to another for greater extensions. A change in magnification is cumbersome to achieve with extension rings and easy to achieve with a bellows unit because it is infinitely variable between its close and far settings (Fig. 13-2). A normal focal length, "standard" (50-mm) lens will usually offer a minimum magnification from about 1/2 lifesize to greater than lifesize on a bellows. A bellows-

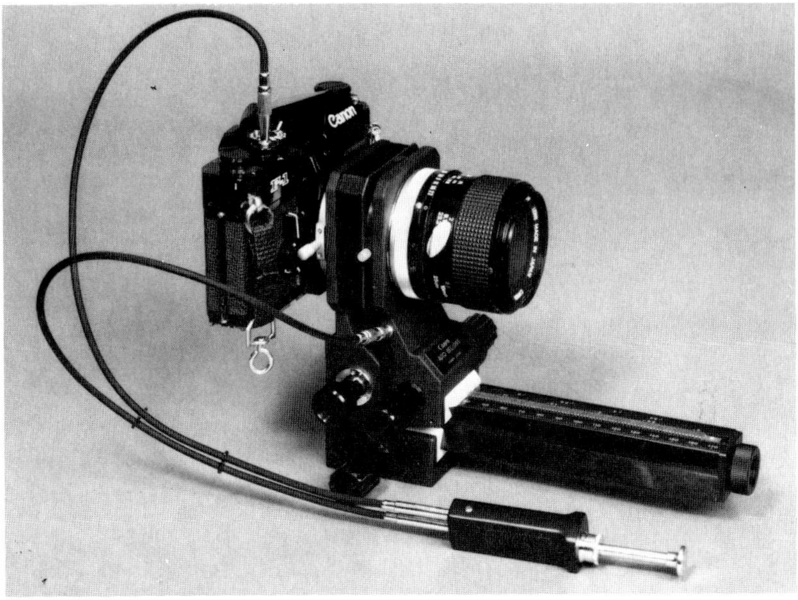

A

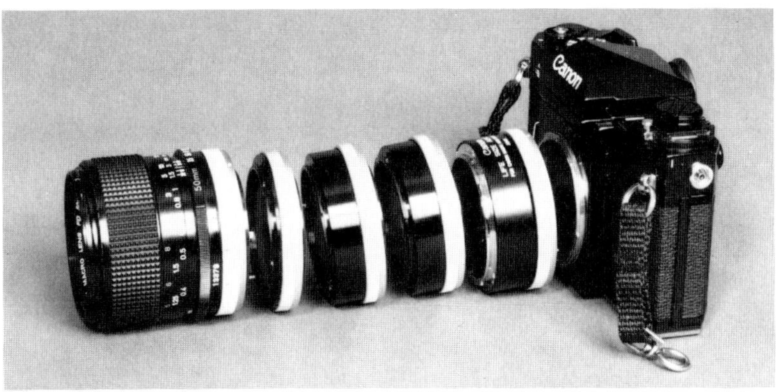

B

Fig. 13-2. (A) *Bellows unit fitted between camera and lens completely compressed illustrating the minimum separation which can be achieved. Magnifications from* ×.8 : 1 *to* ×3.9 : 1 *are possible with the bellows unit shown. A double cable release is used which first stops the diaphragm down to the working aperture and then releases the shutter.* (B) *The lens is separated from the camera to achieve higher magnifications using any combination of different thickness extension rings* (*tubes*).

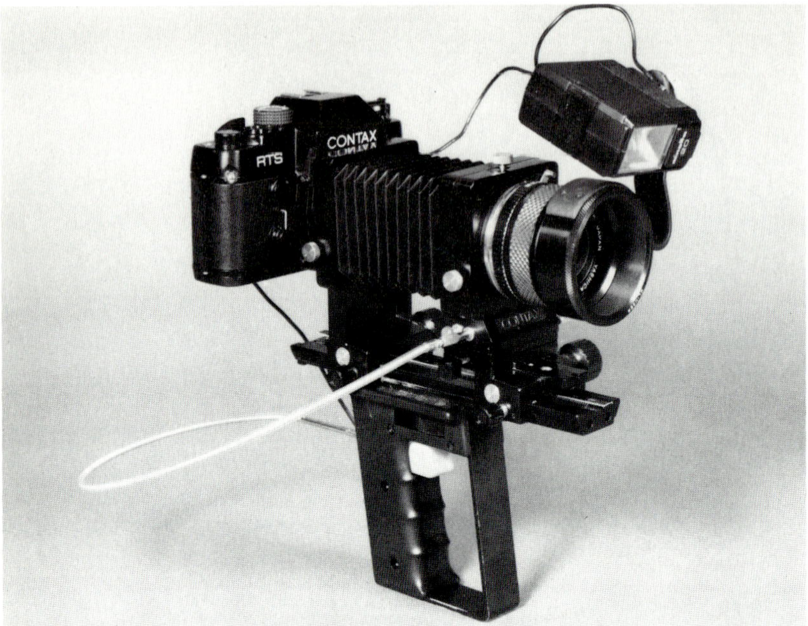

A

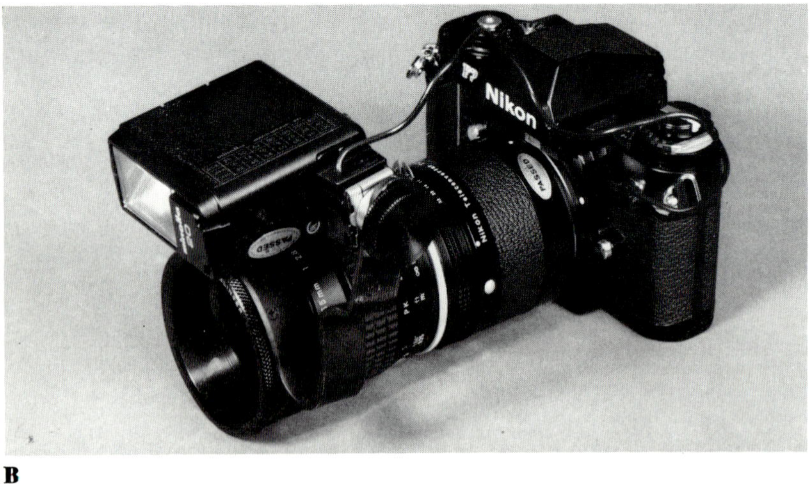

B

Fig. 13-3. (A) *Zeiss Contax camera with Contax Auto bellows and Yashica 100-mm bellows lens, a manual flash, and a Klinger bracket. The system is steadied and triggered by a hand grip allowing one-handed operation of the camera after the magnification is determined and set.* (B) *Nikon F3 with a Nikon TC200 Teleconverter and 55-mm f/2.8 Micro-Nikkor. The manual flash is affixed by a hot-shoe to PC adapter to a Klinger flash bracket. This system can focus from infinity to 1 : 1 and has a 110-mm focal length which provides several inches of working distance to the subject at 1 : 1 magnification. This compact and convenient system provides photographs of high resolution.*

mount lens is more convenient since it is designed to be used with a bellows which becomes the focusing mechanism providing a range of focus from infinity continuously to greater than 1 : 1 (Fig. 13-3A). The primary drawback to using a bellows system is that the total package (camera, bellows, lens, and light source) is very heavy.

A lens' aperture diaphragm is coupled to the camera body in such a way that the aperture is stopped down to the working aperture just before the shutter opens. When the lens and camera are separated to achieve higher magnification, the automatic diaphragm mechanism no longer is coupled. The lens diaphragm needs to be opened completely to focus and then stopped down manually for photography unless the extension tubes or bellows are automatic. Automatic rings and bellows incorporate either a diaphragm-actuating device, which maintains the coupling of the diaphragm between the camera and lens, or a double cable release, which stops down the lens diaphragm to the working aperture and then triggers the shutter (see Fig. 13-2A).

Close-Focusing Lenses

A lens that continuously focuses from infinity to very close, providing high magnification, greatly facilitates external eye photography. This wide range of focus eliminates extraneous manipulations required to switch from one setup to another for different magnifications, as would be necessary when using extension rings or a bellows with a 50-mm general-purpose lens. The close-focusing "macro-micro" lens provides the easiest and most convenient system for external eye photography. These lenses generally focus from infinity to 1/2 lifesize and, with the inclusion of a special extension tube, are able to focus additionally from 1/2 lifesize to lifesize. The extension rings designed for use with these lenses enable automatic diaphragm coupling. Close-focus lenses, like bellows-mount lenses, are designed to provide sharpest photographs in close-up (high magnification) situations, whereas the general-purpose 50-mm lenses are designed to provide sharpest photographs when focused at or near infinity.

Close-focusing lenses are available in normal (50- to 55-mm) focal lengths and telephoto (90- to 105-mm) focal lengths (Fig. 13-4). Longer focal length lenses are more desirable in external eye photography for several reasons. At a 1 : 1 magnification, a 100-mm lens will provide greater distance between the subject and the front of the lens than a 50-mm lens, allowing more satisfactory lighting arrangements. Because a light source can be positioned farther away from the eye, there is a smaller corneal reflection of the light. In addition, the longer focal length lens renders a more natural perspective.

Teleconverters

Recently, teleconverters have undergone a resurgence in photography. Camera manufacturers have begun offering a much improved version

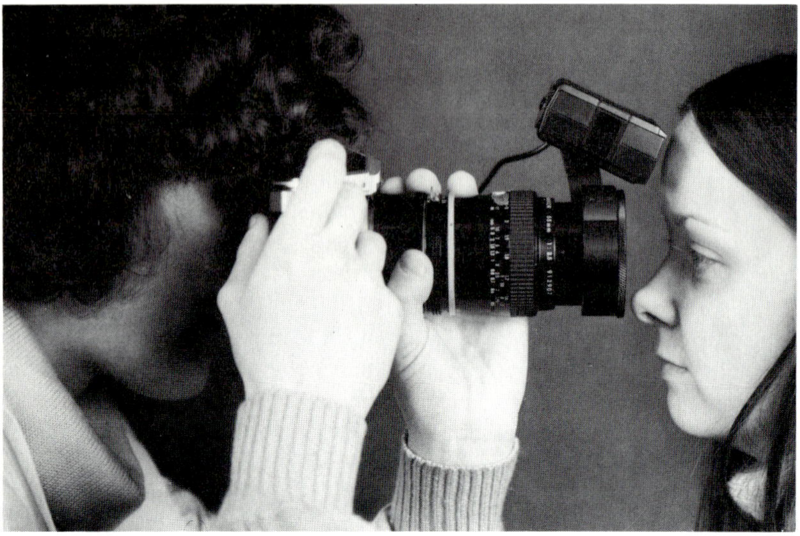

A

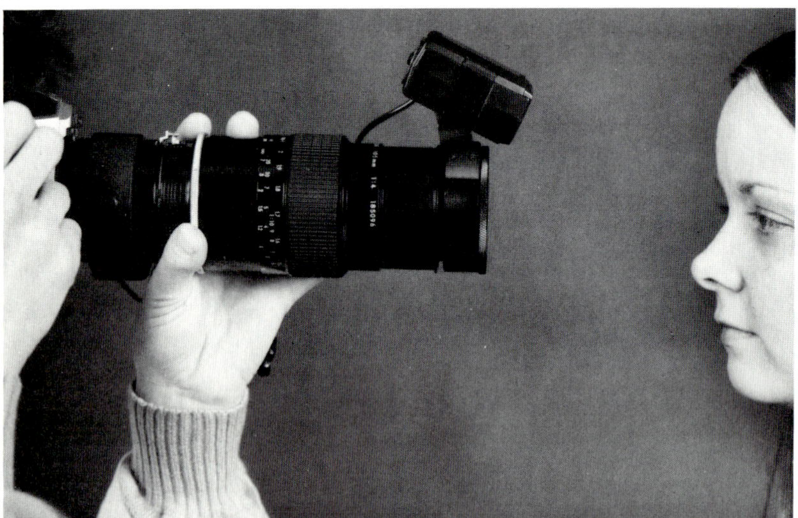

B

Fig. 13-4. (A) *The close working distance of a 55-mm Micro-Nikkor focused at 1 : 1 magnification with a Klinger flash bracket.* (B) *The greater working distance at 1 : 1 magnification with the longer focal length 105-mm Micro-Nikkor. The longer focal length provides sufficient distance to allow the Klinger flash bracket to be used successfully.*

(for their respective cameras) over those offered in the past by independent lens designers. When older versions were used, image quality was compromised; the new versions are of such good quality that results with a ×2 teleconverter and a normal focal length (50-mm) close-focusing lens are hard to distinguish from those with a long focal length (100-mm) close-focusing lens used by itself.

There are several benefits to using a 50-mm close-focusing lens with a teleconverter. The magnification is doubled (with a ×2 teleconverter) at the same camera to subject distance, resulting in a lifesize magnification at the close focus limit instead of only 1/2 lifesize magnification. Focus is continuous from infinity to a magnification of 1 : 1 without the need for the inclusion of an extension tube. The benefits of using a long lens are realized, and a 50-mm lens is accessible when it is needed (e.g., for copy work or full-body photographs). The 50-mm lens with teleconverter is less cumbersome, lighter, and smaller than the 100-mm lens (see Fig. 13-3B).

The disadvantage to using a teleconverter is that the f/stops in use are doubled. A lens is focused at its largest opening. While focusing at a maximum aperture of f/3.5 or f/2.8 is not difficult, when these values are doubled to become f/7 and f/5.6 respectively, focus becomes more difficult. The numbers on the aperture ring have to be mentally doubled: An f/8, which is indicated, is actually an f/16.

Reversing the Lens

For greater magnification than 1 : 1 (lifesize), better optical performance might be obtained by reversing the orientation of the lens so that the front of the lens faces the camera body and the rear of the lens faces the subject. Not all lenses offer better imaging in a reversed mode. Reverse mounting of a lens can be achieved with a reversing ring, offered by most camera companies. Often the reverse mounting of a normal focal length (50-mm) lens will provide a magnification of 1 : 1. Bellows or extension tubes, or both, can be used to achieve even higher magnifications. The automatic mechanism for stopping the lens down to the working aperture no longer is in proper position with the camera to function, and the diaphragm has to be manually set just before the exposure. Some camera manufacturers offer a special device that attaches to the automatic diaphragm and is used with a double cable release, which eliminates the cumbersome problem of manually stopping down the diaphragm after focusing and before exposing the film. From a practical standpoint, unless extensive or extremely critical photography is done at greater than lifesize magnification, reversing the lens is not necessary.

Supplementary Lenses

Supplementary ("plus") lenses are another method of achieving higher magnification but are the poorest option to choose. The resolution of these lenses is acceptable only centrally, and best results require very small apertures. These lenses are affixed to the front of the lens and do not alter exposure. Plus lenses are offered in powers ranging from +1 to +10, and shorten the focal length of the lenses to which they are attached.

Lighting

Although close-up photography can be performed with available light, the procedure is not recommended. With available light, a slow shutter speed often has to be used to permit a small aperture setting (to allow for adequate depth of field). Motion has to be stopped, and, with high magnification, any motion is exaggerated. A slow shutter speed will not halt this motion sufficiently: Motion is seen when either the camera is moved by the photographer or the patient moves during the exposure. Often a blurred picture is the result of both subject motion and camera shake.

Auxiliary light has to be employed to provide adequate depth of field and halt motion. Electronic flash and tungsten photo floods are two sources of illumination which can be used.

The illumination level of a tungsten light source has to be extremely bright to allow a fast shutter speed with a small aperture. When this extremely high light level needs to be maintained for a period of time through the course of a series of photographs, the patient has to endure a heat build-up from the high-intensity illumination source and often cannot avoid squinting or tearing.

Electronic flash units are the preferred illumination source. An electronic flash unit is small, lightweight, very portable, and the power source is self-contained. Because it offers high-intensity illumination of extremely short duration (generally about 1/1000 second), it is not debilitating for a patient, and any camera or patient motion is effectively stopped. A slow, fine-grain, high-resolution film can be used with electronic flash units because of the high level of exposure possible; whereas a faster, large-grain, low-resolution film has to be used with either available light or tungsten illumination sources.

Electronic flash units are offered both in manual and automatic versions. For close-up photography, a manual flash unit fills the need very adequately: An automatic flash unit is not necessary and, for a number of reasons, not a good choice for use in a close-up system. Most automatic flash units will function in either a manual or automatic mode. An automatic flash unit works by shortening the duration of light emitted as it is moved closer to the subject. Reciprocity failure, which results in a color shift of the film (a bluer than normal picture is usually seen), can occur in an extreme close-up situation where the flash duration is very short. The flash duration from a manual flash unit is constant for every flash, and reciprocity failure is not a problem.

If a manual flash unit is mounted directly to the front of the lens, exposure will not have to be modified. As a lens is focused closer to the patient, the aperture effectively becomes smaller, and less light reaches the film. The additional requirement of light is provided since the flash is moving closer to the object as the lens is focused closer. The closer a light is moved to an object, the more intense the illumination becomes (inverse square law of light), offsetting the change in the effective aperture. Effectively, this then is an "automatic" flash system with a manual flash unit within a range of approximately 2½ feet to 4 inches. A manual electronic flash unit that has a guide number between 28 and 32 with an ASA 25 film, will provide sufficient illumination for an f/stop of f/16 or f/22 with an ASA 64 film. When a photograph has to be taken beyond the range of 2½ feet, the f/stop has to be computed by using the exposure calculation scale on the flash unit, a straightforward and fairly simple procedure. An automatic flash unit can be used beyond the range of 2½ feet, eliminating the need to calculate exposures. An important consideration when selecting an electronic flash unit is that it have a short recycling time (less than 5 seconds). A long recycling period might cause patient discomfort when extensive photography is to be done.

The flash unit can be affixed to the front of the lens by several types of brackets, including those offered by Adolph Gasser, Jones, Klinger, and Novaflex (Fig. 13-5).* All of these brackets attach to the front filter threads of the lens and have a flash shoe-mount to hold the flash in place. The flash can be positioned 360 degrees around the front of the lens and directed toward the patient at various angles. In this way, the reflection of the light on the cornea, which cannot be eliminated, can be positioned out of an area that would interfere with the recording of corneal pathology.

Some manual flash units are designed to be used in the hot-shoe of a camera and do not have a flash cord. A hot-shoe to PC cord attachment can be used, allowing the flash to be positioned away from the

* The Gasser custom rotating flash bracket, models 1, 2, and 3, are available from Adolph Gasser, Inc., Medical Systems Dept., P.O. Box 420, San Francisco, CA 94101. Attention: Dan Rosowsky, (415)751-0145.

The Jones retainer ring flash bracket (J-16) is available from Jones Photo Equipment, 10816 Burbank Blvd., North Hollywood, CA 91601, (213)766-7189.

The Klinger bracket is available from Klinger Precision Instruments, 3402-I W. MacArthur Blvd., Santa Anna, CA 92704, (714)641-5878. The Klinger bracket used by the author has been modified by Csaba L. Martonyi, Assistant Professor and Director of Ophthalmic Photography, University of Michigan, Parkview Medical, 1000 Wall St., Ann Arbor, MI 48105. The modified bracket can be rotated freely and is held in place (by click stops) at various positions around the lens. This modification is well worth the additional investment.

The Novaflex flash bracket is comprised of an adapter X-ring plus X-shoe flash bracket, and is available from Kalt Corporation, 2036 Broadway, Santa Monica, CA 90404.

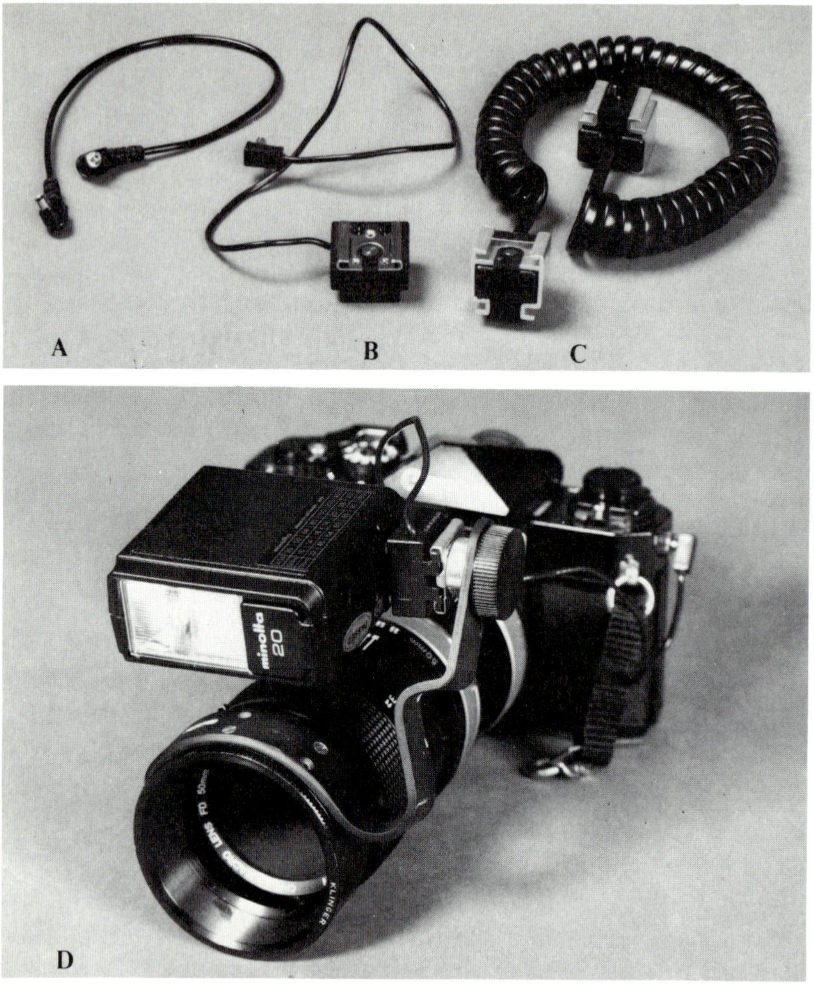

Fig. 13-5. (A) *Different flash connections are shown. A flash cord extender is used between the present flash cord and the flash connection on the camera and is available in different lengths (10-inch cord shown).* (B) A hot-shoe *to PC connection uses the flash positioned in the shoe and the flash cord attached to the flash connection on the camera. This allows the flash to be used away from the camera's own hot-shoe.* (C) *A Duo-synch cord has one end affixed to the hot-shoe of the camera, allowing the other end (with the flash mounted in the other shoe) to be positioned up to several feet away; it is known as a hot-shoe to hot-shoe connection.* (D) *Hot-shoe to PC cord is used with the Klinger flash bracket.*

hot-shoe. If a flash unit's flash cord is too short, a PC-PC extension can be used (Fig. 13-5).

Lester Dyne offers a combination ring light and point light source, which is affixed to a bracket that is attached to the front filter threads of a lens. A major drawback to the Lester Dyne unit is that it has an AC power transformer requiring proximity to an AC outlet, making it less portable and practical. This unit has a switch allowing a choice between the ring light or the diffuse point light source. Ring lights are *not* recommended for ophthalmology. They cause a distracting circular reflection of the ring flash centered on the cornea, and a shadowless illumination which eliminates the effect of depth. Apparent depth is important to discern pathology in eye photography. A single diffuse-point light source is all that is necessary for soft, even-shadowed illumination providing a three-dimensional effect. More than one unit will soften the contrast and eliminate the shadowing, which is necessary to illustrate relative depth.

Determination of Magnification

Before Patient Photography

Several formulas are necessary to calculate magnification. The following can be used when a certain magnification needs to be achieved before patient photography:

$$M = \frac{\text{Extension}}{\text{Focal length}}$$

EXAMPLE A. A 50-mm lens focused on infinity with a 25-mm extension between the lens and the camera body would result in a ×.5 magnification, or 1/2 lifesize magnification.

$$M = \frac{25}{50} = \times.5$$

EXAMPLE B. A 50-mm lens focused on infinity with 100 mm of extension between the camera and the lens results in a ×2 lifesize magnification.

After Patient Photography

After the picture has been taken, this formula will be useful to determine the actual magnification:

$$M = \frac{\text{Image size}}{\text{Object size}}$$

EXAMPLE. An area from one side of the limbus to the other limbal edge photographed on the film is 34.5 mm. In real life, this area is only 11.5 mm. With the formula just given,

$$\frac{34.5\text{mm}}{11.5\text{mm}} = \times 3$$

The size of the image on the film is divided by the actual size of the object.

Focusing
When extreme close-up photography is performed and the magnification needs are predetermined, the camera is simply moved to and from the object until the image is sharp in the viewfinder. Since any movement is amplified under higher magnification, better pictures will result if the patient can be steadied while focusing. The addition of an autowinder or motor drive will prove beneficial by allowing a one-handed operation of the camera, freeing the photographer's other hand to steady the patient's head or to hold open an eyelid.

Determination of Exposure

Exposure Compensation
If exposure has to be calculated, a table can be used to determine the amount of aperture correction required at various magnifications:

Magnification	Aperture Correction Required
×.1	.28
×.5	1.17
×1.0	2.00
×1.5	2.67
×2.0	3.17
×2.5	3.61
×3.0	4.00
×3.5	4.34
×4.0	4.64

Aperture markings on the lens barrel no longer are accurate with magnifications greater than 1/10 lifesize. The effective aperture is now smaller than indicated and more light has to be provided.

EXAMPLE. A lifesize (1 : 1) magnification requires that two additional f/stops of light be provided to the film for an accurate exposure. If the aperture marked is an f/8, in actuality, the aperture value is equivalent to f/16.

Effective Aperture
The effective aperture can be calculated with this formula:

Effective aperture = Aperture on lens × (Magnification + 1)

EXAMPLE. The following example shows that, with a ×2 lifesize magnification, an aperture marked on a lens as f/16 actually becomes f/48. Irregardless of what the lens opening reads at a magnification of ×2 lifesize, the aperture must be opened an additional 3.17 f/stops to equal the exposure when the lens is focused at infinity:

$A_e = A\ (M + 1)$
$A_e = f/16\ (\times 2 + 1) = f/48$

It was pointed out earlier in the text that the problem of the effective aperture is automatically remedied when a manual flash unit is mounted to the front of the lens. It is very important that a series of test exposures be performed with any camera system at various magnifications. Film is the least expensive component of any system. An inexpensive guarantee is to bracket exposures, taking pictures one f/stop above and below the normal exposure.

Conclusions
The decision of which close-up system to select should be based on the equipment available for the particular camera to be used. Unquestionably, the poorest choice and least expensive method of achieving higher magnification are supplementary lenses. Extension tubes used with a standard (50-mm) lens are the least expensive method to achieve satisfactory results at higher magnification. Extension tubes and bellows are available to fit most cameras, with bellows units costing considerably more than extension tubes. As stated previously, bellows lens–bellows combinations and close focusing macro-micro lenses offer the most convenience, and provide the highest resolution in close-up situations.

Not all camera manufacturers offer bellows-mount lenses or close-focusing lenses in various focal lengths. Nikon and Canon do not offer long focal length bellows-mount lenses but choose to market close-focusing lenses in several focal lengths. Olympus and Zeiss Contax manufacture only normal focal length close-focus lenses and provide longer focal length bellows-mount lenses. The bellows lens–bellows combination and longer focal length close-focusing lenses are comparable in expense. For example, the Olympus bellows lens and bellows combination will cost about the same as the Nikon 105 mm Micro-Nikkor. Prices for systems will vary between manufacturers.

Longer focal length close-focusing lenses cost more than normal focal length close-focusing lenses. The cost of a teleconverter and a normal focal length (50-mm) close-focusing lens will be similar in price to the long focal length close focusing lens. Presently, Nikon, Canon, and Minolta are the only major camera manufacturers that offer teleconverters for their lenses. A number of independent lens makers also provide high-quality ×2 teleconverters for use with the more popular cameras. As was pointed out earlier, there are a number of advantages to using a teleconverter and normal focal length (50-mm) close-focusing lens combination without a significant sacrifice in image quality.

The teleconverters provided by Nikon and Canon work remarkably well with their respective close-focusing lenses. The mating of a camera manufacturer's lens with an independent lens maker's teleconverter should be tested to discern how well they work together. It is recommended that any lens combinations be tested extensively before purchase.

Not one system is all-inclusive, and situations will undoubtedly arise that require photography beyond the limits of a system. Additional extension rings, a bellows, a reversing ring, or lighting equipment can be added as necessary to any system. The benefit of using a 35-mm single-lens reflex camera system is that it is readily modified: Replacement components can be fitted quickly, and, as newer equipment is offered, the external eye photography system can be updated. The 35-mm single-lens reflex camera system is the most cost-effective system for external eye photography.

References

Basic Scientific Photography. Kodak Publication No. N-9. Rochester, N.Y.: Eastman Kodak Co., 1970.

Clinical Photography. Kodak Publication No. N-3. Rochester, N.Y.: Eastman Kodak Co., 1972.

Close-Up Photography and Photomacrography, (Vol. II). Kodak Publication No. N-12B. Rochester, N.Y.: Eastman Kodak Co., 1974.

Cooper, J. D., and Abbott, J. C. *Nikon Handbook Series: Close-Up Photography and Copying.* Garden City, N.Y.: American Photographic Book Publishing Co., 1979.

Justice, J., Jr. (Ed.). *Ophthalmic Photography.* Boston: Little, Brown, 1976.

Korn, J. (Ed.). *Life Library of Photography (Photographing Nature).* New York: Time-Life Books.

Mason, R. G. (Ed.). *Life Library of Photography (Photography as a Tool).* New York: Time-Life Books.

Mason, R. G. (Ed.). *Life Library of Photography (Special Problems).* New York: Time-Life Books.

Mindlin, A., and Lamberts, D. Inexpensive External Disease Camera. *J. Ped. Ophthal.* 12(4) : 270–271, 1975.

Slit-Lamp Biomicrography

LEE ALLEN

Photography through the biomicroscope must be highly recommended over the laboriously written descriptions and rough sketches commonly used for recording appearances of eye tissues illuminated by the slit-lamp beam. It is not simply that "a picture is worth ten thousand words," as the old Chinese proverb states, since, conversely, many important abstract words are worth more than ten thousand pictures. Rather, it is recommended because a fine photograph is at least as specific and exact as direct visualization of the subject eye; even more important, it is much more accurate in form and detail than memory. Pictures, belonging to the first level of abstraction, come much closer to meaning the same thing to different persons than do words, which usually belong to much higher levels of abstraction.

If properly used, photography is a consistently repeatable means of making clinical and research records. Because of the special complexities and subtleties of slit-lamp biomicroscopy, photography is considerably more accurate in this process than drawing, which has been used most commonly in the past for illustrations in journals, textbooks, and atlases. Of course, photography is also far more economical than fine detailed drawings, once the initial cost of the photographic equipment has been amortized.

Evolution of Slit-Lamp Photography

Several technical advances made during the past 45 years have been combined to bring slit-lamp photography to its present high level of excellence.

The first major advance was the introduction of a practical color film, Kodachrome, in 1939. Before that time, only black-and-white slit-lamp photography was possible, and it was not widely used because color has always been so important in studying and recording changes in eye tissues.

The next advance was the perfection of electronic flash illumination in the 1940s. An important advance in this area was reported by Herman J. Norton [3] from the University of Rochester, School of Medicine and Dentistry, Rochester, New York at the 1965 annual meeting of the American Academy of Ophthalmology and Otolaryngology. He described the combined use of an incandescent lamp and an electronic discharge tube in order to furnish enough light for short exposure times. The photographic transparencies he showed in a scientific exhibit at the same meeting were very impressive. Also, in addition to single-frame pictures, he showed examples of stereoscopic slit-lamp biomicrography, in good color, for the first time.

Another very important advance was the introduction in 1966 of the Photo Slit Lamp by Carl Zeiss, Oberkochen, Germany. Dr. Hans Littmann and coworkers brought together a fine slit-lamp biomicroscope (for regular visual examination), a 35-mm camera body (or bodies), the electronic flash illumination, and the color transparency film. All these and a fixed common focus of slit-lamp beam and biomicroscope were combined with the simplicity of "joystick" focusing. With the Photo Slit Lamp, hundreds of fully accurate slit-lamp pictures can be taken in the time needed to do just one detailed drawing. This is the system that will be discussed in this chapter.

Applications

All parts of the eye viewable with the slit-lamp biomicroscope and all types of slit-lamp illumination (with the possible minor exception of color rendition of faint aqueous flares) can be recorded in color with the Photo Slit Lamp. Thus, it can be said of this system, "If you can see it, you can photograph it."

Accessory lenses or prisms that cancel or modify the optical power of the anterior corneal surface allow visualization and photography of the anterior chamber angle, peripheral lens and zonule, vitreous, and all parts of the fundus.

Stereoscopic photography is made possible by accessory beam-splitters, twin camera bodies, and side-arm camera adapters for the Photo Slit Lamp. Only the least accessible regions of the eye, such as some parts of the peripheral fundus and ciliary body, cannot be pictured in stereopsis and, therefore, must be photographed in only two dimensions.

Information of a dynamic nature, such as the cumulative knowledge gained by scanning the eye with the oscillating slit-lamp beam, cannot reasonably be collected into one still photograph. Cinematography, especially with 16-mm or larger film, and television recording can accumulate for later perusal and communication information about motion and changes with position and time.

The Photographer

Consistently good slit-lamp photographs cannot be taken without special training. Slit-lamp biomicrography is an art that combines anatomic and medical knowledge of the eye with photographic artistry and technical know-how.

The ophthalmologist who aspires to becoming his or her own photographer must take time to learn certain details of photography and use of the special camera equipment. He or she must learn which magnifications are most effective in recording various kinds of subjects, and how to apply knowledge of slit-lamp illuminations specifically to photography. The ophthalmologist must learn, for efficient recall, the relationships among types of subject, types of illumination, aperture settings for the lens openings, and the intensity settings for the electronic flash. By doing all these things well, the ophthalmologist can be his or her own best photographer, since no one else knows as well what should be recorded on the film.

On the other hand, the hired photographer who expects to be of practical help to the ophthalmologist cannot succeed simply with a traditional fund of knowledge about photography. It is important to know as much as possible about ophthalmic terminology and the anatomy of the eye and orbit, as well as common appearances of diseases and other abnormalities as they are revealed in the eye.

The photographer also must learn the principles of slit-lamp biomicroscopy in order to apply them effectively in biomicrography. It is necessary to know all the different types of slit-lamp illumination, how to apply them, and which type is most applicable and effective in any given condition in any specific part of the eye. The photographer would not be worth hiring if it were always necessary for the ophthalmologist to find the subject area, set the magnification and manipulate the slit-lamp beam for best effect, and merely call on the photographer to snap the shutter.

The two volumes by Berliner [1] on slit-lamp biomicroscopy of the eye are recommended as a good source of knowledge of the slit lamp technique, principles of types of illumination, and typical appearances of many conditions of the eye. A two-volume atlas of stereoscopic slit-lamp pictures by Braley and associates [2] gives some background of visualization of numerous eye conditions and suggests technical approaches for such procedures as alignment and illumination.

The Zeiss Photo Slit Lamp

In this chapter, the Zeiss Photo Slit Lamp (with which this author is most familiar) and accessories that make stereoscopic photographs easy and effective, will be described, together with the types of illumination and common uses of each.

The Camera

The Photo Slit Lamp shown in Figure 14-1 has the original single-view 35-mm camera, *a,* mounted in its place above the lens barrel, *b,* of the biomicroscope. An objective lens and prism arrangement, *c,* projects forward and downward to a point just between the viewing paths of the objective lenses, *d,* of the biomicroscope. One such lens-prism offers ×1 magnification of the image on the film; another, available and interchangeable with the first, offers ×2. In addition to the

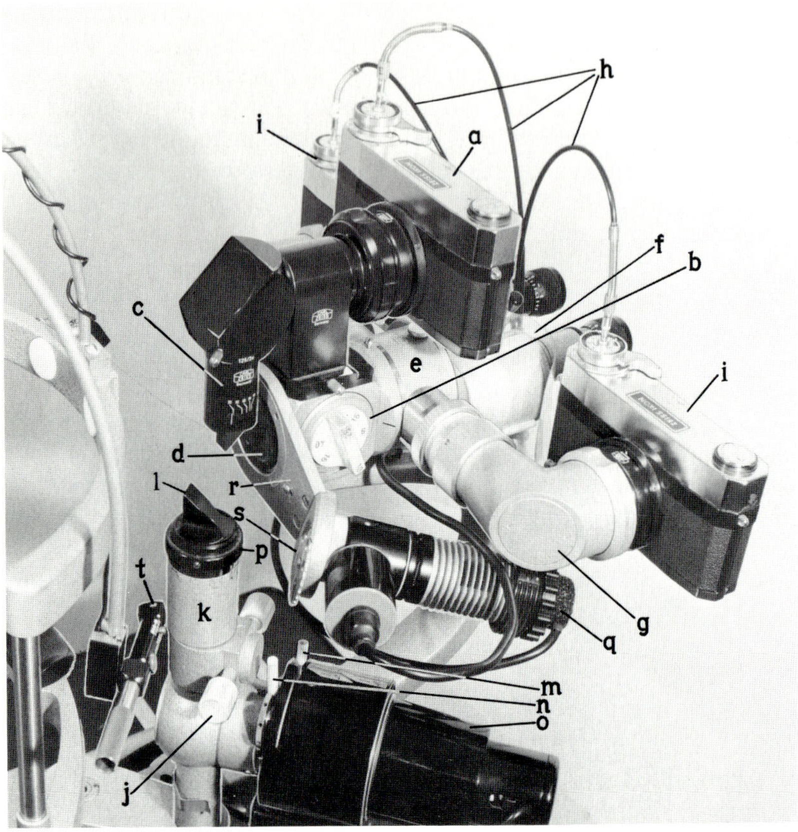

Fig. 14-1. Photo Slit Lamp with stereoscopic accessories. a = *top-mounted single camera body;* b = *barrel of lenses (magnification changer);* c = *lens and prism for top camera;* d = *objective lenses for stereoscopic cameras;* e = *beam-splitter for viewing and stereophotography;* f = *viewing binoculars;* g = *one of two side-arm stereo camera adapters;* h = *triple cable release;* i = *side-mounted cameras for stereography;* j = *knob for horizontal deviation of slit-lamp beam;* k = *tube supporting illuminating prism;* l = *illuminating prism;* m = *lever for changing sizes of circular apertures (and height of slit);* n = *lever for changing width of slit;* o = *slit-lamp house;* p = *ring regulating depth of focus of slit beam;* q = *fill-in lamp house;* r = *rotatable bracket supporting fill-in lamp house;* s = *aperture wheel for varying intensity of fill-in light;* t = *Haag-Streit fixation target device (added substitute for Zeiss target).*

latter, a ×2 accessory magnifier can be inserted just in front of the camera body to give a final magnification of ×4. Since the optical axis of this camera is not in line with either visual axis in the biomicroscope, the various aspects of photographs taken through it cannot be predicted accurately. There can be an unexpected and blinding reflection of the electronic light source from the anterior corneal surface. Because occasionally its angle of view is different from that of either ocular of the biomicroscope, a picture might not serve its intended purpose. In spite of the limitations and slight inconveniences of the center-mounted camera, most of the photographs taken with it are excellent and make fine 35-mm transparencies (2- by 2-inch slides) for lecture hall projection. However, even more dependable results can be achieved by taking the pictures through the objective lenses of the viewing biomicroscope, as follows.

An accessory beam-splitter (Fig. 14-1 *e*) is inserted between the lens barrel housing and the ocular assembly of the biomicroscope, *f*. There is a split prism in the path of each viewing optical axis so that a little less than one-half the amount of light goes to the photographer's eyes and more than half reaches the photographic films by way of the side-arm adapters, *g*, to each camera body. The adapters contain the camera lenses for bringing the image into focus at the film plane. They also contain adjustable lens diaphragms for varying the exposure, calibrated in f/stop numbers from 14 to 64. Dividing the light between the viewing oculars and the cameras makes it necessary to use a faster film in the side-mounted cameras than in the top, center camera, as will be detailed later in this chapter.

For the particular camera shown in Figure 14-1, three 18-inch shutter-release cables, *h*, have been fastened together so that the three camera shutters, set on bulb exposure, are opened in rapid succession—the last to open firing the electronic flash. (The shutters must be opened and shut as rapidly as is humanly possible because the bulb exposure will allow a faint recording of the yellow focusing light within less than one second.) Electronic (solenoid) shutter releases are available from Zeiss.

The two cameras on the side-arm adapters record exactly the disparate views seen by the respective eyes of the photographer. Therefore, the photographer is able to recognize any distracting flares of light or other photographic artifacts and avoid them in the photographs by readjusting the camera and realigning the illumination before making the photographic exposure.

The pictures from the side-arm cameras may be mounted and viewed separately as single slides, or mounted and viewed as stereograms. Single exposures may be made by releasing the shutter of only one side camera. These singles usually are superior to those taken with the central camera for lecture hall projection because they are relatively free from artifacts and allow a greater choice of magnifications. However, the stereograms are the best possible still visual records. Because there is no change or movement, they can be better for study than the living subject, and they may be studied in depth for as long as desired.

Magnification of the image is changed in steps by rotating the lens barrel, *b,* just ahead of the beam-splitter on the Photo Slit Lamp model pictured in Figure 14-1. Newer Photo Slit Lamps can be equipped with the zoom lens originally designed for the Zeiss examining slit-lamp biomicroscope.

The magnifications on the film with the older Photo Slit Lamp are different on the photographic film from the viewing magnifications. The relationships are given in Table 14-1.

The Illumination

The slit-lamp illumination unit is mounted on an arm that rotates around the same axis as does the arm supporting the biomicroscope and cameras. The slit-lamp beam is parfocal with the biomicroscope, no matter how the two are rotated around the axis of the supporting arms, unless there has been damage, such as dropping of the instrument.

A white knob, *j,* at either side of the base of the upright tube, *k,* supporting the illuminating prism, *l,* will shift the slit-lamp beam sideways across the area of the pictures for special purposes.

The height and width of the slit-lamp beam are changed for different lighting requirements by rotating two levers, *m* and *n,* mounted between the lamp housing, *o,* and the upright tube.

The lamp housing contains both the focusing light bulb and the electronic flashtubes, arranged so that their illuminating beams are coaxial and parfocal. As a result, they illuminate exactly the same part of the eye in the same manner. The flash is much brighter than the focusing light, to offer very short photographic exposures. The electronic flash contains a broad spectrum of color similar to daylight, while the focusing lamp produces very little in the blue end of the spectrum. If the latter were used alone for photography with daylight-type film, the resulting pictures would appear too yellow or yellow orange.

Near the top of the upright illuminating tube is a variable aperture, *p,* that can increase and decrease the depth of focus of the slit-lamp beam; it also decreases and increases the brightness of the beam in inverse proportion, that is, the narrower the aperture, the greater the depth of focus but the dimmer the illumination. The calibrations are numbered from 1 to 9; number 1 gives the greatest depth of focus but the least light, and number 9 gives the least depth of focus and the brightest illumination. Because color film usually requires fairly intense illumination, some photographers find it advantageous to place the setting of the adjusting ring at 9, the brightest illumination, and tape it in fixed position on the tube. As a result, one variable that must be checked off before making the photographic exposure is eliminated.

Table 14-1. Relative Visual and Photographic Magnifications

Lens Number and Viewing Magnification	Aperture Range (Effective F/stop)	Magnification on Film Without Accessory Lens	Magnification with ×2 Accessory Lens
6	14–64	0.69	1.38
10	14–64	1.09	2.18
16	18–64	1.76	3.52
25	22–64	2.84	5.68
40	32–64	4.5	9.0

At the very top of the upright tube, the illuminating prism, *l*, redirects the light into a horizontal direction toward the eye. An accessory prism that can be substituted for the regular prism is available for use when a horizontal inclined slit-lamp beam is required. The cylindrical mount for the regular prism slides off vertically and is replaced by the horizontal prism in its similar mount. When the latter is being used, the lamp housing must be rotated into a horizontal position to align the lamp filament and the axis of the flashtube with the horizontal prism.

An accessory fill-in lamp, *q*, is supported on the front of the biomicroscope with a bracket, *r*, which allows the light to approach the subject from the front at an angle of 30 degrees at any of a number of points on either side or above or below. Both a flashtube for the photographic exposure and an incandescent lamp (coaxial) are located in the lamp housing. A ground-glass diffusing disc in the front of the unit, with which the lamp comes equipped, is intended to spread the fill-in light over a large area. This disc does not fill the edges of the field of view when one is photographing through the ×6 lens, and, most important, it does not give enough fill-in light for pictures taken through the ×25 lens. The ground glass has been removed in the instrument pictured in Figure 14-1 and must be removed from others if fine descriptive pictures are to be made at all magnifications.

An aperture wheel, *s*, on the front of the fill-in lamp unit makes it possible to increase or decrease, independently, the amount of light relative to the intensity of the light in the slit-lamp beam. The method of balancing the amount of light furnished by the lamp and beam will be described later in this chapter.

It is important in many instances that the subject eye be held very steady during photographic exposure. For example, small but diagnostically important details such as cysts in a macular degeneration may show only when the very narrow slit-lamp beam is directed exactly upon one small area. If the eye is allowed to shift even one degree away from the optimal position, the photograph may fail to pick up such a small detail. Therefore, good fixation of the subject eye must be maintained.

The fixation light supplied by the manufacturer on the Photo Slit Lamp is not adequate because it presents an out-of-focus light so large that neither the subject's fixating eye nor the subject eye remains steadily aligned. Therefore, the original light should be replaced by a better device, such as the Haag-Streit slit-lamp fixation target, *t,* in Figure 14-1. This is the target with which we have equipped our slit lamp. It presents a bull's-eye target that can be focused for each fixating eye. The target is first seen by the patient through a small opening at the side of a small tube, and then through a system of such small lenses that it must be carefully aligned for the patient's view. The photographer can see a lighted area on the eye, projected from the fixation device. This light spot must be centered within the iris and must fill the pupil before the patient can see the bull's-eye centered within his view.

To ensure accurate focusing of the photographic image, the oculars of the biomicroscope must be adjusted until the cross hairs in the right-hand ocular are in sharp focus and the same details are seen clearly and simultaneously with both eyes. Then, as with any subject that is to be aligned and focused, care must be taken that the subject details and the cross hairs are seen in sharp focus simultaneously at the instant the photographic exposure is made.

Patient Comfort and Camera Alignment

The height of the slit-lamp table and the height of the patient's stool or chair should be adjusted carefully for the comfort of the patient if full cooperation and good photographic results are to be achieved. The photographer should be made comfortable for the same reasons. All moving parts of the Photo Slit Lamp should be positioned properly so that they are either in their "click-stops" or at typical effective angles, and so that the focusing lever, the "joystick," is initially in an upright position while the base of the slit-lamp biomicroscope, per se, is in midposition of movement in all directions on the table.

The vertical adjustment knob should also be turned to midpoint to allow movement upward and downward for vertical scanning across the eye. With the knob in proper position, the height of the patient's head within the headrest can be adjusted until the subject eye is at the same level as the objective biomicroscope lens and so can be seen with the biomicroscope.

Direction of gaze of the subject eye can be changed in all directions by moving the fixation device to any position, and the Photo Slit Lamp can be moved to achieve the desired view and angle of view toward the subject. As a result, very little of the eye is beyond view and, therefore, very little of the eye cannot be photographed. Novices with the slit lamp need to be impressed with the fact that neither the patient's eye nor the parts of the slit-lamp biomicroscope are glued in one place. If one arrangement is not good, others should be tried.

Films and Exposure Factors

It is not practical to use slow color film with the Photo Slit Lamp because of the limitations on intensity of the electronic flash illumination and the small effective apertures in the higher-power (×25 and ×40) biomicroscopic lenses. Even in the camera mounted on top of the biomicroscope, color film must not be slower than DIN 19 : ASA 64. The new Kodachrome 64 and Agfachrome 64 serve equally well. The choice between them will depend entirely on personal prejudice regarding factors such as color saturations and contrast.

Color film in the side-mounted cameras must be high-speed Ektachrome daylight type with a rating of ASA 160 : DIN 23 because the beam-splitter in the biomicroscope divides the illumination between biomicroscopic oculars and the cameras. By coincidence, when the top and side cameras are loaded with the recommended films, ASA 64 and ASA 160 respectively, all the lens aperture pointers must be set on the same numbers (Table 14-2). For example, if a situation calls for an aperture of f/32 for the top camera, the aperture sleeves on the adapter arms of the side cameras must also be set at f/32.

Some subtle, minute subjects requiring very high magnification for proper viewing, such as the endothelial mosaic of the cornea in specular reflection, can be recorded only on high-speed black-and-white film, such as Tri-X. Exact exposure factors can be determined by experimentation after calculating the differences between factors for the films. The same rules apply for the slit lamp as for any common camera: For example, if the black-and-white film is twice as fast as the color film, only half the amount of light is required.

It is desirable for each person to run a number of test exposures for each general type of situation, both to confirm the function of the particular power supply unit and to determine personal satisfaction with types of exposures. However, the following general outline of light and camera settings should provide helpful starting points in the beginning. (Incidentally, the intensity settings of the viewing and electronic flash knobs should always agree in order that the effects in the photograph will be identical to the view through the biomicroscope during focusing.)

Very Narrow Slit

In a typical case with a very fine slit-lamp beam, 0.05, 0.1, or 0.2 mm wide in transparent media (except vitreous), namely, cornea, aqueous, or crystalline lens, light intensities should be set at 4 and IV. The lens aperture should be f/22 if no fill-in light is used. If fill-in is used,

Table 14-2. Suggested Slit Lamp and Camera Settings for Color Film Rated ASA 64-19 DIN in Top-Mounted Camera, and for Color Film Rated ASA 160-23 DIN in Side-Arm Adapter-Mounted Cameras

Type of Subject	Biomicroscope Magnification Lens Number	Slit Width (Aperture 9)	Flash Intensity Setting	Fill-in Lamp Aperture	Camera Lens Aperture
Cornea, anterior chamber, lens, iris	×16	0.05, 0.1, or 0.2	IV	0, 4, or 5.6	f/22 or f/32
	×16	0.5	II or III	0 or 4	f/32
	×16	2.0 or 3.0	III	0	f/32 or f/44
	×16	Full and tangential	III (or II)	0	f/64
	×25	0.5	III	0	f/22 or f/32
	×40	0.2 or 0.5	IV	0	f/22 or f/32
Vitreous	×16	0.2	IV	0	f/22
	×16	2.0	III	0	f/22 or f/32
Sclera, conjunctiva	×16 or ×25	0.05 or 0.2	II	0 or 4	f/32
	×16 or ×25	Wide and tangential	I (or II)	0	f/64
Iris retroillumination against fundus glow	×16	Round spot 4.0 or 5.6 through pupil	III	0	f/32 or f/44

the lens aperture can be either f/22 or f/32, and the aperture in the disc of the fill-in lamp can be either the number 5.6 or 4, respectively. (The numbers represent millimeters of diameter of the openings.)

The photographer can experiment with the effects of different balances between the illumination intensities of the slit-lamp beam and the fill-in lamp during the adjustment of the general effects of illuminations, the alignment, and the focusing. This experimentation is done by making changes in the various knob settings, the width of the beam, and the fill-in aperture disc and then turning the rheostat knob (located just to the left of the "off-on" switch under the table at the right-hand corner) full on to judge the effect. (It is not desirable to keep the rheostat always full on: Low light levels are more comfortable for the patient.) The effect of balanced illumination in the view will be reproduced exactly in the photographic transparency.

Even after the ground glass has been removed from the front of the fill-in lamp, the apertures in the disc smaller than number 4 are of absolutely no use in color photography. In black-and-white photography on fast film, the apertures 3 and 2 might furnish adequate low-background lighting.

Moderately Narrow Slit

A slit-lamp beam 0.5 mm wide can be used to show patterns and details of corneal pathology. As the slit is widened, the intensity of the light increases. Therefore, if one is photographing through the ×16 lens, the knob settings on the power supply unit may be reduced to 2 and II, or the camera apertures may be reduced slightly. A common setting is f/32. Usually it is not good to use fill-in light for such pictures. Often it is best to take such pictures with the side-mounted cameras through the ×25 biomicroscope lens. Because of the smaller aperture of this lens, the light intensity settings frequently are increased to 3 and III.

When the vitreous is being photographed with a narrow beam, the illumination intensities always must be set at 4 and IV.

Moderately Wide Slit

Some corneal and lenticular subjects are best illuminated with a slit-lamp beam 2 or 3 mm wide. When one is photographing through the ×16 biomicroscope lens, the illumination knobs may be set at 3 and III and the apertures set somewhere between f/32 and f/44, depending on the reflectance of the subject.

Wide-Open Slit

Behind the lever that controls the width of the slit is another identical to it (as indicated previously), which moves circular openings of different diameters into the illuminating beam. The lever for the width of the slit may be moved to the farthest wide-open position, at which point the full circle of the widest opening can be seen. Then, the smaller circular apertures may be brought successively into place to illuminate only the area desired. Of course, each successively smaller beam reduces the lux so that the camera apertures or the light intensities, or both, must be increased in counteraction.

Many subjects involving the entire expanse of the cornea are best photographed with the slit at the fully open position, the largest circular aperture in place, and *without the accessory diffusion disc*. The collimated light can reveal details that diffuse light cannot show. Usually, the corneal pathology will show best against the darkest possible background. Therefore, the beam should approach the cornea at an extreme tangent, striking the cornea but passing in front of the iris and lens. When carefully adjusted, this type of illumination substitutes for and improves on the type called *sclerotic scatter*.

The focusing light through the largest opening is so bright that it is often painful to the patient, making it necessary to reduce the brightness with the rheostat knob below the table edge.

The ×16 biomicroscope lens with the side camera and the ×2 lens unit with the top camera nicely encompass the entire cornea. The illumination intensities may be set at either 2 and II or 3 and III, depending on the relucency of the corneal details; all camera apertures must be set at f/64.

When one is photographing the scleral or conjunctival areas with the widest slit, the illumination must be reduced to a setting of 1 and I or 2 and II, and the camera aperture must be set at f/64.

Principles of Slit-Lamp Illumination

Diffuse Illumination

As diagramed in Figure 14-2A and exemplified in Figure 14-2B, diffuse illumination merely illuminates all features in a broadly inclusive view. It does not define details or form as well as focal illumination does. Ordinarily, another type of camera could be used with diffuse illumination for single-frame pictures with equally good results. While it is convenient to have the capability of diffuse illumination and stereopsis in the Photo Slit Lamp, it should be noted that the Donaldson stereoscopic anterior segment camera can provide these also.

Direct Focal Illumination

As shown in Figure 14-3, direct focal illumination consists of nearly collimated light, with the image of an aperture within the lamp housing parfocal with the focal point of the biomicroscope. The focused image of the aperture can be a round spot of light, 8.0 mm in diameter, that nearly covers the area of the cornea and iris; a very broad rectangle; or a vertical line as narrow as 0.01 mm, depending on the adjustment of the slit aperture.

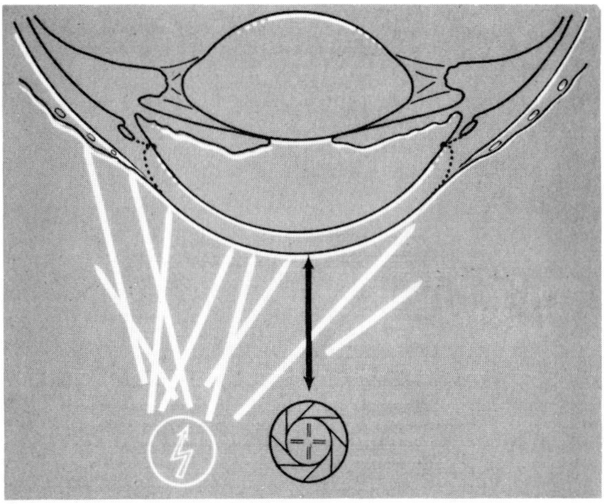

A

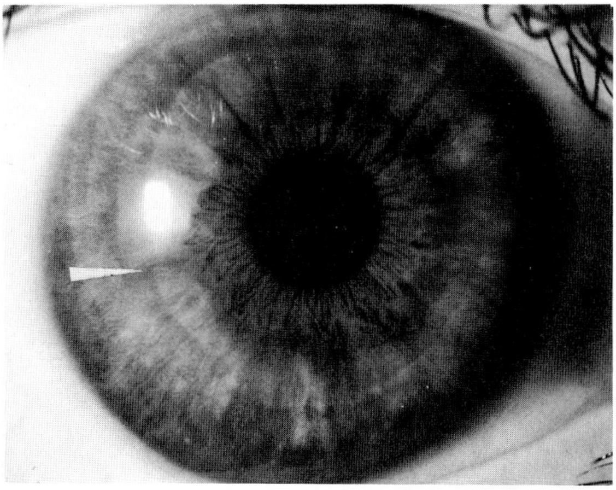

B

Fig. 14-2. (A) *Cross-section of anterior segment of eye and schema for illumination position* (white) *of cameras and biomicroscope. At* bottom, *drawing of camera shutter and focusing cross-hairs for diffuse illumination.* (B) *Example of diffusely illuminated anterior segment.* White wedge *points in direction of approach of light toward subject.* Note: All symbols in this chapter's succeeding figures will follow this scheme.

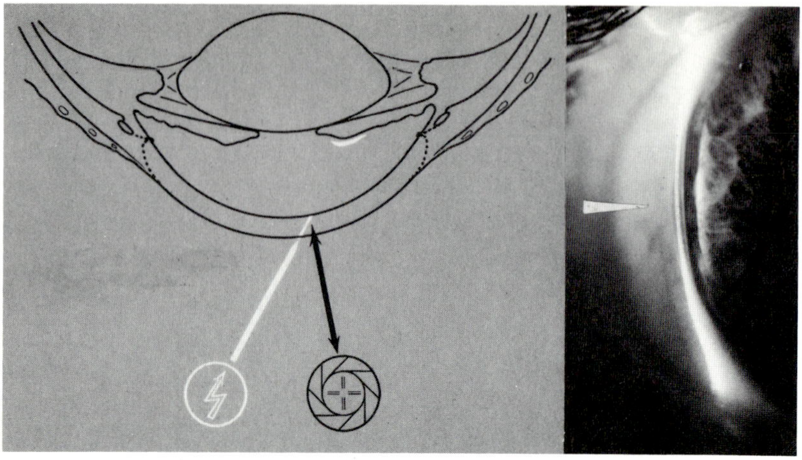

A B

Fig. 14-3. (A) *Focal illumination with fine slit-lamp beam and camera focused at exactly the same point.* (B) *Use of very fine slit beam to record depth of peripheral anterior chamber.*

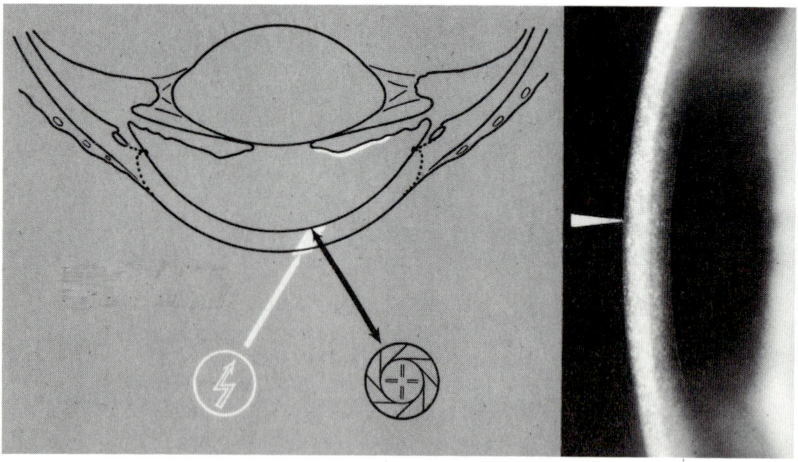

A B

Fig. 14-4. (A) *Focal illumination with moderately narrow slit beam.* (B) *Corneal "parallelepiped" in a case of multiple myeloma.*

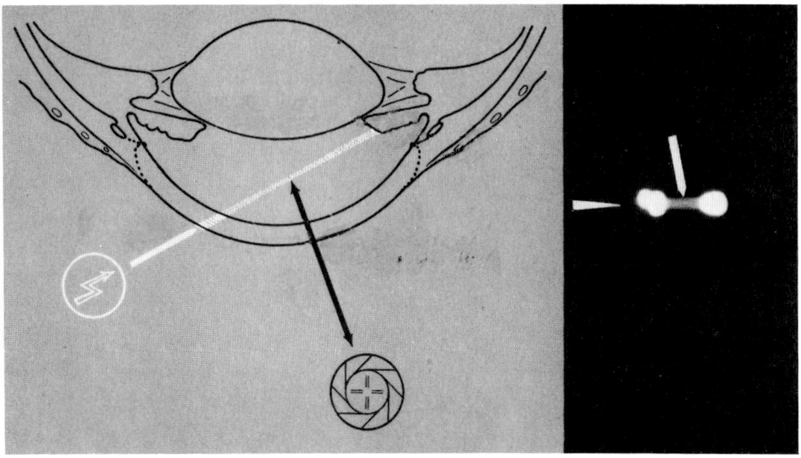

A B

Fig. 14-5. (A) *Method of photographing aqueous flare* (*Tyndall's phenomenon*). (B) *Example of aqueous flare in patient with uveitis. Illuminated through smallest circular aperture in slit lamp, glowing aqueous is seen silhouetted against dark background of the pupil.*

The narrow vertical slit beam must be angled in from one side in order to be effective in its major roles: (1) revealing thicknesses of transparent or translucent tissues, (2) indicating depths of features, and (3) demonstrating contours.

The slit beam, adjusted to intermediate widths (Fig. 14-4), can reveal illuminated details because tissues in front of and behind the details remain dark.

One advantage of focal illumination is that the collimated light causes sharply outlined shadows, which help to define structures.

Tyndall Phenomenon (*Aqueous Flare*)

The smallest circular aperture of the aperture disc (changed by lever *m,* as shown in Fig. 14-1) is used to demonstrate changes in the transparency or translucency of the aqueous. For instance, with increasing severity of uveitis, the aqueous often shows increasing cloudiness. In normal aqueous, the thin pencil-like beam of light will not cause any glow, but in cloudy aqueous it will create an effect similar to that of a focused flashlight beam penetrating fog or a smoke-filled room. The degree of glow is commonly described verbally in a scale of 1-to-4-plus relucency. If black-and-white film were to be used to record these levels photographically, much more accurate and meaningful comparison might be possible. The principle of the illumination is diagramed in Figure 14-5A. A black-and-white copy of a Kodachrome II

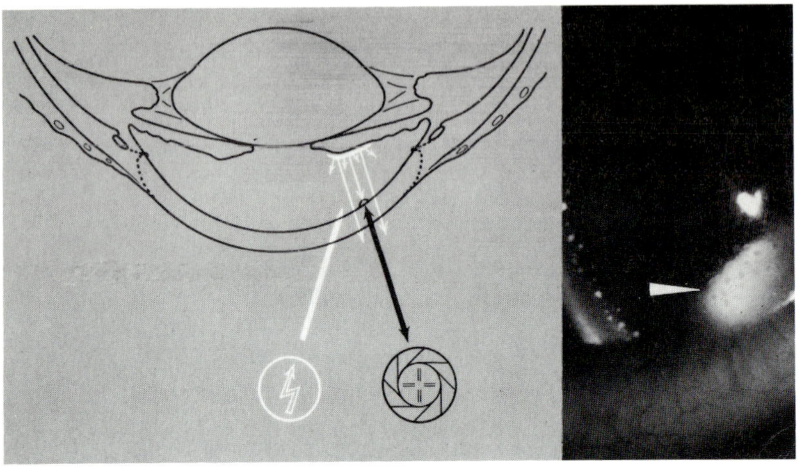

A B

Fig. 14-6. (A) *Direct retroillumination.* (B) *Keratitic precipitates on posterior corneal surface seen at* left *as light spots in the direct focal slit beam, and at* right *as translucent, slightly dark spots silhouetted against an area of illuminated iris.*

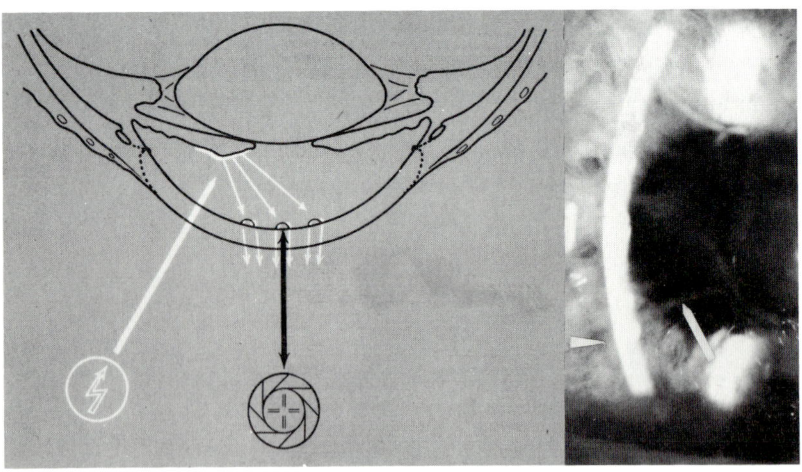

A B

Fig. 14-7. (A) *Indirect retroillumination.* (B) *A case of lattice dystrophy of the cornea;* white arrow at right *indicates direction of light reflected from iris toward refractile streaks in posterior corneal surface.*

transparency showing one example of aqueous flare is reproduced in Figure 14-5B. In order to have a large aperture, the ×16 lens was used, and the strobe illumination was set at IV.

Retroillumination

Retroillumination can be divided into direct and indirect types. For direct retroillumination (Fig. 14-6), the biomicroscope is focused on a feature and the slit beam is moved sideways so that it no longer illuminates the feature from the front. Instead, the field directly behind the object is lighted so that it is seen silhouetted dark or translucent against a light background. For indirect retroillumination (Fig. 14-7), the subject is not illuminated or silhouetted against a light field. Instead, an area just to the side of the immediate background is lighted. From this off-axis point, the light approaches the subject from an angle and, after striking it, is dispersed and refracted toward the biomicroscope. This kind of illumination tells something about the characteristics of the subject, such as whether there are elevated or depressed gel-like areas or relucent streaks.

Iris atrophy, lens changes, and vitreous opacities can be transilluminated against the fundus glow, as shown in Figure 14-8.

Proximal Illumination

As shown in Figure 14-9, proximal illumination is useful in locating small, dense objects just below surfaces and studying changes of density in translucent tissues. Sometimes a small foreign body within a structure such as the iris is seen only by illuminating the tissues around and behind it. Proximal illumination penetrates and disperses within the iris stroma, revealing any cystic and solid masses present.

Tangential Illumination

In various forms, tangential illumination can be one of the most valuable tools in biomicrography, as it can also be in biomicroscopy. However, it must be focal: Only a collimated slit beam will give the helpful value contrasts. As the light strikes elevations and depressions or suspended features, sharply defined shadows are thrown, which greatly enhance the visualization (Fig. 14-10). This technique is helpful in revealing subtle conjunctival and iris lesions.

Tangential illumination of the cornea has proved invaluable in showing subtle pathology. The principle is diagramed in Figure 14-11A and exemplified in Figure 14-11B. In our hands, this technique achieves the same aim as sclerotic scatter, but with far more success. The collimated light strikes the anterior corneal surface so tangentially that it barely penetrates, and so it does not illuminate the iris or lens beyond. Nevertheless, enough light reaches the corneal stroma to reveal differences in tissue structure, expressed as dark and light areas. With most other types of illumination, these tissue differences cannot be seen.

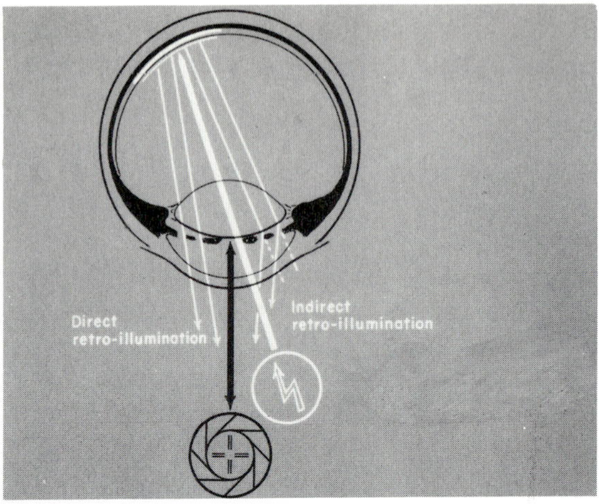

A

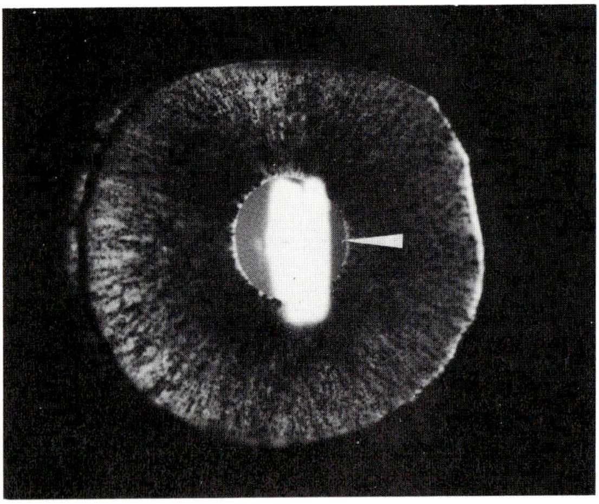

B

Fig. 14-8. (A) *Retroillumination of anterior segment features by light returning toward the cameras from the fundus of the eye.* (B) *Example of retroillumination of albino iris* (*human*).

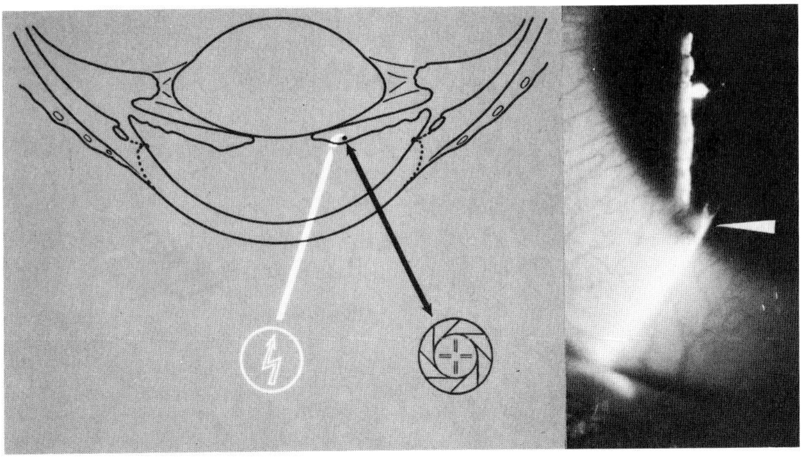

A B

Fig. 14-9. (A) *Proximal illumination.* (B) *Foreign body behind limbus seen best by proximal illumination.*

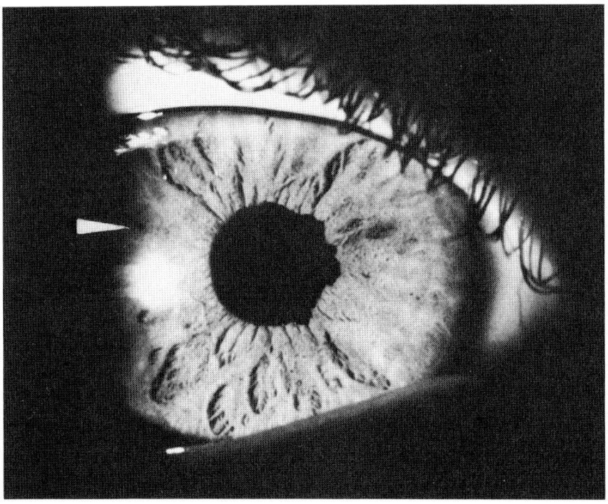

Fig. 14-10. Tangential illumination of iris, demonstrating excellent revelation of crypts and elevations.

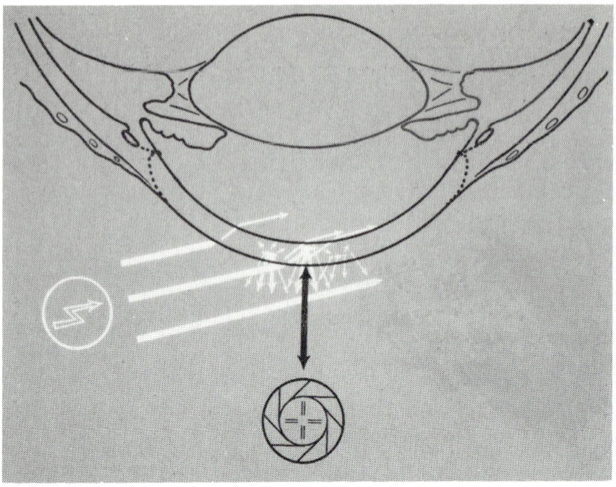

A

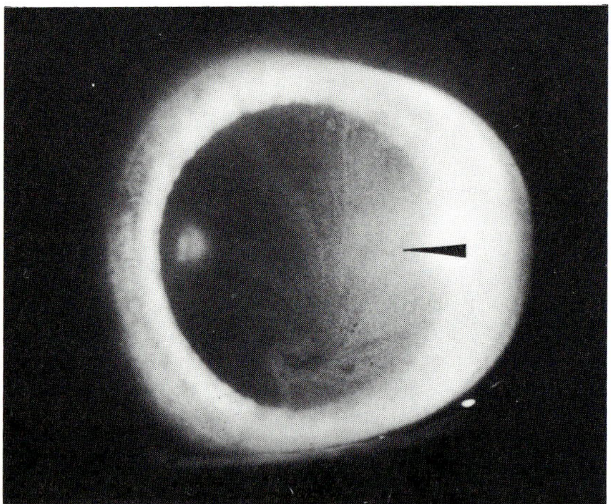

B

Fig. 14-11. (A) *Extremely tangential illumination of corneal tissues with wide focal slit beam.* (B) *Almost imperceptible superficial corneal changes in a case of Fabry disease made visible by tangential focal illumination. In this instance, light approaches from right* (black wedge).

Black-and-white photographs taken by this method can make very good illustrations for articles and books. Thus, it should not always be necessary to do drawings to depict what is seen in subtle corneal changes.

Sclerotic Scatter

Sclerotic scatter is achieved by directing the focal slit beam at right angles to the surface of the sclera just behind the limbus. The fibrous character of the sclera disperses the light in all directions, as shown in Figure 14-12. The light that emerges into the lamella of the cornea is reflected internally between the anterior and posterior surfaces, traversing the entire cornea to the opposite limbus. If the light strikes an area within the corneal stroma, which can interfere with and disperse some light toward the viewer and camera, that area appears to glow faintly. This method has been described in textbooks, for photography, however, the special type of tangential illumination discussed in the previous section is of greater practical value.

Specular Reflection

Specular reflection is one of the most difficult types of biomicrography (as well as biomicroscopy). It can be demonstrated on any highly reflective surface (*specular* refers to "mirrorlike"). Thus, it can be done on the anterior corneal surface or the posterior corneal surface, as diagramed in Figure 14-13A and exemplified in Figure 14-13B. It also can be done on the anterior lens capsule (Fig. 14-14), and it is easily seen on the posterior lens capsule (Fig. 14-15).

While specular reflection is difficult, the basic concept is very simple. The slit-lamp beam and the biomicroscope must be aligned so that their optical axes approach the surface of the subject from opposite sides of a plane vertical to the surface, striking that surface at exactly equal angles. Thus, the light from the slit lamp reflects from the cornea directly into the biomicroscope. The reflection from the anterior corneal surface is so overwhelming that it must be discounted as much as possible when one is studying the specular reflections from deeper surfaces. For instance, when it is desirable to photograph the cells of Descemet's endothelium, the alignment referred to is made: It is absolutely essential that both the focal slit-lamp beam and the biomicroscope be focused exactly upon the endothelium. The light from the anterior corneal surface at first appears blinding, but it is necessary only to rotate either the slit-lamp housing or the binoculars slightly to one side to reveal just the reflection from the mosaic of the endothelial cells (see Fig. 14-12). The reflection of these cells is the color of burnished copper, in contrast to the blinding white reflection from the anterior cornea and tear film.

It is necessary to use the ×25 or ×40 lens in order to magnify the

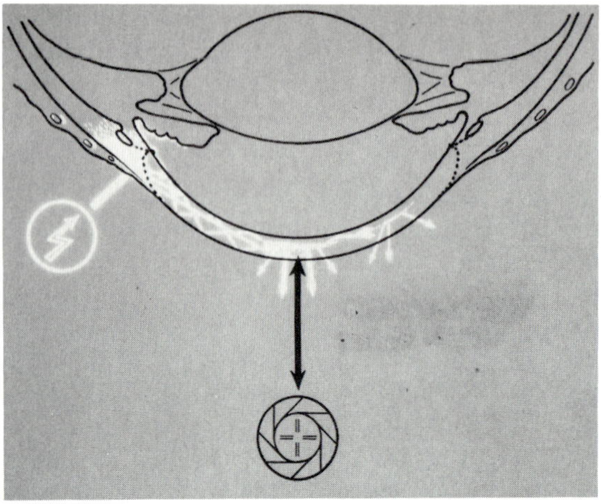

Fig. 14-12. Sclerotic scatter from focal illumination of distant sclera, effective for revealing tissue differences not seen otherwise with the biomicroscope.

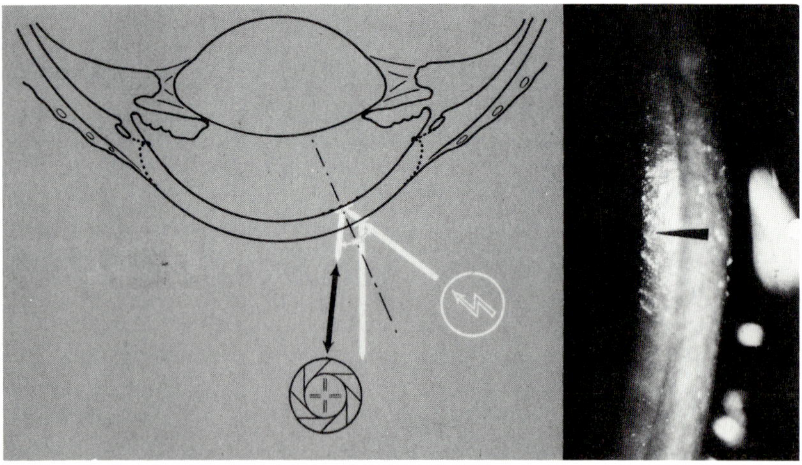

A **B**

Fig. 14-13. (A) *Specular reflection.* (B) Black wedge *indicates direction of focal illumination and also points to reflections from the disturbed mosaic of corneal endothelial cells in a case of posterior polymorphous dystrophy.*

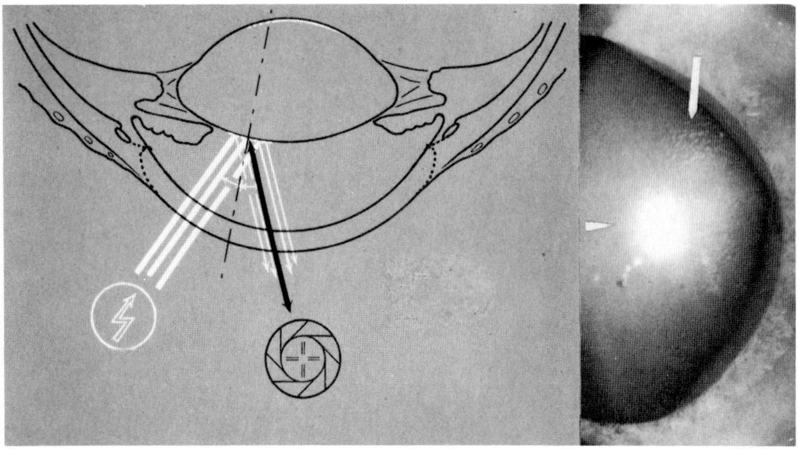

A B

Fig. 14-14. (A) *Specular reflection from the anterior lens capsule.* (B) White vertical arrow *points to area of specular reflection, the shagreen of the lens.*

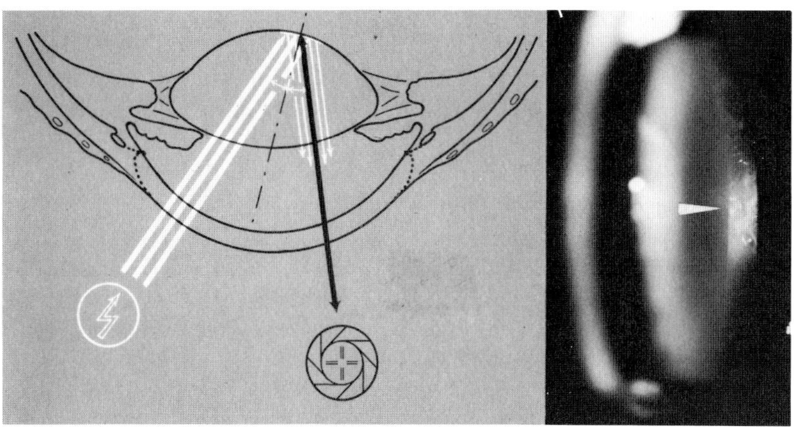

A B

Fig. 14-15. (A) *Specular reflection from the posterior lens capsule.* (B) *Specular reflection from a posterior capsular plaque.*

image enough to see individual cells clearly. Best results are achieved with the ×2 accessory lens used in conjunction with either the ×25 or ×40, giving magnifications of ×5.68 and ×9.0, respectively.

The camera settings for two types of film are: (1) for High Speed Ektachrome, daylight type, ×16 or ×25 microscope lens alone, camera aperture f/22, electronic flash intensity III or IV, and (2) for Tri-X (black-and-white), ×40 microscope lens plus the ×2 accessory magnifier, camera aperture f/22 or wider (the aperture of the lens mounting is less and, therefore, the limiting factor), flash intensity setting III or IV. Both types of film should be developed normally.

If black-and-white prints for publication are to be made from the resulting negatives, it will be found that different bits of information can be revealed by printing lighter or darker on papers of different contrast. Likewise, different information is shown on positive transparency slides by printing lighter or darker.

Photography of Fluorescence

Either fluorescein staining of the anterior segment tissues from topical application of the dye or angiography from intravenous injection of the dye can be performed by placing a blue filter over the front of the illuminating prism (see Fig. 14-1, 1). An example of fluorescein staining of a dendritic corneal ulcer is shown in Figure 14-16; only a Kodak Wratten (blue) filter was used and no barrier filter (yellow) was needed for color representation. If magnification is with the ×16 lens, the camera aperture can be f/22 and the light intensity setting IV, and the widest focal light beam can approach the cornea fairly tangentially.

Fluorescein angiography requires use of an interference filter (blue), such as is best for angiography of the fundus. A yellow barrier filter, such as Kodak Wratten filter No. 15, must be used in front of the film. The camera apertures must be wide open and the flash at full intensity. In order to have pictures at 1- or 2-second intervals, it is necessary to place a rapid booster in the power supply system. Just as for fundus fluorescence, Tri-X film must be used and development time extended.

OSCILLATING OR SCANNING SLIT BEAM. The oscillating or scanning slit beam is of no value in still photography, but it is useful in cinematography and television recording.

Stereoscopic Slit-Lamp Photography

As stated at the beginning of this chapter, stereography adds information not available at all in single two-dimensional pictures. At the present time, it is by far the best and most practical means of recording visual information. Even holography does not yet equal stereophotography in important ways.

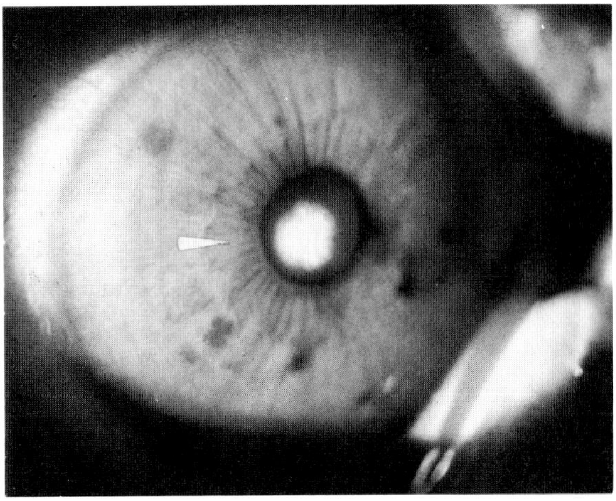

Fig. 14-16. Example of photography of fluorescence in a case of dendritic ulcer of the cornea. Ulcer has stained deeply and glows brightly in focal blue light, using a Kodak Wratten 47A filter in the slit beam, but no yellow filter in the cameras.

Taking pictures with the photo slit-lamp has already been covered in the preceding general outline of photographic methods. When simultaneous pictures have been taken with the two side-mounted cameras, the developed transparencies need only be mounted correctly in stereomounts and either viewed in a hand viewer, such as the Realist, or projected with a stereoprojector onto a metalized screen and viewed through Polaroid glasses.

It should not be necessary to adjust the two transparencies vertically in the stereomounts. Horizontal adjustments are simple. The most sharply focused identical points of the two pictures—usually those at the same distance as the sharply focused slit beams—should be separated 62 mm. This distance is closer than stereo landscape photographs are set, simply because the viewer's eye should be required to converge toward near objects.

Transparent plastic covers are available for protection of the stereos.

Cinematography and Television

Motion picture and television cameras can be attached to either side of the beam-splitter by adapter arms especially designed for each use and available from Zeiss. The adapters contain lenses of specific focal lengths. Lens apertures from f/7 to f/32 give an adequate range of exposures. Only the focusing illumination is used, and adjustment can be either with the knob on the power supply or the rheostat knob, or both.

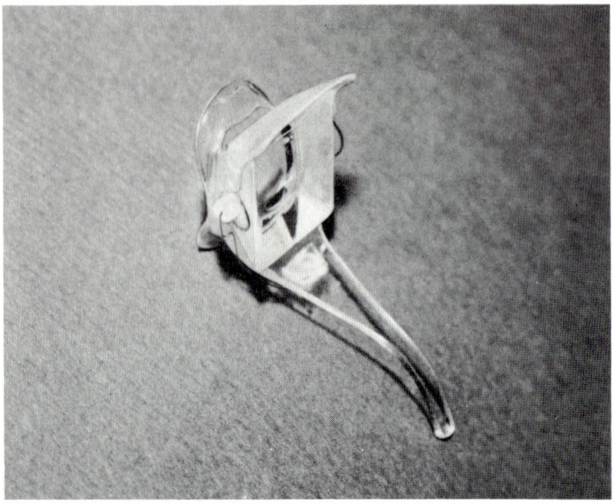

A

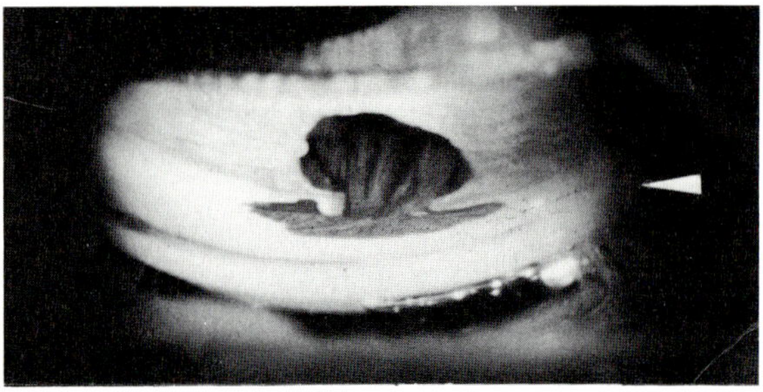

B

Fig. 14-17. (A) *Gonioprism. Curved flange at* left *fits behind the eyelids, upper shelf supporting upper lid with base of handle below resting against lower lid margin. This speculum supports, on fine stainless steel wire springs, the optical element—a truncated pyramid with a flat front surface, four angled mirrors at the sides, and a concave surface to contact only the cornea of the eye.* (B) *Right-hand frame from a stereoscopic transparency goniophotograph in a patient with old trephine and iridectomy for congenital glaucoma. Ciliary processes were accidentally displaced at the time of surgery. In the succeeding 20 years, pigment has been seen to proliferate onto the posterior corneal surface.*

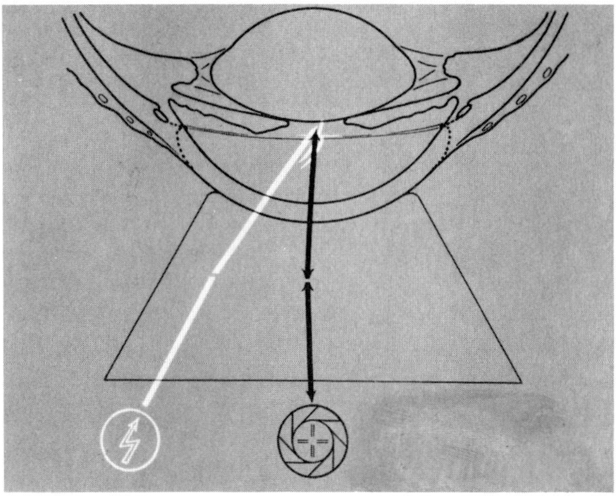

Fig. 14-18. Goniophotography of the upper and lower portions of the anterior chamber with the gonioprism. When photographing upper angle, lower mirror is used; for lower angle, upper mirror is used. The Goldmann contact glass for gonioscopy works in the same manner, except that the one mirror for gonioscopy must be rotated into correct position.

When using a Bolex H 16 camera and Ektachrome EF film (ASA 160), light intensity should be in the higher range for slit photography, but it can be reduced for wide openings.

Television presentation and recording can be monitored so that the best exposures can be reached by adjustment during direct visualization. Different makes and models of cameras have different response characteristics. Many will not leave a dark field when the slit-lamp beam is narrowed down; thus, all surrounding details are lost. Color cameras undoubtedly will overcome this shortcoming.

Use of Accessory Instruments

Gonioscopy

An integral part of slit-lamp biomicroscopy and biomicrography, gonioscopy must be done through an accessory contact glass that has a plano or nearly plano entrance surface and a mirror or mirrors, such as the Goldmann lens or the Allen-Thorpe gonioprism. The latter is shown in Figure 14-17A. An example of a goniophotograph taken through the bottom mirror is given in Figure 14-17B.

Nearly all types of illumination can be used, and each has its special value. Except for possible transillumination, illuminating and viewing must be accomplished through the same mirror. Figure 14-18 is a top plan view showing the disparity of angulation between the axis of the illumination and the axis of the biomicroscope across a mirror for

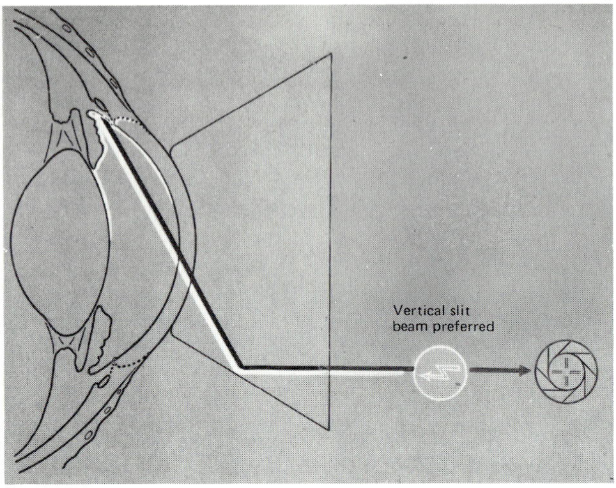

Fig. 14-19. Goniophotography: side view of Fig. 14-18.

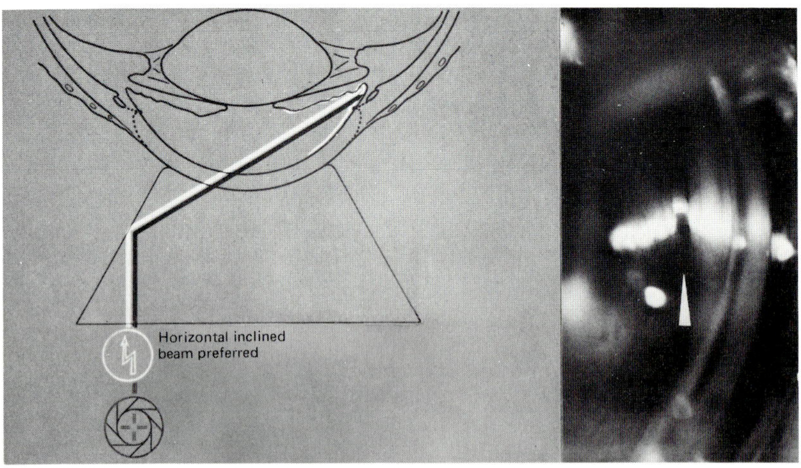

A **B**

Fig. 14-20. (A) *Goniophotography of the lateral portions of the anterior chamber. Note that here, the illuminating prism of the slit lamp must be located between the objective lenses of the biomicroscope in order to be coaxial along a vertical plane.* (B) *Horizontal inclined slit beam penetrating back and upward into a traumatic cyclodialysis cleft. The beam "bumps" across the peripheral iris at the left as it "flows" more smoothly along cornea and sclera at the right. Note that example does not agree with diagram in that this chamber angle was actually viewed in right-hand mirror* (*the mirrors always reverse the images in one plane only*).

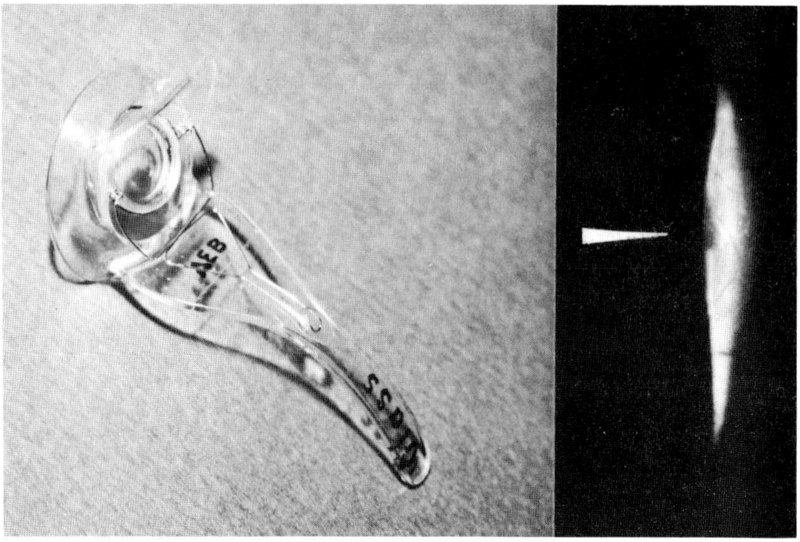

A B

Fig. 14-21. (A) *The Allen-Braley central fundus lens. Curved flange at left fits against the globe, under the eyelids, with upper shelf and handle placed as for the gonioprism. A wafer-thin contact glass with plano front surface and concave posterior surface to contact the cornea is supported upon fine stainless steel wire springs from the top of the speculum handle.* (B) *The right-hand frame from a stereoscopic transparency photograph showing a 0.2-mm wide slit-lamp beam penetrating the very central area of a cystic macular degeneration.*

either the upper or lower chamber angle. Figure 14-19 is a diagram of the same arrangement seen from the side.

The lateral chamber angles are viewed with mirrors from across the cornea, as shown in Figure 14-20A. An example of the use of the lateral mirror and the horizontal inclined slit beam is shown in Figure 14-20B.

The gonioprism can be manipulated across the cornea or rotated in any desirable way to bring the specific subject into optimal position. The eye also may be rotated to some extent under the prism for further improvement of the view. For the best resolution of the images, the biomicroscopy should be directed as nearly as possible at right angles (normal) to the front surface of the prism. Reflection of the light source from the surface must be avoided by proper alignment.

Peripheral Fundus Photography

Slit-lamp photographs may be made of the entire fundus of the eye. Peripheral fundus photography can be carried out far into the periphery, even without indentation. The Goldmann three-mirror lens or the gonioprism may be used for this entire examination.

Central Fundus Photography

The ideal device for central fundus photography with slit-lamp illumination is the Allen-Braley lens, which consists of an extremely thin "wafer" contact lens with a plano front surface. This device minifies the image of the fundus less than any other, without destroying the resolution of the finest slit-lamp beam. It gives a larger effective entrance-exit pupil, for greater angulation of the slit beam, and more effective pupil expanse, for concurrent stereoscopic viewing and photography, than any other instrument. It is pictured in Figure 14-21A, and one example of a slit beam in the central fundus is shown in Figure 14-21B.

The central portions of the Goldmann three-mirror glass or the gonioprism can be used looking directly through the pupil for photography of the central fundus. However, as indicated earlier, the entrance-exit pupil is smaller and the image of the fundus is minified more than with the Allen-Braley lens.

References

1. Berliner, M. L. *Biomicroscopy of the Eye,* Vols. 1 and 2. New York: Hoeber, 1943, 1949.
2. Braley, A. E., Watzke, R. C., Allen, L., and Frazier, O. *Stereoscopic Atlas of Slit Lamp Biomicroscopy,* Vols. 1 and 2. St. Louis: Mosby, 1970.
3. Norton, H. J. Stereography of the slit-lamp optical section. *Trans. Am. Acad. Ophthalmol. Otolaryngol.* 69 : 1965.

A Camera Adapter for Slit-Lamp Photography

JOSEPH W. SOPER

This chapter describes a camera attachment (PhotoMont) designed to be used with the Haag-Streit, the A. O. Campbell, and the Zeiss slit lamps. It can be modified for use on other "joystick"-controlled instruments.

Adapting the Attachment to the Haag-Streit 900 Slit Lamp

The slit lamp's guide plate used for preset lenses is removed from the central hole of the supporting pillar. The PhotoMont is attached by inserting the forward stem into this central hole. The steps that should be followed are:

1. A reflex camera with a detachable lens system is positioned on the camera stage in the same manner as if the camera were being placed on a tripod.
2. The lens system is removed, and a bellows or extension tube capable of 160 mm of extension is added and the lens is replaced. The advantage of a bellows is the ease of changing magnification. Extension tubes, however, can provide equally good final results (Fig. 15-1).
3. The fixation lamp support of the slit lamp is swung to the center of the instrument and a narrow slit beam is then focused on the metal housing. Using the joystick of the slit lamp and observing through the microscope, the operator brings the beam into fine focus and locks the slit lamp in this position. This locking is maintained until the camera has been completely positioned and focused.
4. The camera table is elevated or lowered by gross estimation to align the center of the lens with the height of the slit beam. This change in elevation is permitted by a knob that controls the upward and downward movements of the camera table.
5. The camera is then focused by forward or backward movements of the focusing system of the PhotoMont, using the horizontal adjustment knob. The camera lens system is set at infinity and maintained at this position at all times. The focus of the camera is made on the slit beam, which (as described in step 3) is already focused on the fixation lamp housing. A wide slit beam is used at first to locate the fixation housing through the reflex system of the camera, but when final focus is made, the very narrow beam is used.
6. Before accomplishing the final focus, it may be necessary to adjust

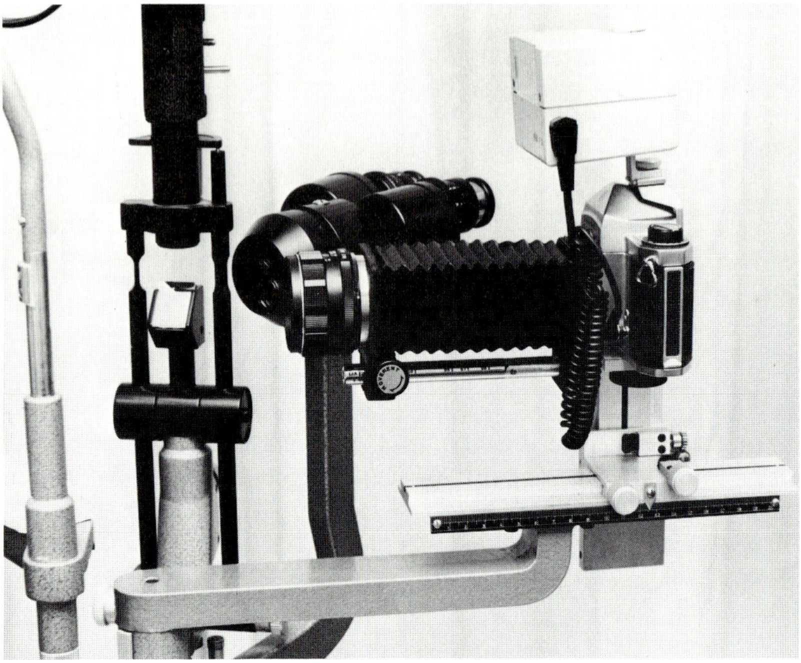

Fig. 15-1. Slit-lamp camera attachment, single lens reflex camera with bellows, and strobe light in position on a Haag-Streit slit lamp.

the vertical height of the camera slightly as well as to swing it into exact centering by loosening and readjusting the body of the camera where it is attached to the camera table.

7. When the camera is considered completely focused, the exactness of focus should be compared between the camera and the microscope. When a satisfactory degree of focus of the camera has been obtained, the slit-lamp table and joystick may be unlocked. From this point the PhotoMont and camera adjustments for focusing are not moved. The slit beam, microscope, and camera are parfocal; as the joystick is moved from one point to another, all three of these elements move simultaneously in prefocused unison.
8. The PhotoMont and the attached camera may be removed as a unit and placed on the PhotoMont stand (Fig. 15-2). When this unit is again placed on the slit lamp, no adjustment will be necessary unless a change in camera magnification is desired; in this case, the extension tubes or bellows are extended or decreased, which will again necessitate a refocusing of the camera by forward or backward movement of the PhotoMont focusing system. Refocusing is accomplished by repeating steps 5, 6, and 7.

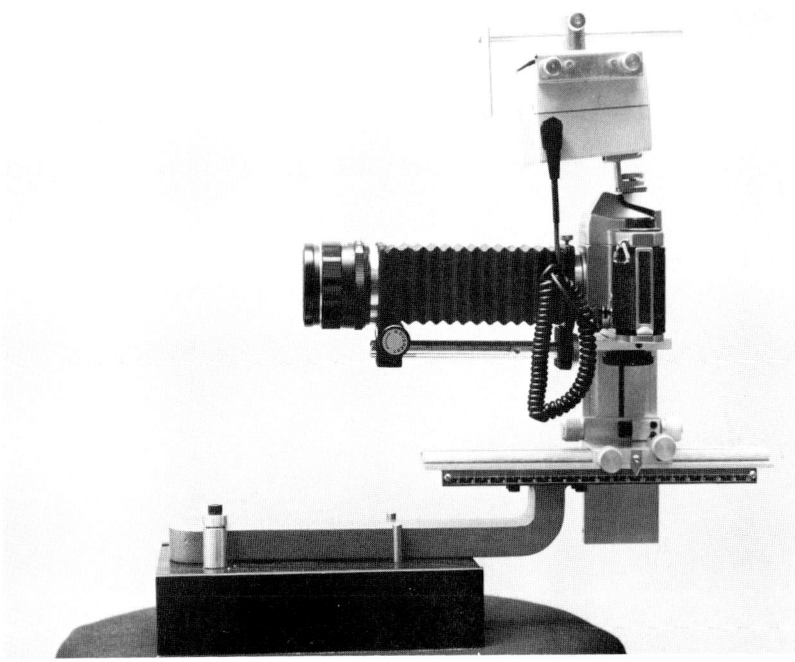

Fig. 15-2. Focused camera on stand ready for immediate placement and use on slit lamp.

9. Movie cameras can be mounted and used with the system, although the camera must have a close-up lens with a focal length within the limits of the focusing system of the PhotoMont. As in the case of still cameras, the movie camera must be of a reflex type.

Attaching the Strobe Light Shield

A strobe light shield (Fig. 15-3) is provided to use with the PhotoMont system. The strobe light is needed to provide "fill" or background light to illuminate the areas surrounding the slit beam for identification. This background light is desirable because the intensity of open, direct light makes patient cooperation difficult, especially in eyes demonstrating marked photophobia. The shield is provided to mask off or reduce the direct exposures of the strobe on the area of regard; it also minimizes the reflection of the strobe on the cornea.

Measures to take when attaching the shield are:

1. The strobe is most effective when attached directly to the camera, so that the distance from the strobe to the point of regard is constant. A small (miniature) strobe can be mounted directly on most

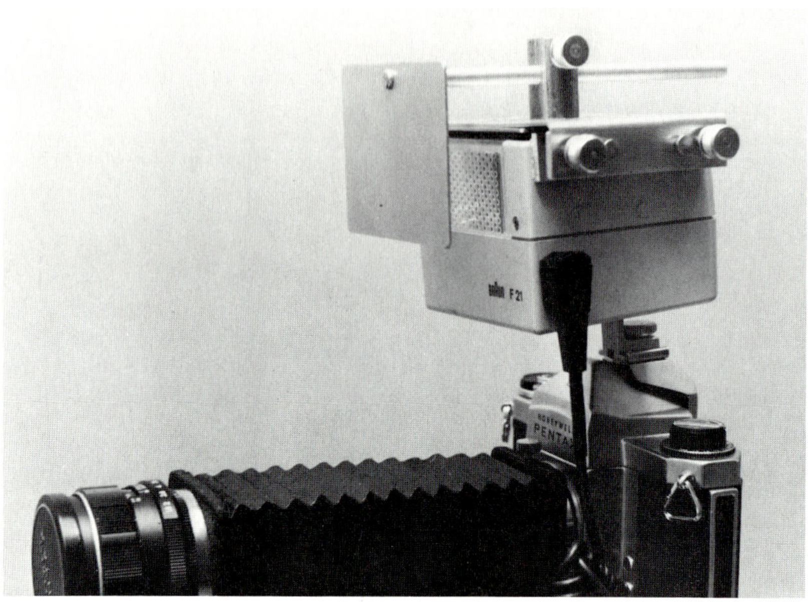

Fig. 15-3. Strobe light and flash shield.

cameras. The PhotoMont strobe shield is adjustable to fit many sizes of strobes. By loosening the center bolt, one may increase or decrease the size of the top of the shield to approximately the size of the top of the strobe. Final fixation is accomplished by tightening two bolts at the side of the shield.

2. The forward screen of the shield can be moved away from or toward the window of the strobe to increase or decrease the amount of illumination. Likewise, the shield can be moved up and down to create the desired amount of exposure.
3. To create fill when using a movie camera, a photo flood is used; it is generally held by an assistant and pointed at the ceiling. The amount of fill is controlled by observing through the reflex system and tipping the photo flood toward or away from the subject.

Taking Pictures

It is difficult to advise the exact f/stops, exposure time, and fill, since these factors will vary greatly from camera to camera of even the same make. The color of walls and clothes also dictates changes in fill. Likewise, the size of the strobe being used will change the strobe shield's location. Each of these factors varies with the amount of magnification (bellows or number of extensions used). It is advisable to shoot a number of experimental rolls of film on a comparative subject (perhaps an assistant) to determine the variables involved. It is recommended

Table 15-1. Recommended Starting Points for Exposure and Speed*

Type of Beam and Light	F/Stop	Exposure (sec)	Size of Extension Tubes or Bellows (mm)	Strobe Shield Displacement (mm)
Narrow beam, white light	f/4	1/8	160	20
Wide beam, cobalt light	f/5.6	1/8	80	10
Wide beam	f/8	1/8	160	30
White light	f/11	1/8	80	15
No beam	f/16	1/30	160	80
External view	f/16	1/30	80	60
	f/16	1/30	20	40

* These suggestions apply to: (1) Pentax H3 camera, 52-mm lens (Asahi Optical Company, Japan); (2) F21 Braun strobe; (3) Bellows (Bellowscope, Kopil, Japan); and (4) Kodak Daylight High Speed Ektachrome (ASA 160).

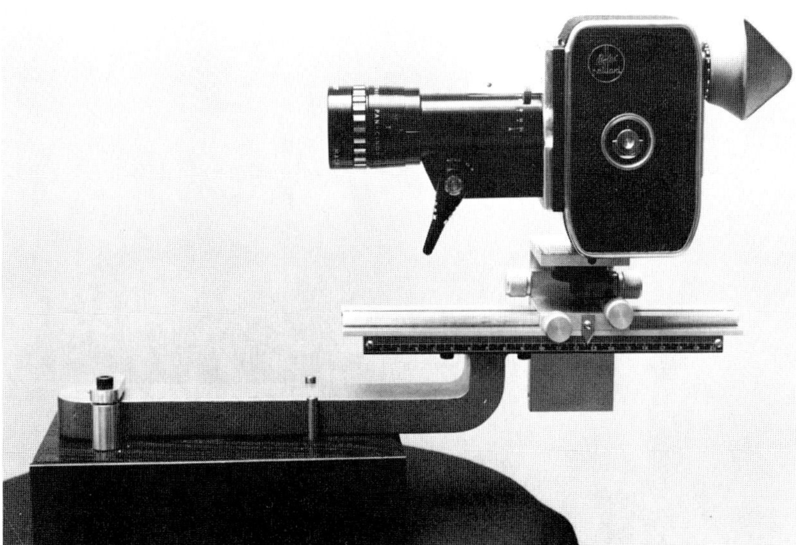

Fig. 15-4. Movie camera on slit-lamp camera attachment.

that all pictures be taken with the bulb of the slit lamp on the highest voltage of the instrument.

The point of regard can be located and final focus accomplished using either the reflex system of the camera or the slit-lamp microscope. It is advisable, however, that framing and a check for undesirable reflexes be made through the camera before the picture is taken.

A bulb cable release is recommended for use and should be held in the same hand as that controlling the joystick of the slit lamp. This gives instantaneous shutter response when exact focus is obtained and also releases the opposite hand for manipulation of the lids.

Starting points for exposure and speed are given in Table 15-1.

Motion Pictures

Motion pictures can be taken with an 8-mm Bolex Zoom P1 reflex camera (Fig. 15-4), using daylight Kodachrome II film and a close-up macro zoom lens.

Suggested Reading

Bitonte, J. L. *Contact Lens Reports.* Contact Lens Society of America. September, 1963.

Dugnani, E. Présentation de deux types d'écrans à fente pour la biomicroscopie et pour la photobiomicroscopie. *Bull. Soc. Ophthalmol. Fr.* 71 : 551, 1958.

Goldmann, H. Spaltlampenphotographie und-photometrie. *Ophthalmologica* 98 : 257, 1950.

Prince, J. H. A new slit-lamp color camera. *Arch. Ophthalmol.* 57 : 49, 1957.

Queiroga, G. Lampe à fente et photographie. *Ophthalmologica* 140 : 9, 1960.

Anterior Segment Fluorescein Angiography

MIZUO MATSUI AND
JOHNNY JUSTICE, JR.

Since Novotny and Alvis [12] first reported its effectiveness in 1960, fluorescein fundus angiography has contributed greatly to the understanding of the pathogenesis of many diseases of the retina, choroid, and optic disc. Soon after this report, the principles and techniques of this method of fundus angiography were applied to the evaluation of ocular anterior segment lesions.

In 1968, Jensen and Lundbaek [5, 6] modified a fundus camera to focus on the iris and published the first paper on iris fluorescein angiography. They added a +200-mm lens to the front of the standard aspherical objective of a Zeiss-Robot fundus camera in order to magnify the image and thereby be able to study the iris and conjunctival vessels in diabetic patients. Since the appearance of their study, numerous other investigators have described methods of fluorescein angiography for studying the anterior segment.

Rosen and Lyons [13], in 1970, utilized fluorescein angiography to delineate microhemangiomas at the pupillary borders; they used a standard Zeiss fundus camera adjusted for anterior segment photography. Mapstone [8] also used this system in his studies. Mitsui and coworkers [11] described a method of iridocorneal angiography in which a Zeiss photo slit lamp with a high speed power supply was used. Amalric and colleagues [1, 2], Wong and Frazier [15], and others employed this same technique. Koh [7] studied the conjunctival vessels angiographically with a low-power binocular microscope using the light source of an Olympus fundus camera. Craandijk and Aan de Kerk [4] used a standard single-lens reflex camera coupled with a macrophotographic objective with a standard Zeiss fundus camera as an illumination device to study anterior segment disease. Cobb and associates [3] used the same method to study vascular tufts at the pupillary margin.

Matsui and colleagues [9] reported further improvements in anterior segment fluorescein angiography after finding certain disadvantages in each of the reported methods. For instance, although a photo slit lamp provides angiograms of good quality, the margins are obstructed. A fundus camera adjusted for anterior segment photography has a limited field, and the peripheral image is out of focus. The usual single-lens reflex camera gives pictures 24 by 35 mm in size, but when a fundus

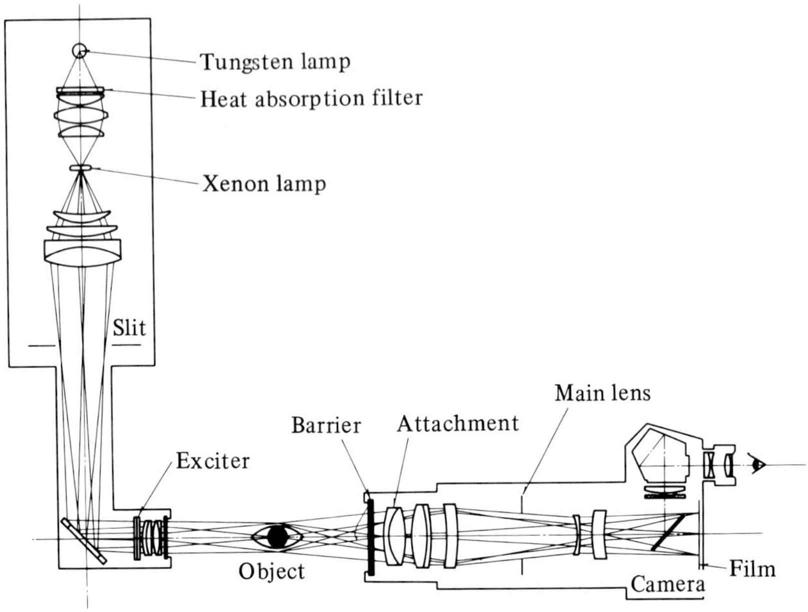

Fig. 16-1. Anterior segment angiography system.

camera is used as a light source, at least 50 percent of the light is lost at each optical interface in the illumination system. To photograph the anterior segment, these investigators coupled a 200-mm medical Nikon lens with a motor-driven Nikon F camera and a light system using a xenon tube powered with a standard Zeiss fundus camera. The camera and the illuminating device were mounted on a Haag-Streit slit-lamp table so that they could both be focused at the same point. This system gives an optimal image size of 24 by 35 mm without obscuring the margins or causing aberrations.

Matsui and colleagues [10] then adapted this system for high-speed serial angiography using a 200-mm Topcon macro lens with an automatic diaphragm coupled with a motor-driven camera body and a power supply for high-speed serial fluorescein fundus photography (Topcon TRC-F3). An optical diagram of this system is shown in Figure 16-1; Figure 16-2 shows a side view of the apparatus.

Applications of Anterior Segment Fluorescein Angiography

Anterior segment fluorescein angiography has been used to study the circulatory dynamics of normal and pathologic bulbar conjunctival vessels, including corneal limbal vessel arcades and aqueous veins. Blue irides can be studied easily by means of angiography; therefore, fluorescein angiography has been used in white patients with lesions of

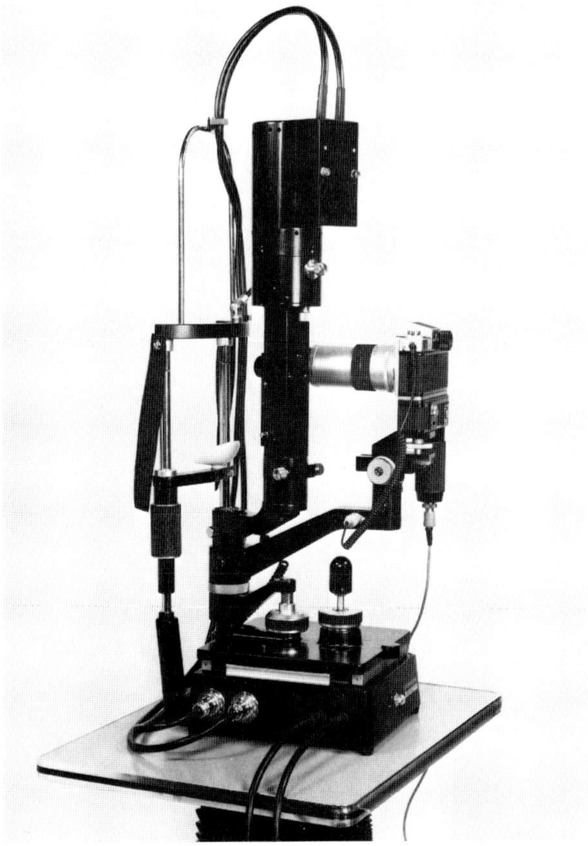

Fig. 16-2. Side view of anterior segment angiography system.

the iris. Figure 16-3 is an angiogram of sector heterochromia iridis; the vessels in the blue portion fluoresced clearly, while those in the brown part did not fluoresce.

Normal Conjunctival Vessels

Several investigators employed fluorescein angiography to study the bulbar conjunctival vessels and the perilimbal vessel arcades. The anterior ciliary vessels fluoresced first, and the posterior conjunctival vessels fluoresced at almost the same time or a few seconds later. Anterior segment angiography revealed that the dye appeared first at the point where the anterior ciliary vessels emerged from the sclera and progressed to the rectus muscles. The dye also entered the small recurrent vessels to irrigate the perilimbal capillaries and then entered the conjunctival venules, which run in centrifugal, straight courses.

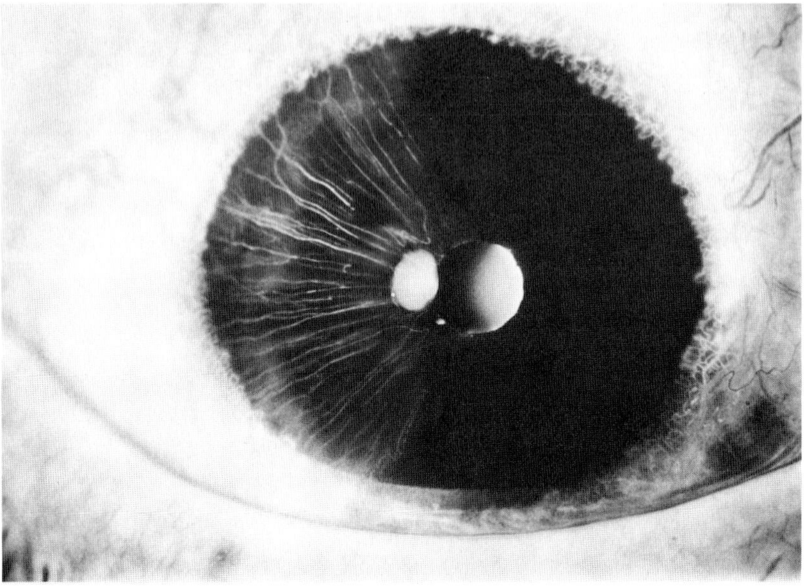

Fig. 16-3. Iris angiogram of sector heterochromia iridis.

Angiography showed that the aqueous veins filled with dye after these two vessel systems fluoresced; this finding was confirmed biomicroscopically.

Normal Iris Vessels

Vannas [14] showed that it was possible to distinguish between radial arteries and radial veins in angiograms of the iris, since the arteries began to fluoresce strongly earlier; the veins filled soon after the arteries. The arteries seemed thicker than the veins. They usually ran in the surface layer of the iris to the pupillary border, where they ramified, sending small branches deep into the sphincter muscle to form a capillary network. The veins appeared thinner and more numerous than the arteries. Fluorescein leakage through the iris vessels seldom occurs in healthy eyes if the patient is less than 50 years old; leakage becomes more common with increasing age.

Clinical Application of Iris Angiography

Wong and Frazier [15] studied iris angiography in two patients with iris melanomas and observed early fluorescence of the vascularized tumor and a discrete focal leakage that is characteristic of choroidal melanomas. In contrast, an iris nevus examined by Craandijk and Aan de Kerk [4] demonstrated diffuse leakage of fluorescein. Figure 16-4 shows angiograms of an iris melanoma.

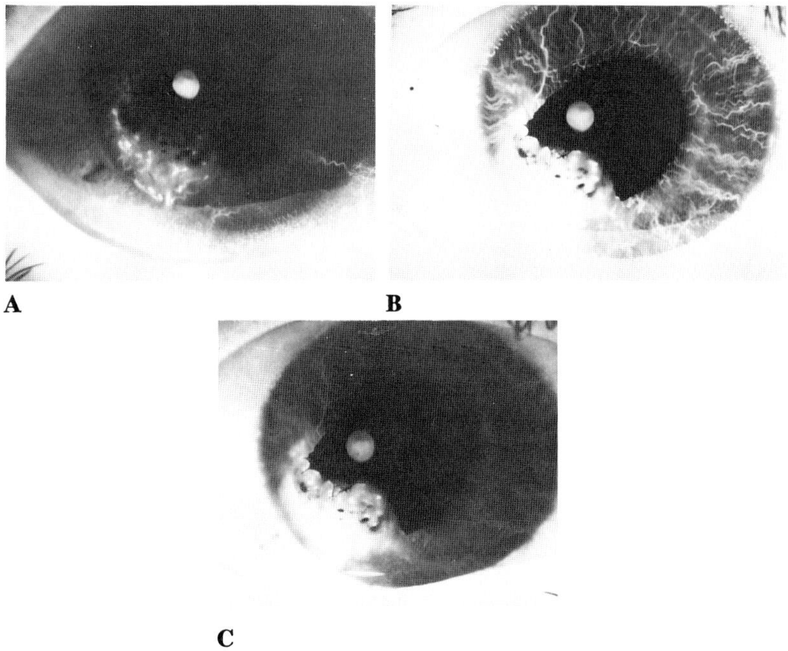

Fig. 16-4. *Iris angiogram of iris melanoma.* (A) *Early phase;* (B) *arteriovenous phase;* (C) *late phase.*

Vannas [14] studied iris angiographic findings in eyes with pseudoexfoliation of the lens capsule, capsular glaucoma, simple glaucoma, and angle-closure glaucoma. He observed vascular changes of varying degrees in the irides of 15 out of 20 eyes with pseudoexfoliation; the changes included gradual loss of the radial vessels and vasoproliferation. In 40 of the 41 eyes affected with capsular glaucoma, vascular changes of the iris, a reduced number of radial vessels, and vascular proliferation were seen. The changes in these eyes were similar but more advanced than in those with pseudoexfoliation. Profuse fluorescein leakage from the pupillary or ciliary portion of the iris, or both, was a regular feature. In 2 of the 33 eyes affected with simple glaucoma, neovascularization and fluorescein leakage were seen in the ciliary portion of the iris. In 8 of the 20 eyes with angle-closure glaucoma, vascular congestion or vasoproliferative changes, or both, appeared. Figure 16-5 is an iris angiogram of an eye with pseudoexfoliation showing marked neovascularization. Figure 16-6 shows the iris of an eye affected with open-angle glaucoma in which neovascularization is present, but to a lesser degree than in the eyes with pseudoexfoliation.

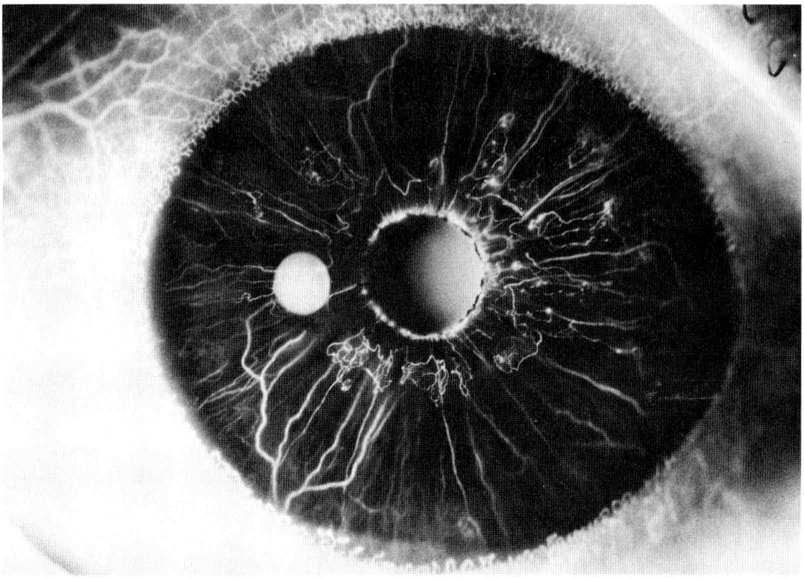

Fig. 16-5. Iris angiogram of eye with pseudoexfoliation.

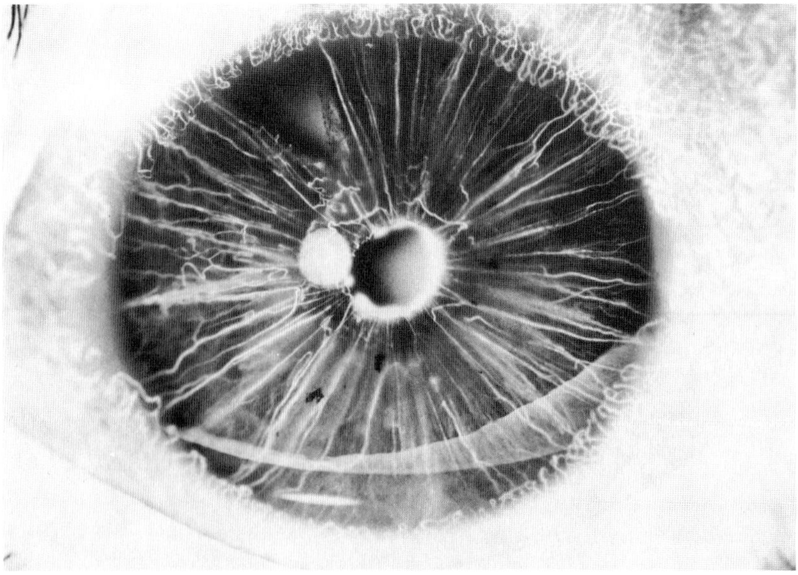

Fig. 16-6. Iris angiogram of eye with open-angle glaucoma.

References

1. Amalric P., and Rebiere, P. Nouvelles indications de l'angiographie fluoresceinique du ségment antérieur de l'oeil: Les veines aqueuses. *Ann. Ocul.* 204 : 469, 1971.
2. Amalric, P., Rebiere, P., and Jourdes, J. C. Nouvelles indications de l'angiographie fluoresceinique du ségment antérieur de l'oeil. *Ann. Ocul.* 204 : 455, 1971.
3. Cobb, B., Shilling, J. S., and Chisholm, I. H. Vascular tufts at the pupillary margin in myotonic dystrophy. *Am. J. Ophthalmol.* 69 : 573, 1970.
4. Craandijk, A., and Aan de Kerk, A. L. Fluorescence angiography of the iris. *Br. J. Ophthalmol.* 54 : 229, 1970.
5. Jensen, V. A., and Lundbaek, K. Fluorescence angiography of the iris in recent and long term diabetes. *Acta Ophthalmol.* 46 : 584, 1968.
6. Jensen, V. A., and Lundbaek, K. Fluorescence angiography of the iris in recent and long-term diabetes. *Diabetologica* 4 : 161, 1968.
7. Koh, K. Studies on the fluorescence photography of the bulbar conjunctival vessels, on the techniques of photography. *Nich. Igaku Zash.* 27 : 386, 1969.
8. Mapstone, R. Fluorescein iridography. *Br. J. Ophthalmol.* 55 : 400, 1971.
9. Matsui, M., Parel, J., and Justice, J. Some improved methods of anterior segment fluorescein angiography: I. Basic system. *Am. J. Opthalmol.* 74 : 1075, 1972.
10. Matsui, M., Parel, J., and Justice, J. Studies on anterior segment fluorescein angiography: II. Improvement of the apparatus. *Jpn. J. Ophthalmol.* 28 : 1347, 1974.
11. Mitsui, Y., Matsubara, M., and Kanagawa, M. Fluorescence iridocorneal photography. *Br. J. Ophthalmol.* 53 : 500, 1969.
12. Novotny, H. R., and Alvis, D. L. A method of photographing fluorescence in circulating blood of the human eye. *Aerosp. Med.* 60 : 82, 1960.
13. Rosen, E., and Lyons, D. Microhemangiomas at the pupillary border demonstrated by fluorescein photography. *Am. J. Ophthalmol.* 67 : 846, 1969.
14. Vannas, A. Fluorescein angiography of the vessels of the iris in pseudoexfoliation of the lens capsule, capsular glaucoma and some other forms of glaucoma. *Acta Ophthalmol.* 105 (Suppl.): 75, 1969.
15. Wong, I. G., and Frazier, O. *Clinical Use of Iris Fluorescein Angiography.* St. Louis: Mosby, 1972. Vol. 3, p. 29.

17

Fluorescein Angiography of the Conjunctiva

CSABA L. MARTONYI

High-contrast fluorescein photographs of the conjunctival vasculature are obtained using the Zeiss photo slit lamp equipped with the anterior segment angiographic flash illuminator powered by the Fundus Flash II power supply, and the Spectrotech SE-40 and SB-50 filter combination.

Although the technique of anterior segment fluorescein angiography was described some years ago [1, 3, 5, 6], it remains a little-used diagnostic adjunct. The informative value of this procedure has been greatly limited by the unavailability of appropriate instrumentation and adequate filtration and, in iris angiography, obscuration of vascular detail by the pigment epithelium [2].

With the use of some more recently available equipment, coupled with the latest interference filter combination [4], scleral pseudofluorescence has been largely eliminated in the photography of circulating fluorescein in the conjunctival vasculature. The object of this chapter is to describe an available method of fluorescein angiophotography of the conjunctiva that yields satisfactory contrast and information.

Materials and Methods

The essential equipment components used in this method are a high-transmission, narrow band-pass interference filter combination, namely, the Spectrotech-Delori SE-40 (excitor) and SB-50 (barrier) filters, and a Zeiss photo slit lamp biomicroscope equipped with a high-output, rapid cycle light source (Zeiss "coffee can") powered by a Zeiss Fundus Flash II power supply. A hand-wound Leica camera back is used to make the exposures on Kodak Tri-X film.

The excitor (SE-40) filter is available in a threaded mount and attaches to the coffee can directly in front of the flash source. The barrier (SB-50) filter is mounted in front of the film in the camera-to-side-arm adapter. The slit illuminator is set at the maximum (No. 9) aperture, with the slit controls set to permit the largest full-circle illumination. A cobalt blue filter is placed over the slit illuminator to allow visualization of the circulating fluorescein during angiography.

The patient is seated at the camera with the head positioned in the usual fashion for slit lamp photography. Preinjection control photographs are taken to show the level of "pseudofluorescence." At ap-

This chapter is reprinted with permission from the *Journal of the Ophthalmic Photographers' Society* 1(1) : 14–15, 1978.

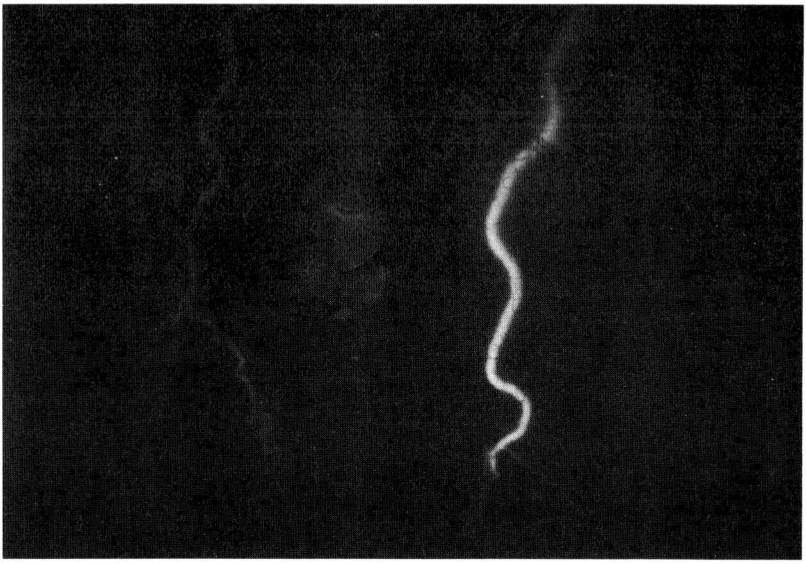

Fig. 17-1. Approximately 14 sec postinjection of fluorescein, deep scleral vessels are initially seen. Their visibility is considerably enhanced by the absence of pseudofluorescence.

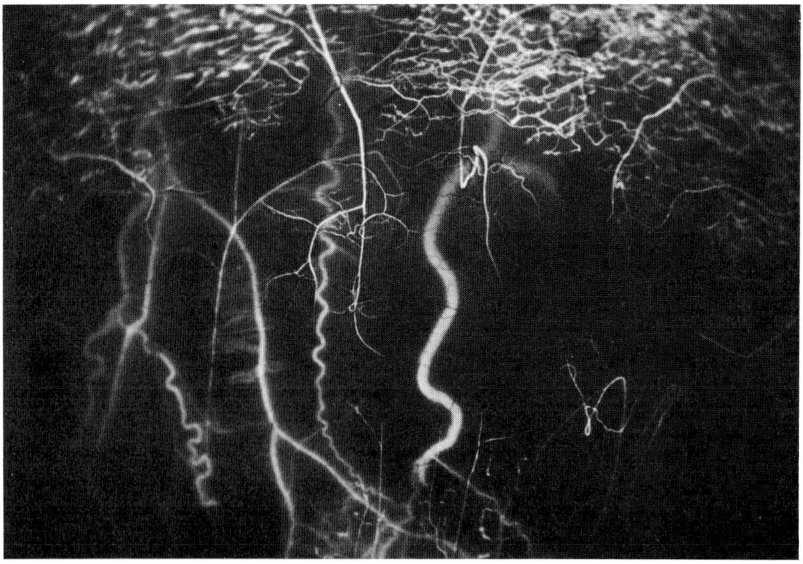

Fig. 17-2. Conjunctival vessels are sharply outlined in the early phase of the angiogram and exhibit prompt leakage of fluorescein.

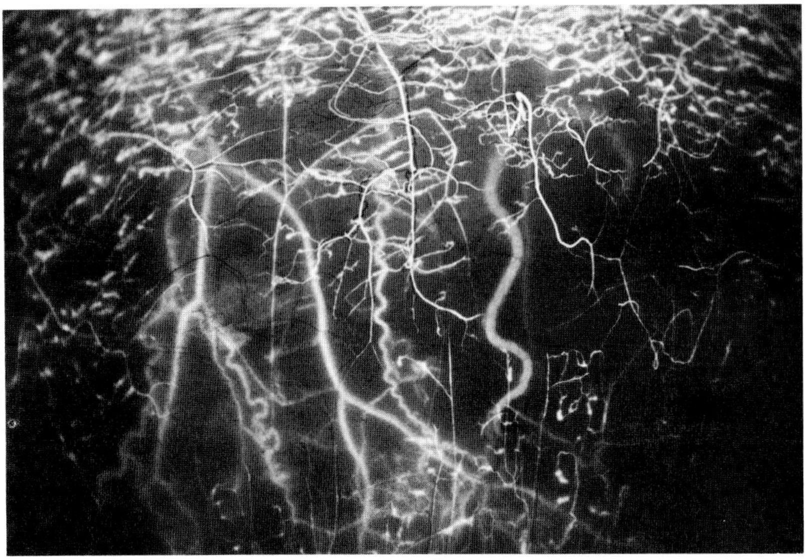

Fig. 17-3. Further filling of the arterial system and early venous filling.

proximately 7 to 9 seconds following the rapid intravenous injection of 3.50 ml of 20% sodium fluorescein*, photography commences at approximately 1 frame per second for 20 to 30 seconds. Since conjunctival vessels fill slowly and circulating fluorescein is often difficult to visualize, the proposed sequencing should provide adequate initial coverage on most patients. Additional exposures are made at 2, 5, and 30 minutes after injection of fluorescein.

The exposed roll of Kodak Tri-X film is processed in undiluted Kodak D-76 developer at 68° F for 11 minutes with normal agitation. Fixing, washing, and drying are performed in the usual manner. The processed film is cut into strips of 6 frames and placed emulsion up on a contact printer and exposed on an 8- by 10-inch sheet of DuPont Cronar S Ortho film. The Cronar is placed in a sheet film hanger and tank processed in undiluted Kodak D-11 developer at 68° F for 3 minutes with a 15-second initial agitation, followed by 5 seconds of agitation at 30-second intervals. Fixing, washing, and drying are carried out in the usual manner.

Results

Figures 17-1 through 17-4 demonstrate the suppression of pseudofluorescence of the sclera and the increased contrast of circulating

* My laboratory uses a specially prepared 20% solution of fluorescein dye for all angiograms, but commercially available 10% and 25% solutions will produce similar results.

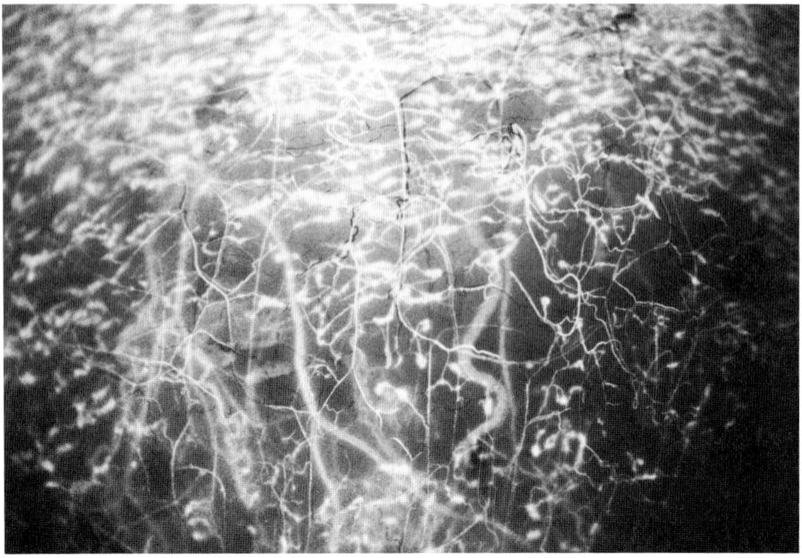

Fig. 17-4. The system is nearly filled.

Fig. 17-5. Considerable leakage of dye from the conjunctival vasculature is seen approximately 2 min postinjection.

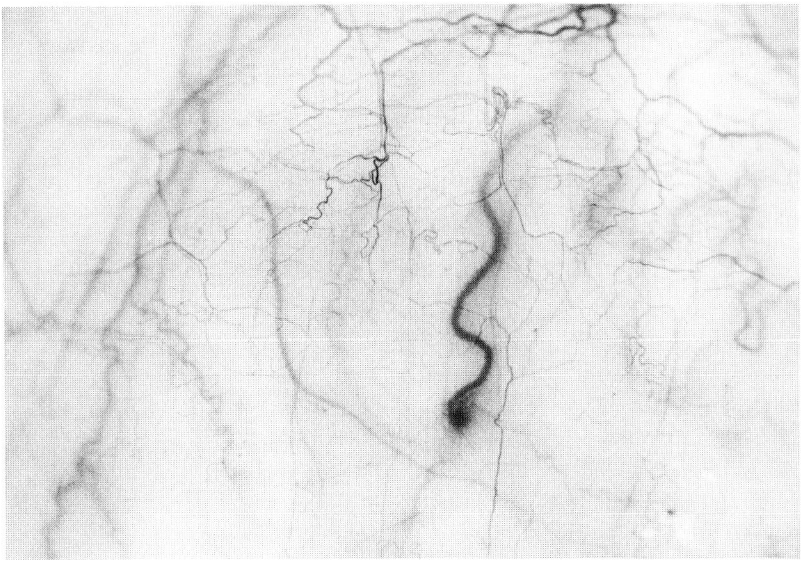

Fig. 17-6. At 45 min postinjection of fluorescein, conjunctival and scleral vessels are seen in relief against a background of fluorescein-stained sclera.

fluorescein. Figure 17-5 shows normal diffusion of fluorescein dye from small conjunctival vessels. Figure 17-6 demonstrates persistent fluorescence of the fluorescein-stained sclera.

Conclusion

The informative content and, I hope, the diagnostic value of fluorescein photography of conjunctival vasculature have been greatly enhanced by the considerable reduction of pseudofluorescence of the underlying sclera through the use of an optimized excitor-barrier filter combination. Although there is available a limited number of modalities for anterior segment angiophotography, the Zeiss photo slit lamp biomicroscope, equipped with the high-output, rapid cycle coffee can illuminator powered by a Zeiss Fundus Flash source, will yield excellent angiograms with little modification. While depth of field is limited, variable magnification and good resolution will provide required detail in most cases. Either a simple camera back can be wound and fired by hand, or motor-driven camera backs, some equipped with data-imprinting devices, can be used, powered by the fundus camera power supply or an auxiliary power source. Angiograms processed and printed as described will yield considerable detail and satisfactory contrast.

References

1. Baggesen, L. H. Fluorescein angiography of the iris in diabetics and non-diabetics. *Acta Ophthalmol.* 47 : 449–460, 1969.
2. Bergstrom, T. J., Roth, M., and Martonyi, C. L. Pigmented iris angiography. *Arch. Ophthalmol.* 94 : 1180–1182, 1976.
3. Craandijk, A., and Aan de Kerk, A. L. Fluorescein angiography of the iris. *Br. J. Ophthalmol.* 54 : 229–232, 1970.
4. Delori, F., Ben-Sira, I., and Trempe, C. Fluorescein angiography with an optimized filter combination. *Am. J. Ophthalmol.* 82 : 559–566, 1976.
5. Justice, J. (Ed.). Ophthalmic Photography. *Int. Ophthalmol. Clin.* 16(2), 1976.
6. Mitsui, Y., Matsubara, M., and Kanazawa, M. Fluorescein irido-corneal photography. *Br. J. Ophthalmol.* 53 : 505–512, 1969.

18

A Simplified Technique for Anterior Segment Fluorescein Angiography

EARL A. CHOROMOKOS

The objects of this chapter are to describe a simple, economical method that can produce high-quality anterior segment fluorescein angiography and to present a variety of angiograms documenting this method's capability and versatility.

In the past, others have described anterior segment angiographic techniques that use modified slit lamp cameras and 35-mm cameras with adapted light sources [1, 4]. The results obtained were excellent but expensive, and exotic equipment was essential.

We use a conventional Topcon TRC-F3 retinal fundus camera [3], but several other fundus cameras can also be used. These fundus cameras do not need modifications. Other benefits of using them are their (1) standard high transmission filters, suitable for fluorescein angiography, (2) rapid sequence capability, (3) built-in time-frame counter, and (4) dual capacity for retinal and anterior segment angiography.

Methods

The pupils need not be dilated for anterior segment angiography. After the patient is in position, the anterior segment lens on the diopter compensator wheel is moved into the optic pathway. Three other lenses (emmetropic, myopic, and aphakic) are also located on this wheel (Fig. 18-1). I use the regular excitor and barrier filters employed for retinal angiography. The room must be dark because the cornea will reflect the unfiltered room lighting. The eyelids should be opened as wide as possible to keep annoying shadows from appearing on the angiogram. Sodium fluorescein 10 ml is injected intraveneously. Exposures should begin 8 to 10 seconds and serial photographs for up to 1 minute postinjection; late photographs are taken 5 to 10 minutes postinjection.

When photographing the cornea or iris, set the flash at 300 watt-seconds. Iris angiography cannot be accomplished on darkly pigmented irides because the pigment obscures the vessels. However, the technique will demonstrate abnormal vessels on the surface of the iris, regardless of pigmentation. Figure 18-2 is an iris angiogram, and Figure 18-3 shows congenital corneal vascularization.

For conjunctival angiography (Fig. 18-4), the power should be set

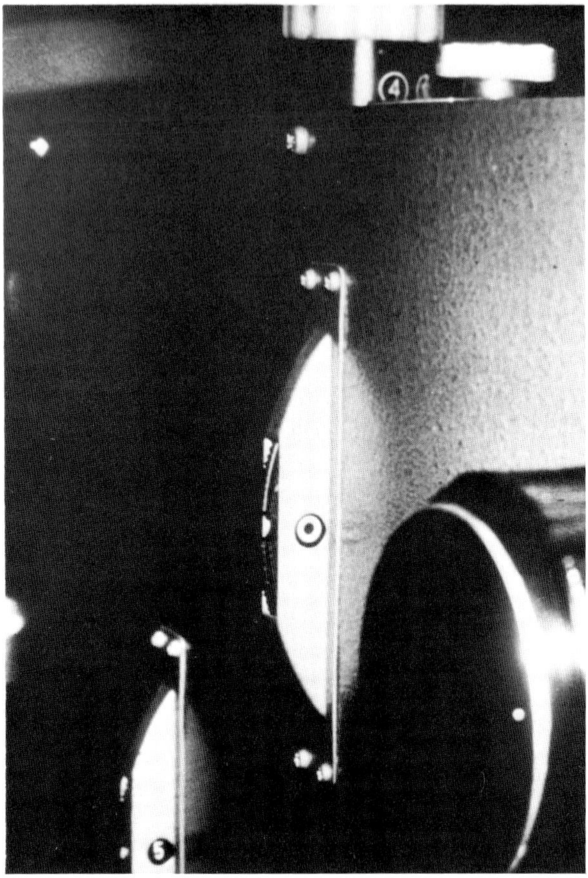

Fig. 18-1. *Diopter compensator wheel.*

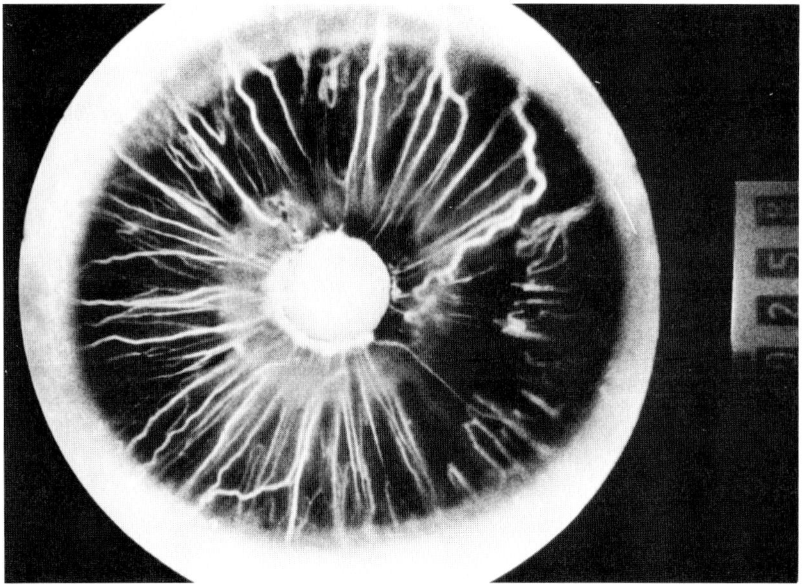

Fig. 18-2. Iris angiogram.

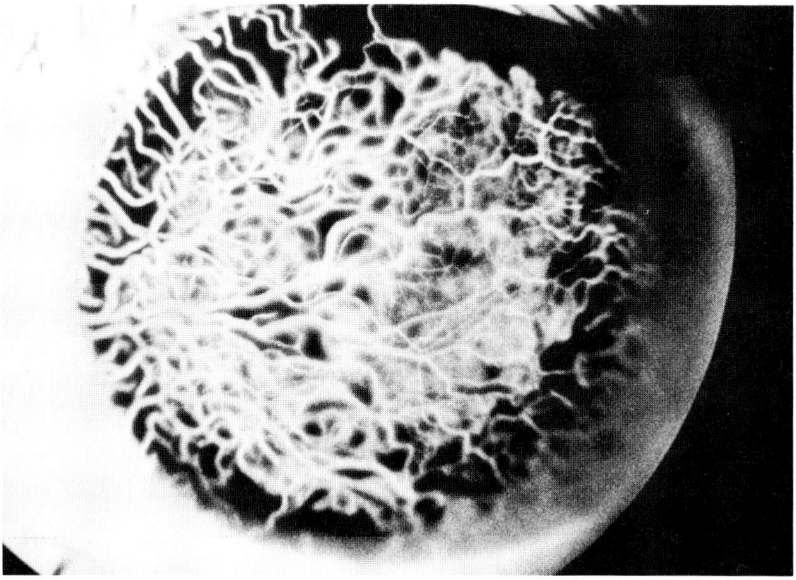

Fig. 18-3. Congenital corneal vascularization.

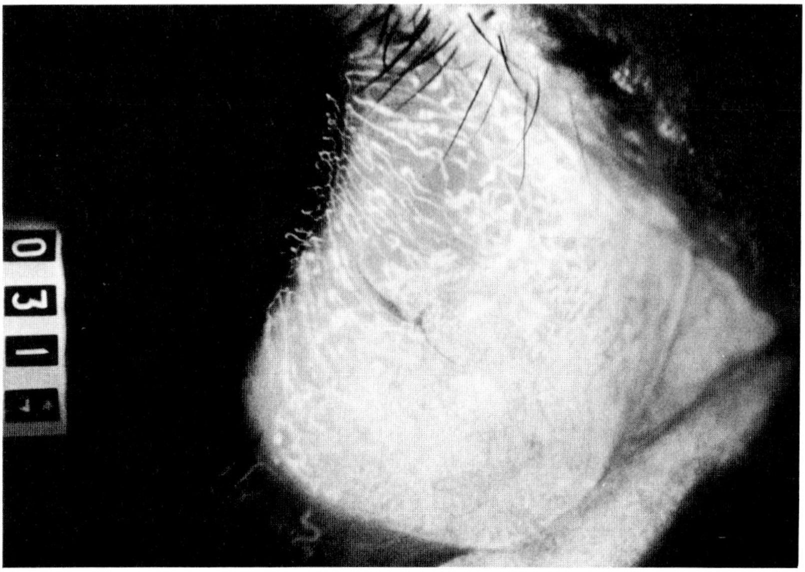

Fig. 18-4. Conjunctival angiogram.

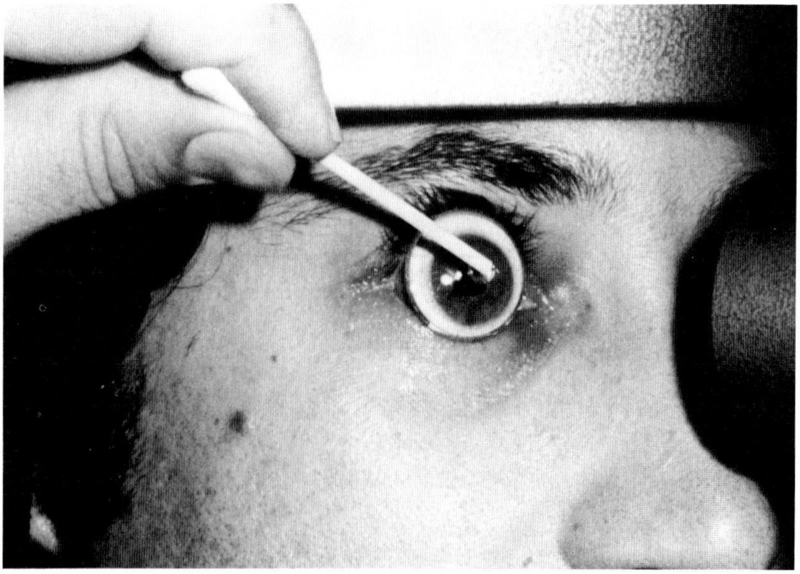

Fig. 18-5. Koeppe lens in position.

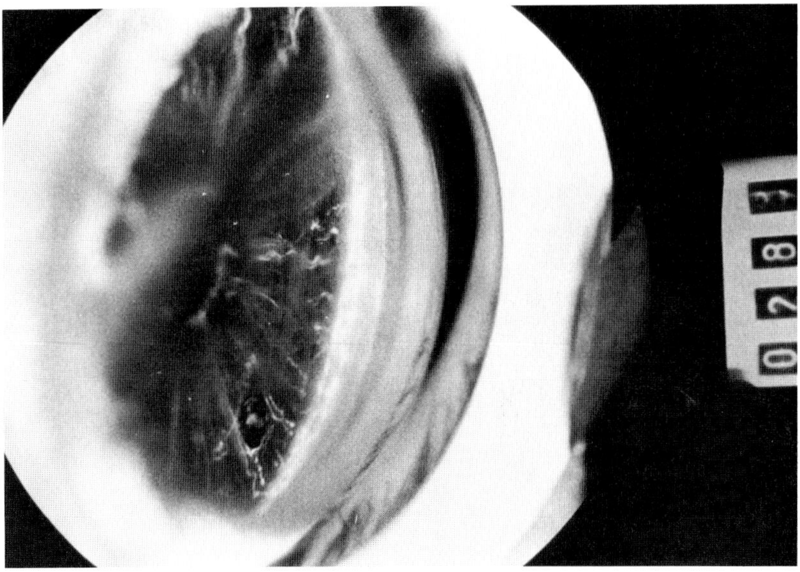

Fig. 18-6. Goniogram.

at 75 watt-seconds. Since the dye rapidly passes through the highly vascular conjunctiva, rapid sequence (3 frames/sec) is desirable.

Anterior segment angle angiography (*gonioangiography*) is performed with a power setting of 300 watt-seconds. A Koeppe contact lens, filled with methylcellulose and held in place with a cotton-tipped applicator, is positioned on the anesthetized cornea (Fig. 18-5). The camera is tilted 45 degrees to view the angle structures (Fig. 18-6).

To conclude, a standard retinal fundus camera can be used to perform anterior segment angiography.

References

1. Bruun-Jensen, J. Fluorescein angiography of the anterior segment. *Am. J. Ophthalmol.* 67 : 842–845, 1969.
2. Delori, F., Ben-Sira, I., and Trempe, C. Fluorescein angiography with an optimized filter combination. *Am. J. Ophthalmol.* 82 : 559–566, 1976.
3. Fetkenhour, C., and Choromokos, E. Anterior segment fluorescein angiography with a fundus camera. *Arch. Ophthalmol.* 96 : 711–713, 1978.
4. Matsui, M., Parel, J. M., Weder, H. J., and Justice, J. Some improved methods of anterior segment fluorescein angiography: I. Basic System. *Am. J. Ophthalmol.* 74 : 1075–1079, 1972.

19

Photography of the Corneal Endothelium

WILLIAM M. BOURNE

Although slit-lamp photography of the cornea has been highly successful, adequate pictures of individual endothelial cells have not been possible with the slit lamp because of the magnification requirement, troublesome light reflexes, and continuous small eye movements. Successful photographs of living endothelial cells were first obtained by Brown [7] in 1970 with a corneal macrocamera that he described. However, more magnification and a clearer view were obtained with a device called a *specular microscope,* first described by Maurice [10] in 1968. This instrument was designed to allow the examination and photography of the endothelium of intact enucleated eyes through a fluid medium. Laing and colleagues [9] added important modifications to this instrument to obtain photographs of endothelial cells in vivo. Bourne and associates [5] made further modifications so that the specular microscope can be used for the routine examination and photography of the corneal endothelium of any patient with a relatively clear cornea. This chapter describes the clinical specular microscope and initial observations made with it in humans.

The Clinical Specular Microscope

Figure 19-1 shows the clinical specular microscope in use, and Figure 19-2 presents a schematic diagram of the instrument. Light from the viewing lamp is directed by mirrors through the objective lens into the cornea. The objective is a ×20 water immersion lens with an attached dipping cone lens (Nikon Corp.). The dipping cone lens is an extension of the objective lens with a flat anterior surface. This surface flattens the cornea, eliminates the air-cornea interface, and dampens the continuous small eye movement. Light is reflected from the endothelium (presumably from the posterior surfaces of the endothelial cells at the interface with the aqueous humor). The illuminating and the image-forming rays pass through different portions of the objective lens, eliminating unwanted reflections. A ×70 magnified image of the endothelial borders is projected onto the film plane of a reflex camera. A high-intensity, short-duration flash unit provides clear pictures despite continuous small eye movements. Several photographs may be taken rapidly with an automatic film advance.

The endothelial image is focused on the viewing screen by adjusting the distance between the dipping cone lens and the objective lens. This adjustment can also provide a direct measure of the corneal thick-

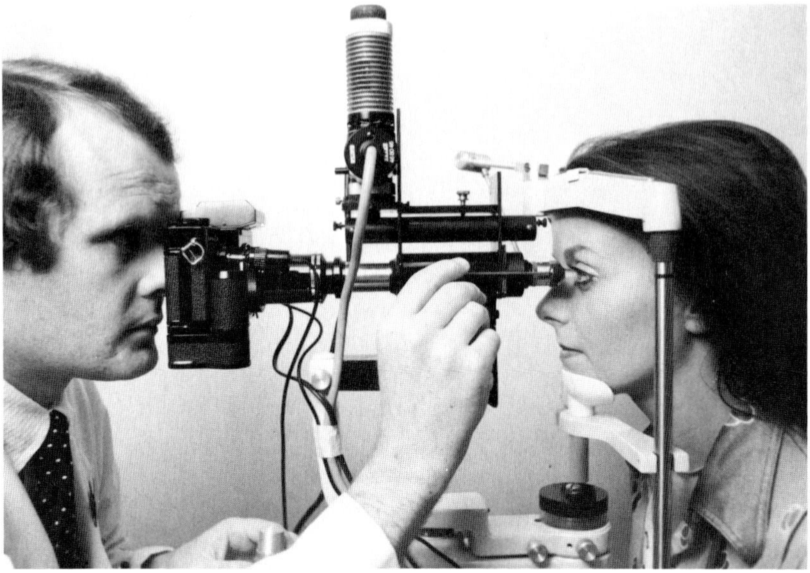

Fig. 19-1. Clinical specular microscope in use. (From W. M. Bourne, B. E. McCarey, and H. E. Kaufman, Clinical specular microscopy. Trans. Am. Acad. Ophthalmol. Otolaryngol. *81 : 743–753, 1976.*)

ness [3]. Endothelial cell density may be computed from photographs by counting the number of cells in a known area. The system is calibrated by photographing through an aqueous medium the surface of a glass slide scored at 10-μm intervals. This picture is projected on a screen to give a total magnification of approximately ×400 (the 10-μm marks are 4 mm apart). Endothelial cell images are projected and counted at the same magnification and in the same position as the calibration slide. The area counted is usually about 0.04 mm^2, and the result is expressed as cells per square millimeter. The error in cell count introduced by variations in corneal thickness or refractive index is less than one percent [3]. Individual endothelial cell sizes may also be measured [2].

Use of the Instrument

Examination with the clinical specular microscope is simple, safe, and rarely takes more than a few minutes. A topical anesthetic is used. Contact of the cornea with the dipping cone lens causes only occasional punctate epithelial irregularities, similar to those seen following applanation tonometry; these disappear within a few hours. Examination and photography can be performed on any relatively clear cornea, even on the first postoperative day, without danger to the eye.

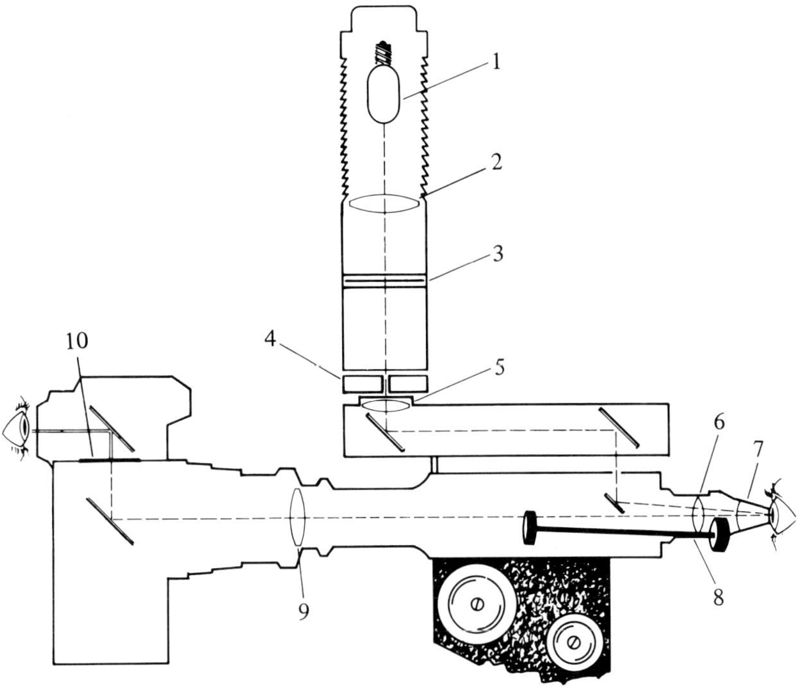

Fig. 19-2. Schematic diagram of the clinical specular microscope. 1 = *viewing lamp;* 2 = *condensing lens;* 3 = *xenon flash tube;* 4 = *slit aperture;* 5 = *condensing lens;* 6 = *objective lens;* 7 = *dipping cone lens;* 8 = *attachment for focusing;* 9 = *eyepiece lens;* 10 = *viewing screen.* (*Published with permission from* Am. J. Ophthalmol. *81 : 319–323, 1976. Copyright by the Ophthalmic Publishing Co.*)

Any portion of the endothelium can be examined. However, all the photographs shown in this chapter are of the central endothelium only.

Normal Corneas

Figure 19-3 illustrates views of the endothelium of normal corneas. Differences in endothelial cell density may not be apparent during individual examinations, but they are readily seen when the photographs are compared. It is obvious in Figure 19-3 that the endothelial cells of the older subject are larger. When a large number of normal corneas were examined and photographed, a statistically significant decrease in central endothelial cell density with increasing age of the patient was found [4]. Variations in cell size and shape are easily discerned from these photographs, in which the borders between cells are clearly shown. However, the contrast obtained with the specular microscope described in this chapter is not sufficient to determine the size or location of nuclei or other subcellular components.

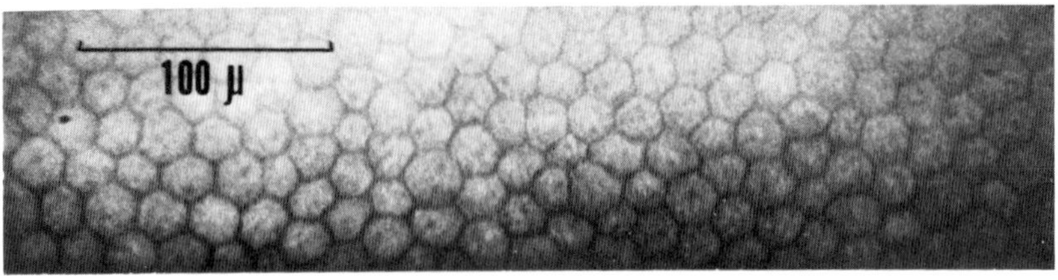

6-Year-old 3015 Cells/mm^2

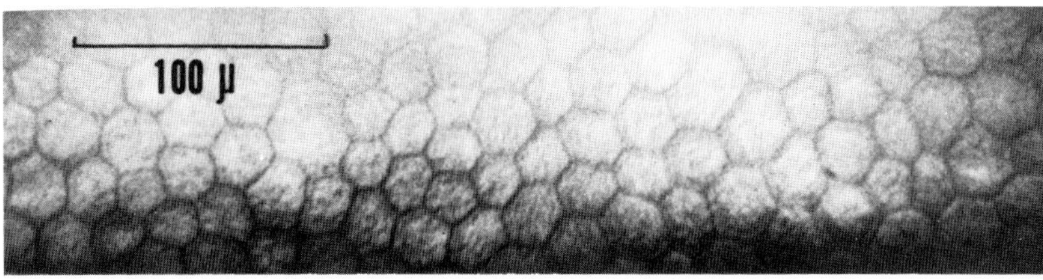

74-Year-old 1944 Cells/mm^2

Fig. 19-3. The central corneal endothelium of two normal patients of differing age. (From W. M. Bourne, B. E. McCarey, and H. E. Kaufman, Clinical specular microscopy. Trans. Am. Acad. Ophthalmol. Otolaryngol. *81 : 743–753, 1976.)*

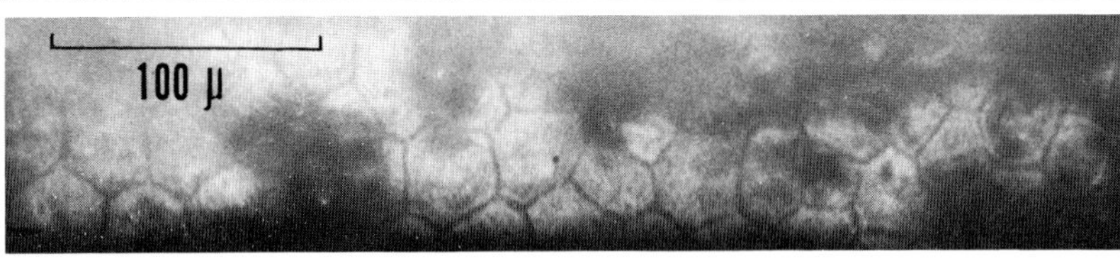

Fig. 19-4. Specular microscopic view of a mild cornea guttata. (From W. M. Bourne, B. E. McCarey, and H. E. Kaufman, Clinical specular microscopy. Trans. Am. Acad. Ophthalmol. Otolaryngol. *81 : 743–753, 1976.)*

Abnormal Corneas

Photography through the specular microscope is especially useful in the study and documentation of endothelial abnormalities. The cornea guttata of Fuchs' dystrophy is readily apparent. Guttate changes can probably be seen with this technique before they are visible by slit-lamp examination. The endothelium of a patient with mild cornea guttata is shown in Figure 19-4; Figure 19-5 illustrates a more advanced case.

Traumatic endothelial damage may not be evident on slit-lamp examination. Figure 19-6 shows the endothelium of both eyes of a boy

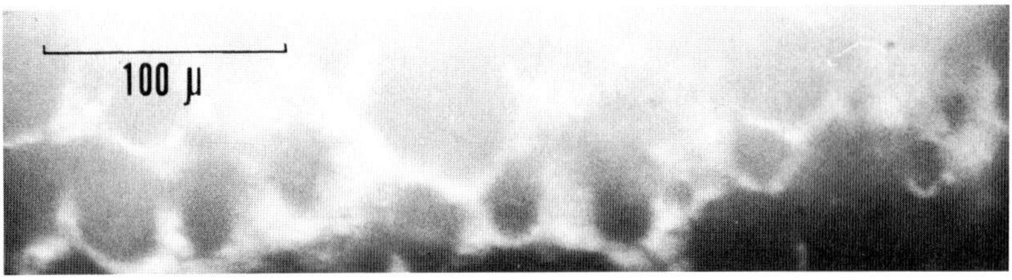

Fig. 19-5. Specular microscopic view of a moderately advanced cornea guttata. (From W. M. Bourne, B. E. McCarey, and H. E. Kaufman, Clinical specular microscopy. Trans. Am. Acad. Ophthalmol. Otolaryngol. *81 : 743–753, 1976.)*

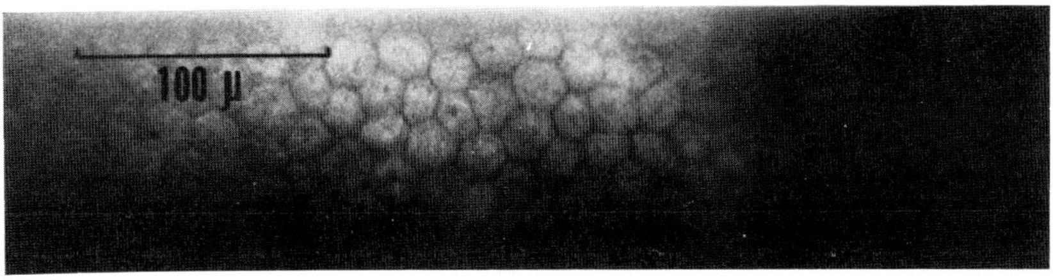

Normal OS 3221 Cells/mm^2

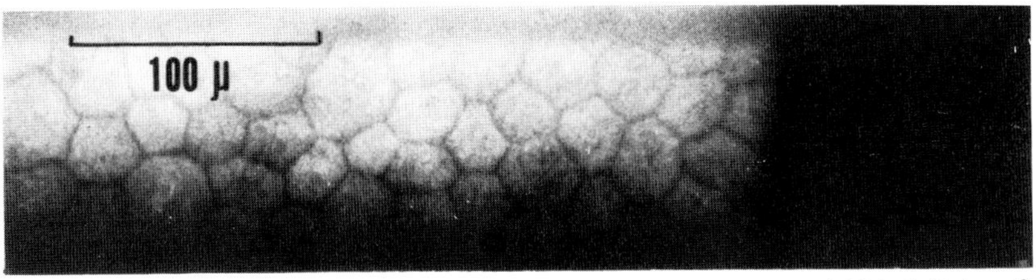

Trauma OD 1498 Cells/mm^2

Fig. 19-6. Endothelium of both eyes two years following blunt trauma to right eye. Half of the endothelial cells have been lost in the right eye. (From W. M. Bourne, B. E. McCarey, and H. E. Kaufman, Clinical specular microscopy. Trans. Am. Acad. Ophthalmol. Otolaryngol. *81 : 743–753, 1976.)*

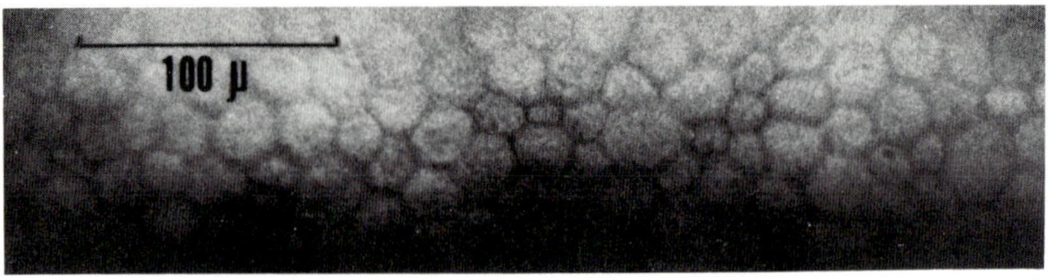

Preoperation 2397 Cells/mm^2

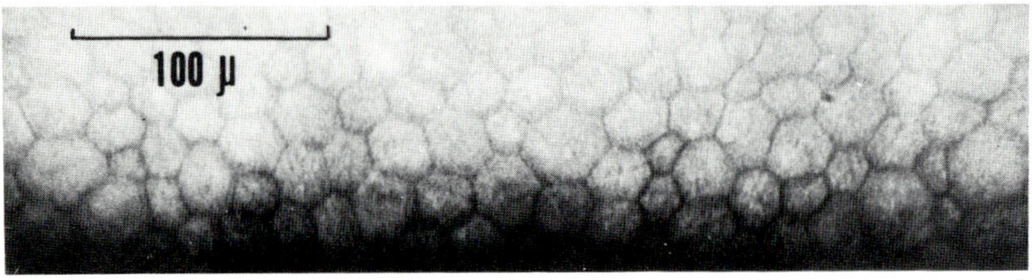

1 Day postoperation 2307 Cells/mm^2

Fig. 19-7. Central endothelium before and after uncomplicated intracapsular cataract extraction. No loss of endothelial cells occurred. (*From W. M. Bourne, B. E. McCarey, and H. E. Kaufman, Clinical specular microscopy.* Trans. Am. Acad. Ophthalmol. Otolaryngol. *81 : 743–753, 1976.*)

whose right cornea had been struck with an air rifle pellet 2 years previously. The cornea had remained thin and clear, and no endothelial abnormality was detected by slit-lamp examination. As shown in the lower photograph, more than half of the endothelial cells in the right cornea had been lost. This cornea is probably more susceptible to the detrimental effects of aging, inflammation, and ocular surgery.

Ocular Surgery

The most practical application of endothelial photography is the evaluation and documentation of the endothelial effects of intraocular surgery. Photographs can be obtained on the first postoperative day without danger or inconvenience to the patient. Figures 19-7 and 19-8 show the corneal endothelium of two patients both before and after intracapsular cataract extraction. The patient shown in Figure 19-7 underwent an uncomplicated cryoextraction; no loss of endothelial cells occurred. Vitreous loss complicated the procedure for the patient in Figure 19-8, but his cornea remained clear and his postoperative course was uneventful. The photographs show that a significant loss of endothelial cells has occurred, however. This cornea is probably more likely to develop endothelial failure and aphakic bullous keratopathy than the cornea in Figure 19-7.

Preoperation 2860 Cells/mm^2

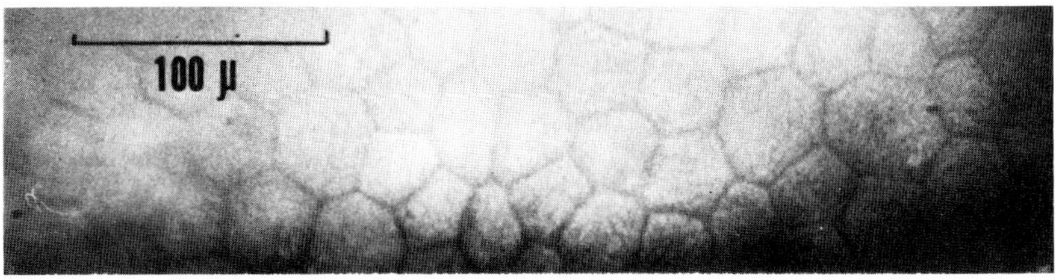

2 Mo postoperation 1110 Cells/mm^2

Fig. 19-8. Central endothelium before and after intracapsular cataract extraction complicated by vitreous loss. A significant loss of endothelial cells occurred. (From W. M. Bourne, B. E. McCarey, and H. E. Kaufman, Clinical specular microscopy. Trans. Am. Acad. Ophthalmol. Otolaryngol. *81 : 743–753, 1976.*)

The extent of endothelial damage from intraocular lenses is relatively unknown and represents an ideal subject for examination and photography with the clinical specular microscope. Figure 19-9 shows the endothelium of a 68-year-old woman both before and after combined extracapsular cataract extraction and intraocular lens insertion. The cornea remained thin and clear. A 70 percent loss of central endothelial cells had occurred, however, which could be documented only by endothelial photography. By comparing the endothelial damage associated with different intraocular lenses and techniques of insertion, one can obtain an objective appraisal of the corneal effects of this surgical procedure.

Endothelial photography with the specular microscope is useful at all stages in the clinical management of keratoplasties. First, a record of the appearance of the donor endothelium can be obtained before transplantation procedures [1, 8]. The effects of various corneal preservation techniques can be studied and documented, and the immediate effects of surgical trauma can be observed and recorded. Figure 19-10 shows the endothelium of a penetrating corneal graft 24 hours after transplantation. The endothelial monolayer is intact. By comparison with preoperative photographs of the donor cornea, endothelial cell loss resulting from the surgical procedure itself can be documented.

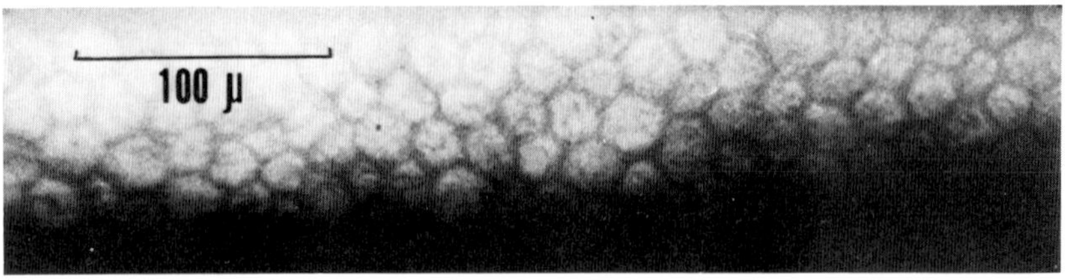

Preoperation 2730 Cells/mm^2

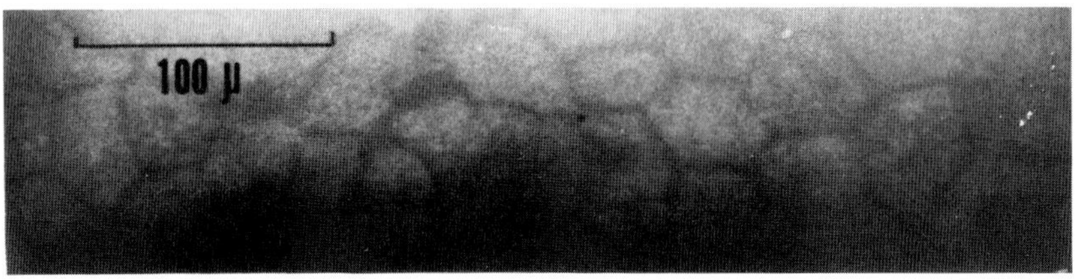

2 Wk postoperation 834 Cells/mm^2

Fig. 19-9. Central endothelium before and after extracapsular cataract extraction and intraocular lens implantation. (From W. M. Bourne, B. E. McCarey, and H. E. Kaufman, Clinical specular microscopy. Trans. Am. Acad. Ophthalmol. Otolaryngol. *81 : 743–753, 1976.)*

Fig. 19-10. Endothelium of penetrating corneal transplant 24 hours following keratoplasty. (From W. M. Bourne, B. E. McCarey, and H. E. Kaufman, Clinical specular miscroscopy. Trans. Am. Acad. Ophthalmol. Otolaryngol. *81 : 743–753, 1976.)*

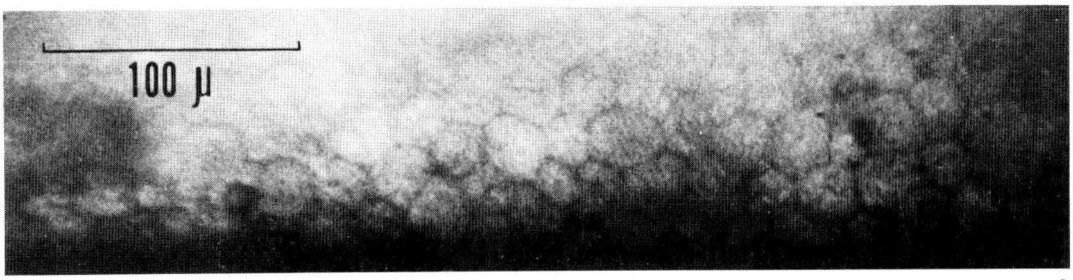

Aphakic, 3 wk postoperation 2444 Cells/mm^2

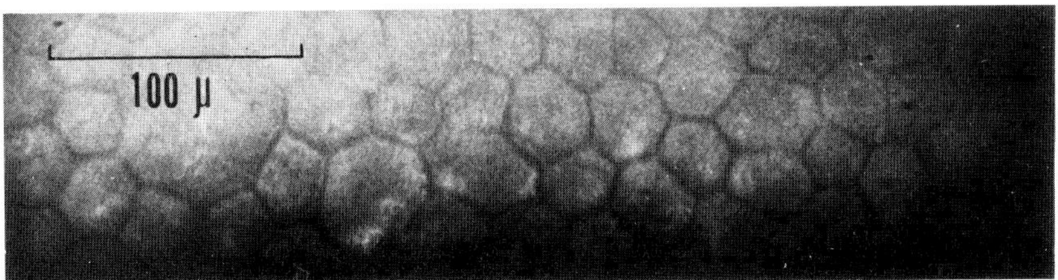

Phakic, 3 wk postoperation 1056 Cells/mm^2

Fig. 19-11. Endothelium of mated donor corneas 3 weeks after transplantation into phakic and aphakic eyes. (From W. M. Bourne, B. E. McCarey, and H. E. Kaufman, Clinical specular microscopy. Trans. Am. Acad. Ophthalmol. Otolaryngol. *81 : 743–753, 1976.)*

It is a clinical impression that endothelial damage to the donor cornea occurs more frequently during transplantation procedures in phakic than in aphakic recipient eyes. Damage is presumed to be caused by contact between the donor button and the recipient iris in the shallow anterior chamber of the phakic eye before the graft is sewn in place. This hypothesis was tested by transplanting corneas from the same donor to a phakic and an aphakic patient on the same day. No operative or postoperative difficulties occurred, and the grafts remained clear. Figure 19-11 shows the endothelium of both transplants 3 weeks following keratoplasty. The endothelial cell density in the phakic graft is much less, thus supporting the hypothesis. A prospective study confirmed that more endothelial cells are lost during phakic than during aphakic keratoplasty [6].

Conclusion

Excellent photographs of corneal endothelial cells may be obtained during clinical examinations with the specular microscope. Endothelial photographs are extremely useful in documenting the corneal effects of ocular trauma, aging, inflammation, and surgery. An objective appraisal of various ocular surgical techniques and their effect on the corneal endothelium is possible. This new photographic technique provides information that can improve both the diagnosis and the therapy of corneal diseases.

References

1. Bourne, W. M. Examination and photography of donor corneal endothelium. *Arch. Ophthalmol.* 94 : 1799, 1976.
2. Bourne, W. M., Brubaker, R. F., and O'Fallon, W. M. Use of air to decrease endothelial cell loss during intraocular lens implantation. *Arch. Ophthalmol.* 97 : 1473, 1979.
3. Bourne, W. M., and Enoch, J. M. Some optical principles of the clinical specular microscope. *Invest. Ophthalmol.* 15 : 29, 1976.
4. Bourne, W. M., and Kaufman, H. E. Specular microscopy of normal human endothelium in vivo. *Am. J. Ophthalmol.* 81 : 319, 1976.
5. Bourne, W. M., McCarey, B. E., and Kaufman, H. E. Clinical specular microscopy. *Trans. Am. Acad. Ophthalmol. Otolaryngol.* 81 : 743–753, 1976.
6. Bourne, W. M., and O'Fallon, W. M. Endothelial cell loss during penetrating keratoplasty. *Am. J. Ophthalmol.* 85 : 760, 1978.
7. Brown, N. Macrophotography of the anterior segment of the eye. *Br. J. Ophthalmol.* 54 : 697, 1970.
8. Hoefle, F. B., Maurice, D. M., and Sibley, R. C. Methods of Evaluating Corneal Donor Material. In J. A. Capella, H. F. Edelhauser, and D. L. VanHorn (Eds.), *Corneal Preservation.* Springfield, Ill.: Thomas, 1973. Pp. 96–108.
9. Laing, R. A., Sandstrom, M. M., and Leibowitz, H. M. In vivo photomicrography of the corneal endothelium. *Arch. Ophthalmol.* 93 : 143, 1975.
10. Maurice, D. M. Cellular membrane activity in the corneal endothelium of the intact eye. *Experientia* 24 : 1094, 1968.

20

Techniques and Applications of Endothelial Specular Photomicrography

JAMIE NICHOLL AND
TERRANCE L. TOMER

Specular photomicrography is a new and important area of ophthalmic photography which uses the principle of specular reflection to observe and photograph the corneal endothelium in vivo. Not only is this technique in demand as a method of evaluating the endothelium but, by providing the basic material for detailed analysis of the living endothelium, specular photomicrographs have led to new areas of corneal research.

Corneal Anatomy

The cornea is the transparent, curved structure covering the anterior portion of the eye. It is composed of five layers, the most anterior of which is the epithelium, followed by Bowman's membrane, the stroma, Descemet's membrane, and, finally, the endothelium, the most posterior surface. Behind the endothelium lies the aqueous of the anterior chamber, which nourishes the not normally vascularized cornea [35]. The endothelium is a single continuous layer of polygonal cells about 4 to 6μ thick; it has an average cell density of 1600 to 4000 cells per square millimeter, with a mean cell density of 2800 cells per square millimeter [30]. Although the endothelium is a rather leaky barrier between the passive hydration pressure of the stroma and the fluid of the aqueous, it also pumps fluid out of the cornea by an active metabolic transport process which maintains normal corneal deturgescence [11, 19].

History of Specular Photomicrography

The function of the endothelium has been known since the late 1800s, but clinical observation was not possible until 1920 when Vogt [32] introduced the technique of specular reflection with the biomicroscope. Previously, only flat preparations could be used to study the endothelium, and these methods were unsatisfactory because the delicate endothelial cells are easily altered by the fixing and staining process

This chapter is adapted from an article that appeared in the *Journal of Ophthalmic Photography* (2[2] : 73–77, 1979) and is published with permission from the Ophthalmic Photographers' Society.
The authors wish to extend a grateful acknowledgment to Vicki A. Berardi for her assistance in the preparation of this chapter.

[29]. For this reason, an instrument to observe endothelial cells in situ was needed.

In 1968, Maurice [18] pioneered the development of the specular microscope for in situ photography of the corneal endothelium. In 1975, Laing, Sandstrom, and Leibowitz [15] published further developments on this microscope for in vivo photography and, in 1976, Bourne and Kaufman [8] modified it for routine clinical photography.

Visualizing the Endothelium by Specular Reflection

The principle of specular reflection makes it possible to visualize and photograph this highly reflective transparent surface. A narrow beam of light is focused on and reflected from the interface of the corneal endothelium and aqueous [28]. The optical axis of the incident and reflected light form a critical angle that is split by a plane vertical to the surface at the point of the focus [1]. Differences in the reflective quality of the endothelium cause the cell borders to appear dark [2].

Specular reflection can be achieved with a slit lamp and is a commonly used technique to examine the endothelium clinically. Photographs can be made using a slit lamp with ×40 magnification and a ×2 accessory lens [1]; however, they do not contain sufficient endothelial matrix detail as a result of low magnification. There are several methods of obtaining specular photomicrographs, the most widely used of which is the contact specular microscope as developed by Laing and associates [15] and modified by Bourne and Kaufman [8] for routine clinical photography.

Optics of the Contact Specular Microscope

A knowledge of the contact specular microscope's optics is important in evaluating photographic results and problems. The instrument is basically a high-power slit lamp that misuses the optics of a microscope objective lens [18]. Incident light passes through an adjustable slit aperture and a condensing lens and is then directed off axis through one side of a ×20 objective lens system consisting of a microscope objective and a water immersion dripping cone lens that applanates the cornea. The slit of light is focused on the corneal endothelium and reflected back through the objective lens system on the side opposite the incident light beam. It proceeds through an eyepiece lens and is then directed either to the viewing system or the film plane of a 35-mm camera at magnifications up to ×200 (Fig. 20-1). The dipping cone lens can be moved back and forth over a range of 2 mm, and the image is focused by varying the distance within the objective lens system between the dipping cone and the objective lenses. All other optical distances are fixed. In this way, variations in corneal thickness are accommodated and measurable. The variation in magnification caused by corneal thicknesses is less than 1 percent [5].

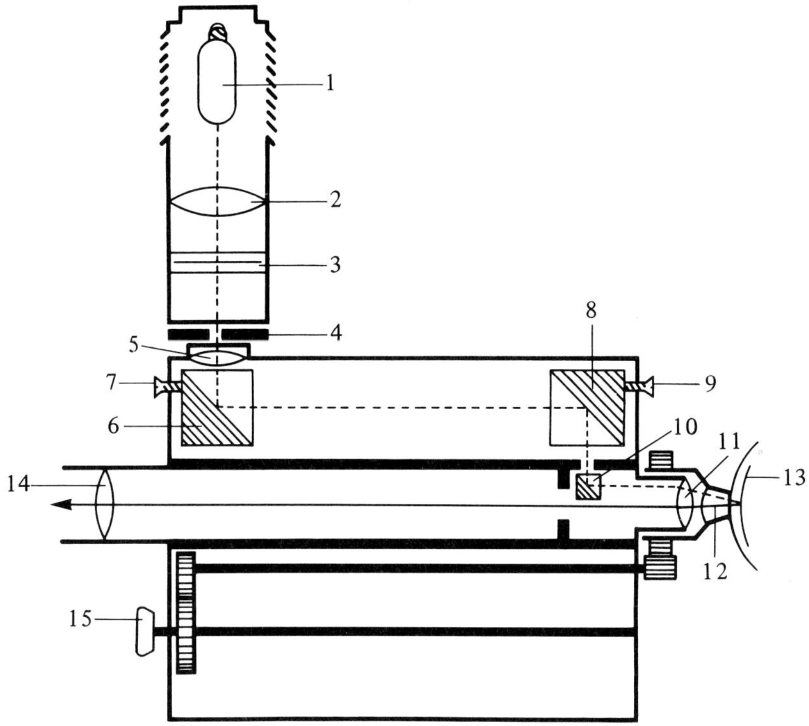

Fig. 20-1. Clinical specular microscope. 1 = *viewing light;* 2 = *condensing lens;* 3 = *flashtube;* 4 = *slit aperture;* 5 = *condensing lens;* 6 = *reflecting prism;* 7 = *prism adjustment;* 8 = *reflecting prism;* 9 = *prism adjustment;* 10 = *reflecting prism;* 11 = *objective lens;* 12 = *dipping cone lens;* 13 = *endothelial aqueous interface;* 14 = *eyepiece lens;* 15 = *fine focusing mechanism.* (*Reprinted with permission from the* J. Ophthal. Photo. *2(2) : 73–77, 1979. Ophthalmic Photographers' Society, Inc.*)

A few adjustments will affect the image (Fig. 20-1). Adjustment screws on the tungsten lamp socket permit its proper alignment with the adjustable slit aperture which must be kept narrow [21]. Widening the slit in an attempt to increase the field will correspondingly increase light scatter from the other corneal layers, fogging the image. Two prisms in the incident light path can be adjusted to move reflections out of the visible field, restoring the critical angle necessary for specular reflection. Masking the eyepiece lens reduces the scattered light and improves contrast [28].

Patient Management and Photographic Procedure

A slit-lamp examination should be performed before the procedure to verify that the cornea is intact. Corneal abrasions, basement membrane dystrophies, and active infections should not be applanated.

As with any type of ophthalmic photography, the photographer should inform the patient what is expected of him or her and explain the procedure, thereby assuring the patient's cooperation. The lens should be cleaned before each patient is photographed. A topical anesthetic is instilled in the eye to permit comfortable contact of the lens with the cornea. Inform the patient to expect to feel a slight pressure as the lens touches the eye.

Properly position the patient's head at the camera and provide a fixation target. Then adjust the camera in relationship to the eye by means of the "joystick" and vertical adjustment. Bring the applanation lens in contact with the cornea. The endothelial image is then brought into focus with the fine focusing mechanism.

Patient cooperation is essential. The photographer must be aware of the patient's movements to avoid excessive applanation because the dipping cone lens is rigid. To avoid abrading the cornea, do not slide the lens across the cornea. Proper applanation with the lens should cause only slight epithelial irregularities.

Specular photomicrographs might not be obtainable on some patients who have stromal edema, which could obscure the view of the endothelium, or on patients with excessive tears, which fog the image and make focusing difficult. Patients fitted with a bandage lens can be photographed as long as the combined thickness of the lens and cornea does not exceed the focusing range of the microscope.

The photographer should be aware of the effects the patient's normal eye movements, breathing, blinking, and lack of fixation can have on obtaining proper applanation. The high magnification amplifies the eye movements and makes it difficult to focus the moving field of cells. Uniform applanation of the dipping cone lens on the curved corneal surface is important. Eccentric applanation can cause dark streaks in the image. These are not areas of cell loss but are shadows possibly caused by wrinkles in the anterior corneal layers [28]. Changing the applanation slightly and keeping the dipping cone lens perpendicular to the cornea can eliminate many of these streaks.

Photographic Technique

Several major problems affect the resulting photographic image produced by contact specular microscopes: The half aperture light path restricts the field size and the high magnification results in low light levels. A flash unit is used with Kodak Tri-X pan film for clinical photography.

The negative density is uneven from edge to edge because the light scattered from the anterior corneal layer fogs the image. This scattered illumination, together with the film characteristics of low contrast and poor resolution, cause these negatives to be of low contrast. Develop the film for contrast in Kodak D-11 stock solution at 70°F for 6 or 7 minutes; this will also increase the film grain. Even well-focused negatives give poor resolution of the endothelial matrix. To study the endothelial cell patterns in detail, either positive transparencies or prints are necessary. The negatives can be copied on Kodak Technical Pan High Contrast Copy Film 2415 and developed in Kodak D-11 1 : 1 at 70°F for 7 minutes. Prints are difficult because photographic papers do not have the same latitude as films. To increase contrast and overcome density variations, use a high-contrast paper and burn in the denser areas of the negative (Fig. 20-2).

Recent Advances

Heyer-Schulte has improved the original design of the Syber specular microscope, modernizing it by making it more compact and easier to operate. The power supply was converted to solid state, which provides a recycling time of less than 5 seconds. A quartz halogen lamp is now used, and an electronic digital pachometer which provides automatic display of corneal thickness has been incorporated into the system. A video system is now offered with electronic printer and Polaroid attachment, and an interchangeable objective lens is available to convert the microscope for eye bank use.

In 1978, McCarey presented a noncontact specular microscope for clinical use [20] that consisted of a macrophotography unit attached to the tonometer mounting post of a slit lamp. The macrophotography unit incorporated a single-lens reflex camera, extension tube, tele-extender and objective lens. It provided a larger viewing area and greater depth of field than a contact specular microscope.

Recently Nikon introduced a noncontact specular microscope. Magnifications from ×10 to ×28 at the film plane with ×60 to ×168 through the viewfinder are obtained using a ×10 objective lens and accessory teleconvertor lenses. The lower magnification permits the use of slower films. A ×2 or ×5 objective lens can be used for macrophotography of the anterior segment [13].

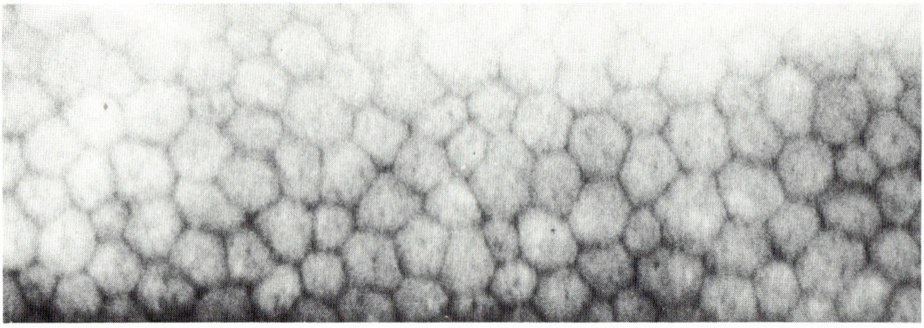

A

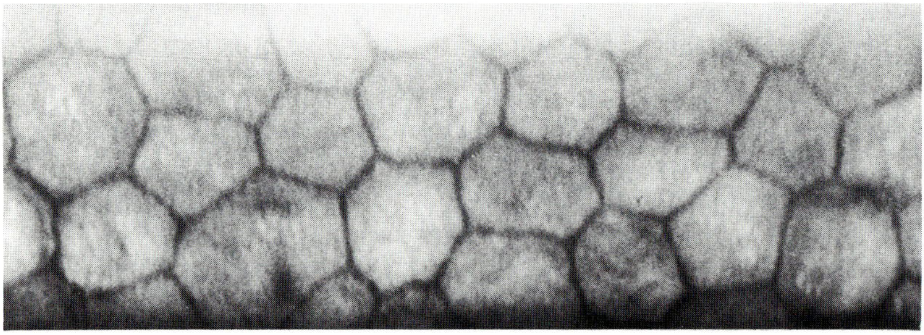

B

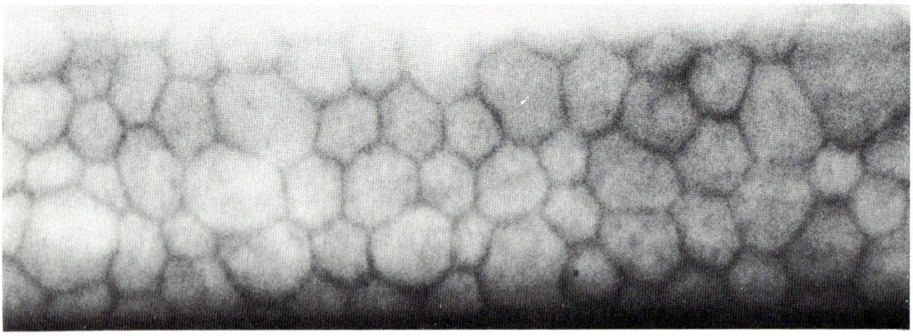

C

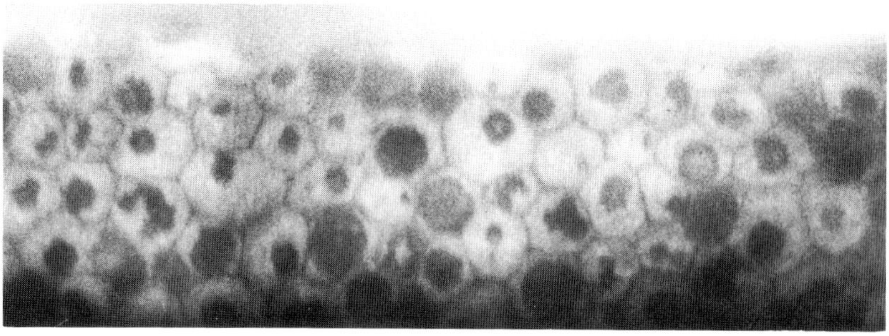

D

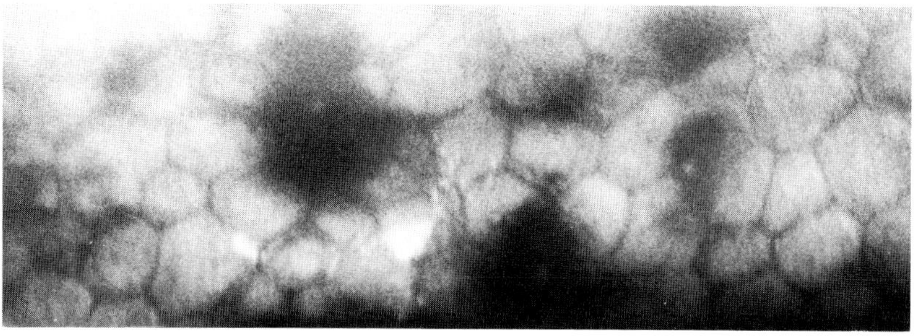

E

Fig. 20-2. Specular photomicrographs showing (A) *endothelial pattern typical of a young normal cornea;* (B) *endothelium of relatively low cell density;* (C) *endothelial pattern exhibiting varying cell size;* (D) *widespread endothelial changes;* (E) *mild guttata in Fuchs' endothelial dystrophy. (Reprinted with permission from the* J. Ophthal. Photo. *2(2) : 73–77, 1979. Ophthalmic Photographers' Society, Inc.)*

Carl Zeiss, Inc. has introduced an "endothelial microscope attachment" for use on its photo slit lamp. A cone-shaped lens fits over the objective lens of the slit lamp. Magnifications of ×14, ×22, and ×34 at the film plane are obtained using the slit lamp auxiliary lens system. Viewing magnifications of ×100, ×160, and ×250 are obtained using ×12.5 eyepieces [34].

These instruments have made endothelial photography readily accessible. The future of specular photomicrography could be influenced by the recent introduction of the scanning mirror microscope [14], a wide-field contact specular microscope developed for in vivo photography. By its use of a multisided oscillating mirror, the scanning mirror microscope's field of view is reported to be 20 to 25 times that of the contact specular microscope [12].

Applications

Specular photomicrography is being used for clinical and research purposes. With specular photomicrography, it is possible to see and photograph early changes in endothelial cell morphology, such as guttatae, before they are evident by slit-lamp biomicroscopy [4].

Specular photomicrographs are used to determine precisely the size, shape, and density of endothelial cells. There are several methods of calculating endothelial cell density [5, 23, 27, 33]. The Heyer-Schulte endothelial microscope has a calibrated grid that can be inserted into the light path and superimposed on every photograph; cell density can thus be determined by counting the cells in a known area. Cell density as well as individual cell size and shape can also be determined by programmable calculator analysis [16] and computerized image analysis [25, 26].

Specular photomicrography primarily serves a documentary function. It permits accurate appraisal and comparison, allowing, for example, study and evaluation of the effects of aging, drugs, disease, trauma, and surgery [31]. In one of several investigations using specular photomicrography of the effects of aging on the corneal endothelium, Laing and associates [16] reported decreasing endothelial cell density and increasingly variable cell size with age in a study of 61 normal individuals ranging from 20 to 89 years. Bourne and Kaufman [8] studied 40 normal individuals ranging in age from 6 to 87 years and also reported a cell density decrease with age that bore no correlation to corneal thickness. Laule and associates [17] supported these findings in a study using noncontact specular photomicrography of 152 normal individuals, 97 females and 55 males ranging in age from 3 to 88 years. Cell densities of both eyes were reported to be similar, with no sex-related differences.

Changes in cell density, size, and shape are evidence that endothelial cells rarely replicate but rather spread and enlarge to cover areas of cell loss. This could indicate that the functional reserve of the endothelium as a whole can be compromised [2].

Through preoperative and postoperative photographs, we can make an objective measurement of cell loss caused by surgical trauma. Bourne and Kaufman [6] found no detectable cell loss following cataract extraction in 12 of 16 patients; cell loss was more likely to occur after complicated surgery. They proposed that specular photomicrography might more accurately predict which corneas could be at risk for surgery. In another study, they reported a high percentage of cell loss following intraocular lens implantation [7]. Binkhorst [2] reported only 6.7 percent decrease in cell density following intraocular lens implantation. Since little is known about the long-term effects of intraocular lenses, specular photomicrography contributes to an objective analysis of this surgical procedure.

One of the most valuable clinical uses of specular photomicrography is in corneal transplantation [24]. The donor corneal endothelium can be photographed before excision [22] or after preservation [3] and can be evaluated for cell density, guttatae, and other features that could reflect its viability. Specular photomicrography allows a more critical evaluation of donor tissue and could ensure greater success in corneal grafting by helping to eliminate unsuitable tissue.

Bourne and Kaufman [9] studied 36 clear corneal transplants that occurred from 1 to 19 years postsurgery. They reported no correlation between cell density and corneal thickness or method of preservation, and that cell density decreased with age, as is expected with normal corneas. Rao and coworkers [26] reported that an amazingly low number of cells, 44 cells per square millimeter, can maintain a clear corneal transplant. These findings suggest that the number of endothelial cells might not be the only factor in the maintenance of corneal transparency.

Conclusion

Specular photomicrography has provided a better understanding of the living cornea and its physiology. Recent advances in instrumentation and technique have firmly established it as a necessary objective tool in the evaluation of the corneal endothelium. The ophthalmic photographer has the opportunity to play a vital role in this challenging new field of research.

References

1. Allen, L. Slit-lamp photography. In J. Justice, Jr. (Ed.), Ophthalmic Photography. *Int. Ophthalmol. Clin.* 16(2) : 145, 1976.
2. Binkhorst, C. D., Nygaard, P., and Loones, L. H. Specular microscopy of the corneal endothelium and lens implant surgery. *Am. J. Ophthalmol.* 85 : 597, 1978.
3. Bourne, W. M. Examination and photography of donor corneal endothelium. *Arch. Ophthalmol.* 94 : 1799, 1976.
4. Bourne, W. M. Photography of the corneal endothelium. In J. Justice, Jr. (Ed.), Ophthalmic Photography. *Int. Ophthalmol. Clin.* 16(2) : 199, 1976.
5. Bourne, W. M., and Enoch, J. M. Some optical principles of the clinical specular microscope. *Invest. Ophthalmol.* 15 : 29, 1976.
6. Bourne, W. M., and Kaufman, H. E. Cataract extraction and the corneal endothelium. *Am. J. Ophthalmol.* 82 : 44, 1976.
7. Bourne, W. M., and Kaufman, H. E. Endothelial damage associated with intraocular lenses. *Am. J. Ophthalmol.* 81 : 482, 1976.
8. Bourne, W. M., and Kaufman, H. E. Specular microscopy of human corneal endothelium in vivo. *Am. J. Ophthalmol.* 81 : 319, 1976.
9. Bourne, W. M., and Kaufman, H. E. The endothelium of clear corneal transplants. *Arch. Ophthalmol.* 94 : 1730, 1976.
10. Bourne, W. M., McCarey, B. E., and Kaufman, H. E. Clinical specular microscopy. *Trans. Am. Acad. Ophthalmol. Otolaryngol.* 81 : 743, 1976.
11. Dikstein, S., and Maurice, D. M. The metabolic basis to the fluid pump in the cornea. *J. Physiol.* 221 : 29, 1972.
12. Gunby, P. Microscopic scrutiny reveals condition of cornea. *J. A. M. A.* 243 : 1320, 1980.
13. Johnson, J. L., and Rosenthaler, T. D. A study of photographic techniques using the Nikon non-contact endothelial/anterior segment camera system. *J. Ophthal. Photo.* 3 : 7, 1980.

14. Koester, C. J., Campbell, C. J., and Donn, A. Ophthalmic optical instruments: Two recent developments. *Jpn. J. Ophthalmol.* 24 : 1, 1980.
15. Laing, R. A., Sandstrom, M. A., and Leibowitz, H. M. In vivo photomicrography of the corneal endothelium. *Arch. Ophthalmol.* 93 : 143, 1975.
16. Laing, R. A., Sandstrom, M. M., Berrospi, A. R., and Leibowitz, H. M. Changes in the corneal endothelium as a function of age. *Exp. Eye. Res.* 22 : 587, 1976.
17. Laule, A., Cable, M. K., Hoffman, C. E., and Hanna, C. Endothelial cell population changes of human cornea during life. *Arch. Ophthalmol.* 96 : 2031, 1978.
18. Maurice, D. M. Cellular membrane activity in the corneal endothelium of the intact eye. *Experientia* 24 : 1094, 1968.
19. Maurice, D. M. The location of the fluid pump in the cornea. *J. Physiol.* 221 : 43, 1972.
20. McCarey, B. E. Non-contact specular microscopy of corneal endothelium. *Invest. Ophthalmol. Vis. Sci.* 17 (Suppl.): 118, 1978.
21. McCarey, B. E. Specular microscopy: Practical aspects for the researcher and clinician. In H. Kaufman and T. Zimmerman (Eds.), *Current Concepts in Ophthalmology.* St. Louis: Mosby, 1979. P. 174.
22. McCarey, B. E., and McNeill, J. I. Specular microscopic evaluation of donor corneal endothelium. *Ann. Ophthalmol.* 9 : 1279, 1977.
23. Olsen, T. Optical principles for estimation of endothelial cell density with the non-contact specular microscope. *Acta Ophthalmol.* 57 : 860, 1979.
24. Polack, F. M. *Corneal Transplantation.* New York: Grune & Stratton, 1977. Pp. 87–89.
25. Rao, G. N., Shaw, E. L., Stevens, R. E., and Aquavella, J. V. Automated pattern analysis of corneal endothelium. *Ophthalmology* 86 : 1367, 1979.
26. Rao, G. N., Waldron, W. R., and Aquavella, J. V. Morphology of graft endothelium and donor age. *Brit. J. Ophthalmol.* 64 : 523, 1980.
27. Schutten, W. H., and Schultz, R. O. A new method for determining corneal endothelial cell density from specular photomicrographs. *Arch. Ophthalmol.* 98 : 552, 1980.
28. Sherrard, E. S. Specular microscopy of the corneal endothelium. *The Ophthalmic Optician.* Oct. 1, 1977. P. 709.
29. Stocker, F. W. *The Endothelium of the Cornea and its Clinical Implications* (2nd ed.). Springfield, Ill.: Thomas, 1971. Pp. 9–39.
30. Stocker, F. W. *The Endothelium of the Cornea and its Clinical Implications* (2nd ed.). Springfield, Ill.: Thomas, 1971. P. 25.
31. Sugar, A. Clinical specular microscopy. *Surv. Ophthalmol.* 24 : 21, 1979.
32. Vogt, A. H. Die sichtbarkeit des lebenden Hornhaut-Endothels. *Albrecht von Graefes Arch. Ophthalmol.* 101 : 123, 1920.
33. Waring, G. D., Krohn, M. A., Ford, G. E., Harris, R. R., and Rosenblatt, L. S. Four methods of measuring human corneal endothelial cells from specular photomicrographs. *Arch. Ophthalmol.* 98 : 848, 1980.
34. Warnicki, J. W. The Zeiss endothelial lens. Presented at the 10th Annual Meeting of the Ophthalmic Photographers' Society, San Francisco, 1979.
35. Wolff, E. *Anatomy of the Eye and Orbit* (7th ed.). Philadelphia: Saunders, 1976. P. 45.

21

Cinematography in Ophthalmology

ARTHUR SMIALOWSKI

Motion picture photography in ophthalmology is usually confined to short-sequence filming of an operation or of a patient in the studio. Cinematography is helpful as an aid in followup care of patients with motility disorders, and it is particularly useful in teaching and research. It is seldom desirable to present lengthy movies to professional audiences since the lecturer usually has a limited time to deliver a presentation. Brief and precise films are used to supplement or clarify a point. The single concept motion pictures are generally silent, and the speaker provides a narration to the movie and can adjust the commentary to meet the needs of the audience. Motion pictures with sound have the advantage that the topic can be understood without the presence of a lecturer.

If publication is contemplated, it is best to have still photographs taken during filming to obtain the best results. When this is not possible, single motion picture frames can be copied and prints of adequate quality made for publication.

In this chapter an outline of the basic techniques of cinematography in ophthalmology will be presented.

Operating Room Cinematography

The filming of surgical operations requires organized planning. Before the operation, the surgeon will give the photographer pertinent information regarding the specific type of movie required. This data includes the type of surgery, length of coverage, and the purpose of the movie. Usually the photographer is notified the day before surgery; however, on occasion, the photographer will be called to record an unusual event at a moment's notice. For this reason the following checklist is invaluable:

1. Name of surgeon
2. Name of patient
3. Consent for photographs
4. Date of operation
5. Time of operation
6. Type of operation

For their help with the manuscript, I would like to thank Ann Smialowski, Linda A. Huett, and Thomas Liesegang, M.D.

7. Right or left eye
8. General views
9. Operating room number
10. Short or long filming
11. Camera and close-up lenses
12. Exposure meter
13. Adequate film
14. Camera stand
15. Lights, spare bulbs
16. Extension cord (operating room approved)
17. Specialized equipment (microsurgery)
18. Notebook, marker pen, tape
19. Still camera (if needed)

Under ordinary circumstances, a surgical operating room consists of sterile and nonsterile areas. The sterile areas include a draped operating table, a draped instrument table, a gowned surgeon, an assistant, and a circulating nurse. Precise information concerning sterile and nonsterile areas must be obtained from the operating room circulating nurse. Before entering the operating room, the photographer is obliged to put on the designated clothing. The camera stand used near the operating table must be draped in sterile sheets. The photographer should conduct himself in a professional manner and not make personal remarks, since many surgical procedures are performed under local anesthesia.

Camera and Lens

Super 8 film size cameras are used for special purposes as well as everyday use. The disadvantage of Super 8 films is that the image quality projected on a large screen is poor. The standard film size for photography in medicine is 16-mm motion picture film because it gives a good quality image on a large screen and the equipment is reasonably priced. The projection equipment for this size film is readily available in teaching institutions and at medical conventions.

The ideal motion picture camera for operating room use should be light, preferably under 10 pounds. The camera must have single-lens reflex viewing and focusing and accept 100- and 400-foot film rolls. A shutter speed of 24 frames per second is necessary for standard filming; slower and faster shutter speeds should be available for special purposes. A slower shutter speed of 16 frames per second is sometimes necessary to gain more light for operating microscope cinematography. Provision for single-frame exposures is useful in making titles, animation, and time lapse photography. There are a number of excellent professional motion picture cameras on the market, such as Bolex, Eclair, Beaulieu, and Arriflex. The Arriflex 16 S/B is the ideal basic camera for the serious 16-mm filmmaker. It weighs approximately 8 pounds and has an excellent shutter speed range as well as through-the-lens focusing and viewing, which are essential in extreme close-up cinematography. The lenses available for this camera are numerous, ranging from several zoom lenses to lenses with fixed focal length. The camera accepts internally 100-foot film rolls and is designed to accept 400-foot rolls.

A worthwhile accessory is the periscopic finder attachment, which is especially useful when filming an operation from an awkward overhead position. This unique finder permits focusing and viewing from several positions, including those that would be almost impossible for the photographer to maintain during filming of some surgical eye operations.

Most ophthalmic cinematography is performed with zoom lenses, but fixed focal length macro lenses are useful for extreme close-ups and for high resolution. Equipped with a proper zoom lens and a set of supplementary close-up lenses, the ophthalmic photographer is ready to record fields ranging from a close-up of one eye to the entire body. A zoom lens of 12- to 120-mm zooming range is ideal for operating room photography. To cover the field adequately, two close-up attachments are necessary: a No. 1 attachment, which will allow coverage of an area of 2 inches in tele-position to 20 inches in wide-angle position, and a No. 2 attachment, which will cover approximately 1 inch in tele-position and 12 inches in wide-angle position. The advantage of a zoom lens is that it permits quick changing of the field size (Fig. 21-1).

Camera Stand

Filming surgical operations requires the use of a sturdy camera support. Tripod stands are not suitable because they take too much floor space. The heavy duty single central support stand, preferably with a horizontal bar, will allow the photographer to approach the operating room table closely. Custom-made ladders and platforms for camera supports are more appropriate for extensive operating room filming. The camera stand must be draped with sterile sheets, a job usually done, according to protocol, by the circulating nurse. The stand must be properly grounded to prevent an accumulation of static electricity.

Film and Lighting

The modern fast speed color films are used to record eye operations; the advantage of using them is that the available operating room lighting is sufficient for good film exposure. Kodak Ektachrome 16 mm and Super 8 film EF 7242 balanced for tungsten 3200° K of ASA 125 are popular films used to record both surgical procedures and studio work. These films permit cinematography of the eyes with lower light levels, resulting in minimal discomfort to the patient.

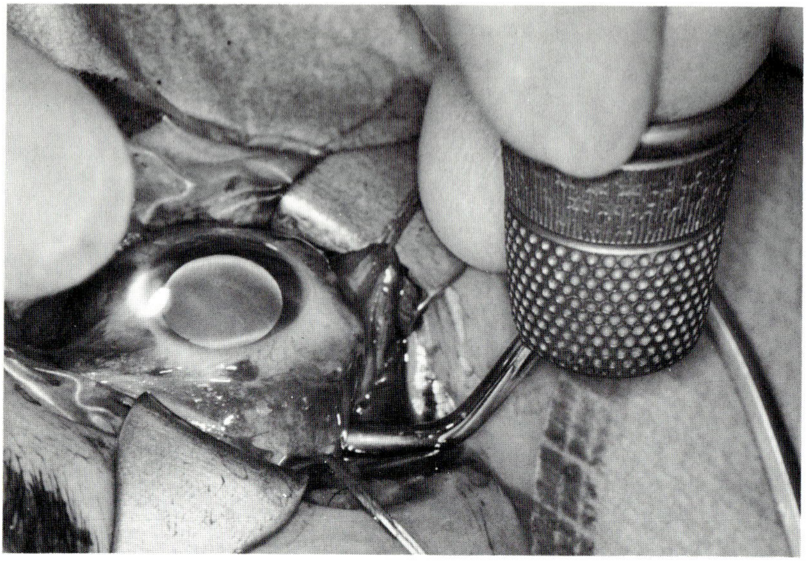

A

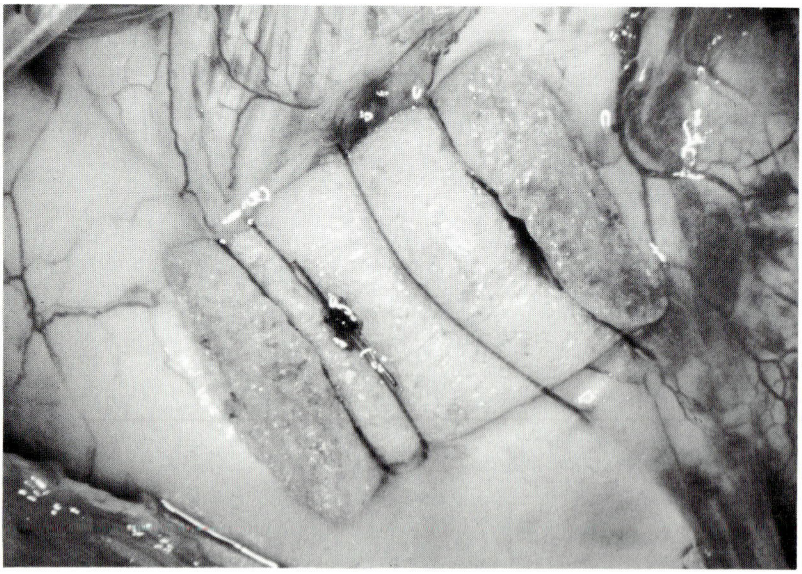

B

Fig. 21-1. Motion picture camera and lens for ophthalmic operating room photography must have single-lens reflex framing and focusing. Standard is a lens with a zoom range of 12–20 mm and close-up No. 1 and No. 2 attachments. With this equipment, it is possible to have a ready choice of several field sizes. (A) *Typical field for eye operations.* (B) *Close-up often necessary to depict details.*

Available operating room light will suffice to photograph most eye operations, but on occasion supplementary illumination is necessary (Fig. 21-2). An excellent operating room light (Bio-light), made especially for this purpose, is available from Art Bodkins of Boston. The Bio-light has a cool beam 650 watt lamp (either 3200° K or 5600° K), with a safety shield, barn doors, and an approved power cable. Other suppliers of good lighting for operating room filming are Color-Tran, Inc. and Mole-Richardson Company. When several light sources are used in operating room filming, it may be necessary to adjust the hue by using appropriate color correction filters.

Film Procedures

Today, there is a departure from the old filming routine of "beginning with the incision and ending with closure." The ophthalmologist is interested in case records, teaching aids, and research films, which usually depict concise information. The filming of eye operations is done with sound speed (24 frames per second) to accommodate later narration. This is a standard projection speed for motion picture projectors. Operating room motion pictures are not made to a scenario but follow the surgery and are made into a story sequence by editing. The exposure determination is calculated by the use of a sensitive spot light meter; the experienced photographer uses judgment in addition to the light meter. Slight adjustments are necessary to compensate for light and dark irides. When photographing the sclera, one should close the diaphragm by one f/stop; otherwise this white area will be overexposed. Before filming the surgical procedure, all pertinent data, such as name of patient, name of surgeon, type of surgery, date, and place, should be recorded. When using several film rolls, one should always identify the sequence. The exposed film is sent to the laboratory for processing, and a color work print is ordered.

Use of the Surgical Microscope

The operating room microscope is now used by many ophthalmic surgeons, and a number of new surgical techniques have evolved from its use. Some of the modern operating microscopes have provisions for a beam-splitter and an adapter for both still and motion picture photography. The earlier surgical microscopes had a separate lens system for photography, with the accompanying disadvantages of fixed magnification and a need for parallax adjustment. Because of the identical image and magnification in modern microscopes, cinematography can be almost completely automated. In spite of automation, however, the photographer still plays an important role: loading the camera, adjusting and maintaining equipment, editing the film, and acting as a liaison between the surgeon and the processing laboratory.

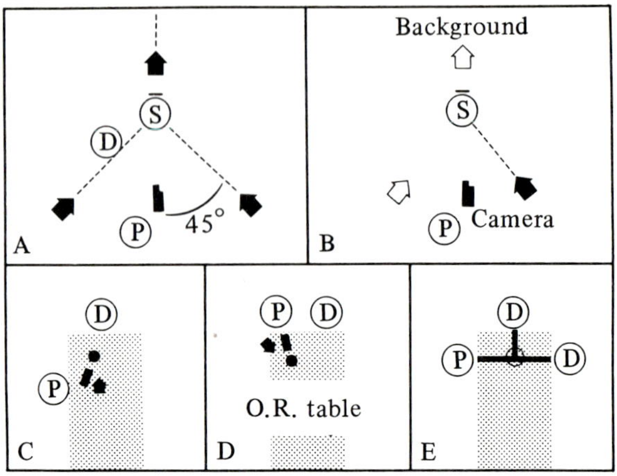

Fig. 21-2. Basic lighting arrangement of ophthalmic cinematography. D = *physician;* S = *patient;* P = *photographer;* arrow = *light 650 watt quartz 3200° K.* (A) *For photography of head and shoulders and close-up of eyes, two lights are used plus a third for background subject separation.* (B) *To photograph one eye, single light source is placed at temporal side.* (C and D) *Surgical operations are photographed with available light, which can be supplemented by one spotlight. Most common positions for filming are beside surgeon or on opposite side.* (E) *Photography through operating microscope can be done by surgeon, assistant, or photographer.*

Studio Cinematography

Cinematography in an ophthalmic photography studio is usually done to record unusual eye movements in patients with neuroophthalmologic problems. Patients with strabismus are followed preoperatively and postoperatively with cinematography to evaluate their progress. Usually, in routine ophthalmic studio cinematography, an outline is composed just before filming. The ophthalmologist or neuroophthalmologist informs the photographer of the pathologic conditions he or she wishes to record, and the photographer makes the appropriate technical arrangements. The camera and film described for use in the operating room are ideal for ophthalmic studio cinematography.

Lighting

Simple, standard lighting techniques are advisable for cinematography in an ophthalmic studio, since the patient may be photographed on several dates. The suggested light source is several 650 watt quartz 3200° K lamp heads on adjustable stands. For close-ups of both eyes, two lamp heads are positioned approximately 5 feet from the patient at a 45-degree angle. A third light can be used for background subject

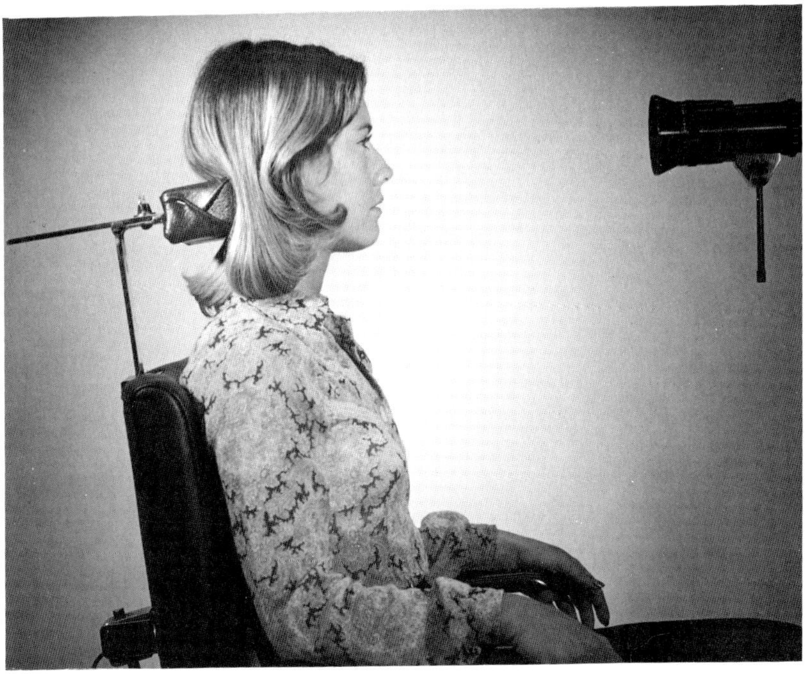

Fig. 21-3. Eye photography in the studio requires sturdy neck support. To maintain sharp focus and exact field, patient head immobilization and sturdy camera support are imperative.

separation. When only one eye is being filmed, the best results are obtained by using one light source placed on the temporal side of the patient. Slight repositioning of the light source will change the highlight emphasis.

Filming Procedure

When filming eye movements, it is desirable to have the ophthalmologist, who may wish to emphasize many subtle features, present. Before filming, the patient's name, diagnosis, physician's name, and date should be recorded. When filming either one or both eyes, one should zoom in to the whole head and finish by zooming out to the whole head. The zoom should be used sparingly; if the zoom footage is not needed, it can be eliminated during editing. The field must be tightly composed. A neck support is necessary; otherwise slight movements by the patient will result in out-of-focus films (Fig. 21-3). Many patients have photophobia with the bright lighting and need time to adjust before proceeding. The photographer should be patient, take more footage than necessary, and then edit the best (Fig. 21-4). He or she is judged not by the difficulties encountered but by the final result.

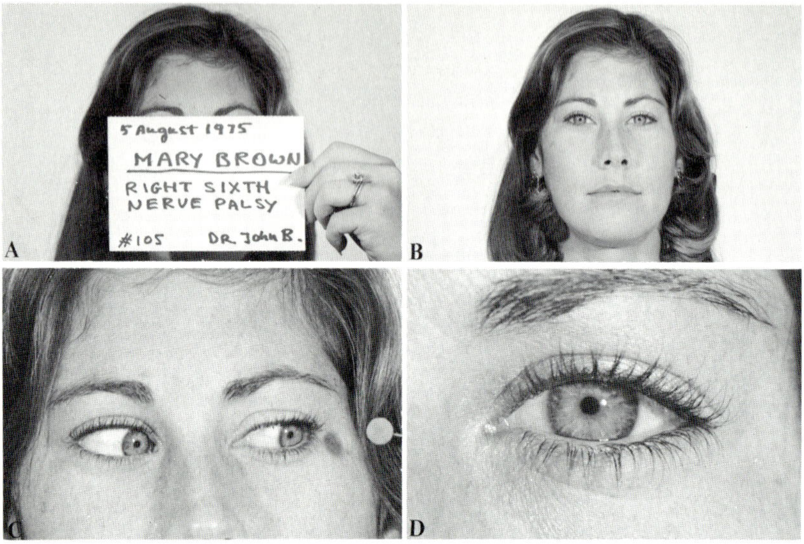

Fig. 21-4. Typical sequence of events in recording eye movements. (A) *Information card;* (B) *head shot;* (C) *zoom to two eyes, have physician direct gaze and include a pointer in the frame;* (D) *zoom to one eye close-up when necessary. Usual footage for eye movements is 100 feet per patient.*

Processing and Editing

On completion of filming, one should make sure that the rolls and boxes are numbered in sequence so that the processing laboratory will splice and develop them in the correct order. When film is sent to the laboratory for processing, special instructions should be given and a color work print ordered. The original film should not be used for projecting because if it is scratched, all subsequent copies will carry the defect.

The photographer should do the initial, rough editing of the work print; for final editing, it is necessary to have the ophthalmologist present. Editing takes an unspecified amount of time depending on subject matter, film length, and complexity of the motion picture. An institutional cinematographer seldom has the facilities for making titles, animation, or sound recording, but there are a number of excellent laboratories that supply these services at a reasonable cost.

The film should be stored in special dust-proof containers in a cool, low-humidity area. Filing and coding of films are critical. An index and cross-index of films will guarantee easy retrievability of material.

Cinematography is a demanding subspecialty of ophthalmic photography that requires dedication, organization, cooperation, and, most importantly, enthusiasm.

22

Television in Ophthalmology

JERRY SEWELL

Television can be a useful adjunct to an ophthalmology teaching program because, in comparison to photographic film, the video image is instantly accessible. There is no need to wait for the film to return from the processing lab to determine whether the exposure, focus, lighting, and color are correct: This information is displayed instantly on the monitor and can be immediately corrected. However, television does not have the range of sensitivity of photographic film and should not be expected to give as good resolution as film under extremely critical circumstances. Video equipment—cameras, camera control units, monitors, carts, and cables—is bulky and requires electricity to operate. The equipment can also be expensive, especially with the addition of a good editing system. Video recording can become cost-effective, however, if tapes of uninteresting procedures are erased and then reused until a sequence worth keeping is obtained [5].

Recording surgical procedures is valuable in the following ways:

1. Normal surgical techniques can be used to train surgeons and operating room nurses.
2. Unusual occurrences and remedial surgical actions can be shown.
3. Residents can review tapes of surgery for self-critique.
4. Portions of tapes can be extracted for production of teaching materials.

The primary instrument used to examine the anterior segment of the eye is the slit-lamp biomicroscope. The biomicroscope portion gives sufficient magnification to show the structures in the eye, and the parallel pipette of the slit illumination source reveals translucencies or semiopaque pathology. In surgery, of course, the operating microscope is essential in enlarging the surgeon's visual field.

It is in conjunction with these two instruments, the biomicroscope and the operating microscope, that the miniature television camera is most useful, primarily because it is small and lightweight. When a miniature camera is adapted for such use, some provision must be made for diverting part of the image from the viewer to the television camera. Usually diversion is achieved with a beam splitter and cine adapter, which take advantage of the optics of the operating microscope or the biomicroscope to achieve the magnification necessary for the final image on the television tube.

There are other circumstances in which television is useful in instruction. Envision a clinical ophthalmology session: The instructor examines the patient and the students crowd in to see the object of the session, the eye. The students must take turns examining the patient with instruments that light and magnify the structures of the eye, often to the patient's distress. A television camera and monitors can serve well in such situations, particularly if squint problems, wherein the dynamics of motility must be seen, are involved.

When using a biomicroscope for magnification, one must consider the limits of television in recording an unanesthetized eye. Color television requires substantial lighting, which the patient does not tolerate well. Likewise, the amount of light required through a fundus camera lens system for color television is prohibitive. Carl Zeiss, Inc. offers the Urban black-and-white television system adapted to a fundus camera for performing fluorescein angiography. There are color camera systems that use the indirect ophthalmoscope with a miniature color camera mounted on a helmet, but the resulting image size and resolution are barely acceptable.

Kowa and Circon Corporation are currently investigating the coupling of a sensitive color television camera with a fundus camera system. Research at the University of Illinois is emphasizing funduscopy, oximetry, blood flow, and dye dilution analysis through computer linkage [2].

The Problems of Magnification and Resolution

Two factors should be considered when selecting a television (or movie) lens for ophthalmic photography: magnification and working distance. A lens capable of 1 : 1 magnification is essential in demonstrating ophthalmic features on a television screen. One can obtain this or a greater magnification only by the use of macro lenses, supplementary + D lenses, extension tubes, or, as mentioned before, a biomicroscope system.

The second factor, the working distance, refers to the lens-to-subject distance. A working distance of 3 to 3½ feet at maximum zoom is recommended: This distance preserves the sterile field and allows the camera to be used over the surgeon's shoulder. Also, supplementary lights can be used in the operating field.

Whereas film resolution occurs at the microscopic level, the level of television resolution might be described as "macroscopic." A television picture is composed of scan lines that move rapidly across the face of the picture tube, giving the impression of a single image. The electronic control of these lines is known as *synchronization,* or *synch.* There are three basic synchronization systems, none of which is compatible with either of the others. The American standard system is called NTSC or EIA and consists of 525 horizontal scan lines. The European system is called PAL and consists of 625 lines. The French and Russians use a system called SECAM [1].

It is important to remember that using scan lines to define television resolution gives only an approximation and serves as a starting point for making comparisons.

Monitors and Monitor-Receivers

Television monitors are designed for picture playback only. The more expensive models (550 lines) are for studio use; they are more complicated than the cheaper monitor-receivers, which, in turn, are more forgiving of substandard video signals. A high-resolution color monitor-receiver has about 350 scan lines, and a black-and-white model has about 600 to 700 lines [1].

A standard television set can serve as a monitor if the video recorder is equipped with a radio frequency (RF) adapter that transmits a very low-power broadcast frequency. This adapter is connected to the television antenna lead by a 75- to 300-Ω adapter, and the video is displayed on Channel 2 [7].

To display a picture on several monitors, coaxial cables are connected from one set to another in a process known as *looping*. When several monitors are looped in a series, the last set must be terminated with the 75-Ω switch placed in the on position; the intermediary sets must have this switch in the off position (Fig. 22-1).

If television sets are used instead of monitors, an RF splitter is used with a 75- to 300-Ω transformer on each set. If more than four to six sets are to be used, or if the video signals are sent over a long distance, a video distribution amplifier, or RF amplifier, must be used to boost the signal (Fig. 22-1).

Television Systems

A television system can assume several configurations, depending on the desired end product (e.g., broadcast, video tape, or closed circuit) and on the amount of money available for equipment and personnel.

Consideration must be given to the quality and compatibility of the system's components: The maxim that the weakest link determines the strength of the chain holds true. For example, consider a color camera with a resolving power of 400 lines, a monitor with a resolving power of 350 lines, and a video tape recorder with a resolving power of 270 lines. The recorder is the controlling factor of quality in the system; in other words, it is a 270-line system. Then consider future components that could be of higher quality but limited by weak links.

The simplest system consists of a camera with a control unit and a monitor for live demonstrations. Add to these a recorder, and you have the potential for ex post facto analysis. For a more efficient presentation, add two editing video recorders and a computer control unit.

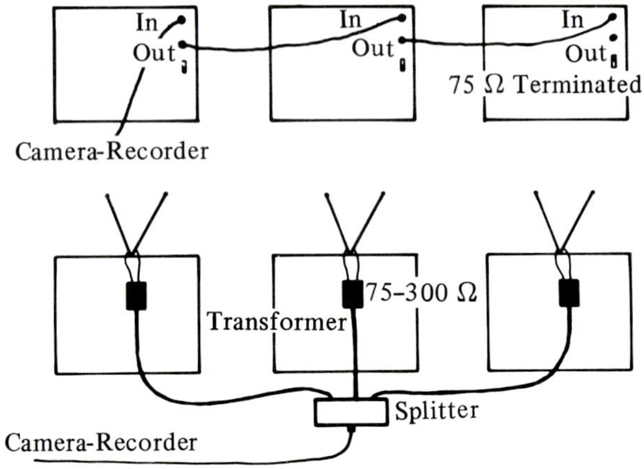

Fig. 22-1. Method of using monitors (top) *and television receivers* (bottom) *for large audiences.*

Other optional equipment for improving quality can include a wave form monitor, an image intensifier, an underscan and pulsecross monitor, a special-effects generator, and a time-base corrector [6].

The wave form monitor enables consistency from one recording session to another where conditions may vary. Its electronic display of the composite video signal serves as a starting point to calibrate color in the television cameras by signal analysis [7].

Among methods of overcoming apparent low resolution in the small-stripe tube video cameras, electronic image enhancement has been successful. In this process, the true resolving power of the system is not improved, but certain portions of the electronic signal are memorized on a time-delay basis and used to reinforce that same portion of the image; thus, you can see what appears to be more detail [6]. The trade-off for electronic enhancement is slightly more noise in the signal, which is also amplified. This may or may not be a problem, depending on whether you use multiple generation tape releases from the original recording.

A pulsecross and underscan monitor allow the technician to see portions of the video signal not ordinarily displayed on a monitor unless malfunctions are occurring; sync, tracking, and skew [7]. Special-effects generators allow the addition of special inserts, superimpositions, and transitions between edited segments. Time-base correctors will be discussed in the section Video Tape Recorders and Editors.

Miniature Cameras

There are many brands of miniature cameras, but one basic component, the striped video tube, is produced by only a few manufacturers worldwide. The question to answer, then, is how the electronics have been altered to improve the television system, if indeed they have been altered at all. It is virtually impossible to determine the quality of a miniature camera just by reading the statistics in the manufacturer's brochure. The camera should be placed in the proper operating environment and tried side by side with other cameras being considered for purchase. Only then can you determine which camera will best suit your needs. Contact people at institutions that use miniature cameras and ask about performance records and which cameras they would buy again. The track record of a camera is extremely important when making a final selection.

Most single-tube color cameras are of the striped-tube type. The stripes across the tube face consist of prismatic filters that separate light into the three primary colors—red, blue, and green. The colors then pass through the striped filter and are inclined by each stripe in such a way that they fall upon the target within the video tube. The separated light components are recombined electronically in a process called *frequency multiplexing,* similar to the signal on an FM stereo radio.

Some features to look for in a miniature camera are:

1. Pedestal control, which is responsible for setting the black level on the television sets.
2. Color correction filters that correct for the color temperature of the basic light source, which should be 3200° (Tungsten) and 5000° (daylight); some units have an additional filter selection for fluorescent lights, 4500°.
3. Color bars, which are used to set up the television monitor and calibrate the television equipment. This display function is usually found in the camera control unit and might not be present on all models.
4. Light level indicator, which indicates whether the camera is being overdriven; it is present on most miniature cameras.
5. Automatic gain control, which protects against overdriving the camera when too much light saturates the video tube.

Collateral equipment that should be purchased separately for use with a miniature color camera are a color chip chart, which displays various hues of color that can be achieved on the television monitor, and a gray scale, which is necessary for the proper setup and calibration of the miniature color camera.

Studio Cameras and Lenses

Studio cameras have a limited use in ophthalmology because of their size, weight, and need for attachment to a magnification system. Also, calibrating the studio camera requires the services of a well-trained technician. These cameras could have special application in orbital and muscle surgery and in demonstrating strabismus problems. When combined with a miniature camera, a broader perspective of the operating room can be shown.

To work together, the sync signals from the two cameras must be compatible, and a switcher is employed to blend the transitions from one scene to another. In live production, a simple switching device (a passive switcher) can be used without breakup noticeable to the audience. Since signal breakup will be recorded on video tape and therefore appear during editing, a more sophisticated switcher (an active or vertical interval switcher) must be used to prevent it if the procedure is to be recorded.

Studio cameras are used in the production graphics for teaching tapes. A simple rear projection screen and Carousel projector serve well for this technique. Remember that video graphics do not have the same format as 35-mm slides, and original materials must be placed in the video width-height ratio. The safe title area in video is a border one-tenth the height and width of the title card [7] (Fig. 22-2).

Black-and-white studio cameras of low-light level are suited for demonstrating strabismus. A single light for illumination and pupillary highlight detail should be used.

Video tubes for cameras come in several price ranges. The Vidicon is the least expensive and requires considerable light. Plumicons and Saticons are more sensitive and more expensive [1]. Any investment in this equipment for an ophthalmologic setup should be made with the advice of a qualified video engineer. For comparison, a broadcast camera has a color resolving power of around 550 lines compared to 250 to 270 lines for a closed-circuit color television camera.

Zoom lenses are standard for studio cameras because they can take a variety of shots. For ophthalmology, a zoom lens with a range of 10 : 1 or 12 : 1, a field of 1½ to 2 inches at maximum zoom, and a working distance (subject to lens) of at least 30 inches is desirable. When required, supplementary close-up lenses of +1, +2, and +3 D will allow greater magnification with a little distortion on the picture edges. Extension tubes permit greater magnification but negate the zooming effects because the focus is constantly changing. Lenses should be capped when not in use to prevent damage to the video tube caused by incidental light.

Video lenses often have a back-focus to adjust the rear lens to video tube distance. However, some cinema lenses might work and should be tried with the simpler cameras. Nikon offers a C-mount to 35-mm adapter that can be used on some of the smaller cameras; it gives a telephoto effect with approximately double the magnification [1].

Television Microscope Attachments

Galilean microscopes use parallel beams of light between components, allowing the attachment of optical beam-splitters that divert light from

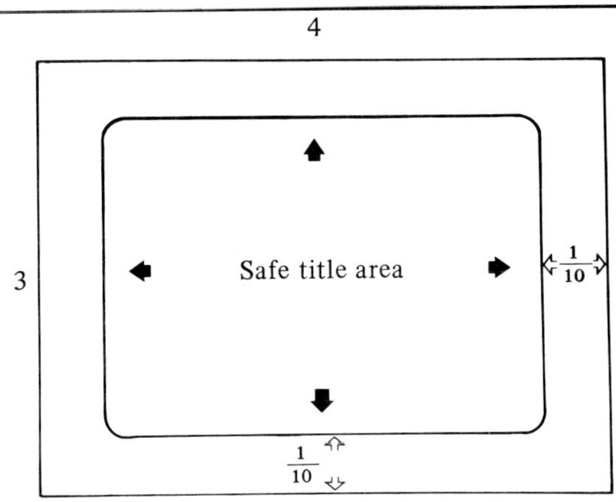

Fig. 22-2. Aspect ratio of 3 : 4 for making television graphics with a safety margin.

the primary observer to a secondary viewer [3, 4] (Fig. 22-3). Carl Zeiss, Inc. offers two beam-splitters that can be used in adapting television to a microscope: One diverts 50 percent of the observation light and the other diverts 70 percent. The surgeon who diverts 70 percent of the observation light to the television camera must be prepared to work at a reduced light level.

The 16-mm cine adapter readily accommodates the striped Vidicon tube and is responsible for imaging on the film plane or video tube. Its iris diaphragm controls the light. An adjustable intermittent C-mount adapter couples the cine adapter with the camera body (Fig. 22-3), and a threading collar brings the light from the cine adapter into sharp focus on the video tube.

House Urban and other manufacturers offer several options in beam-splitters and cine adapters to suit the needs of surgeons who want special configurations on their operating microscopes. A new device from Urban Engineering allows the photographer to focus the television camera by overriding the surgeon's focus. It is employed when the surgeon accommodates and the television picture is no longer parfocal (Fig. 22-4).

A cine adapter of 137-mm focal length is an f/8 system and produces an image of the same relative field seen by the surgeon. A 105-mm cine adapter is an f/7 system, and a 74-mm adapter is an f/5.6 system that requires about one-half the light as a 137-mm cine adapter but has a substantially reduced monitor field, with vignetting at the lower magnifications and high f/stop settings. When lighting is critical, as in some vitrectomies, it can be of value; for demonstration, however, the surgeon might have to use a higher magnification than is comfortable.

Sometimes it is desirable to have an image slightly larger than that

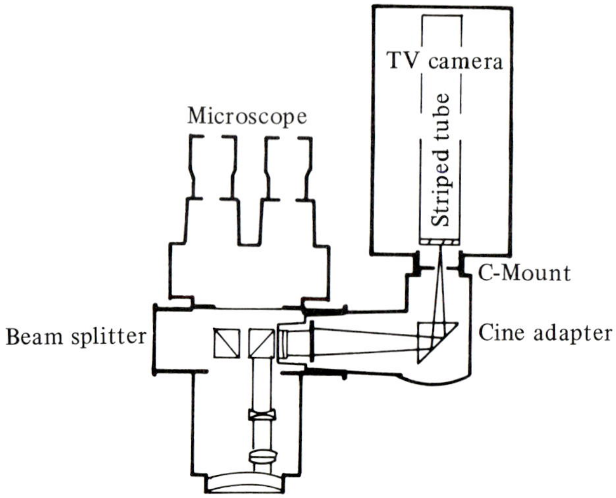

Fig. 22-3. Galilean microscope with beam-splitter, cine adapter, and C-mount adapter on miniature camera.

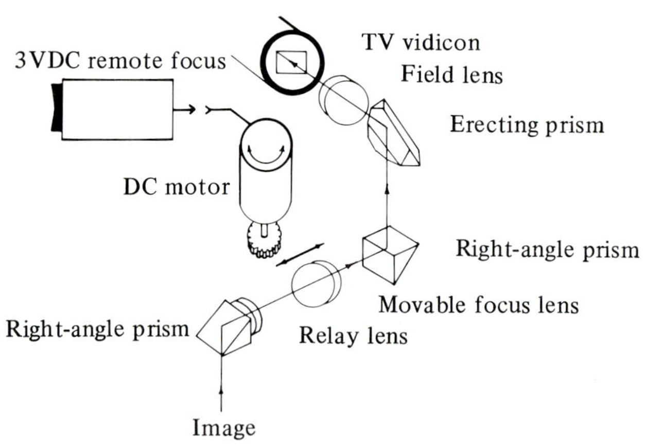

Fig. 22-4. The Urban Engineering focusing relay. A technique to control focus on surgical microscope independently.

seen by the surgeon. For example, the surgeon might want to operate at a slightly lower magnification to gain greater depth of field, but, in order to televise the procedure, sufficient magnification to show structural detail is needed.

Setting Up the Operating Microscope

Traditionally, the surgeon is responsible for the quality of the picture through the operating microscope. A few preliminary steps can ensure that the physician obtains a sharper image on the television monitor. First, the microscope's focusing mechanism must be set at midpoint in its range. If there is no tare mark at the midpoint of focus, make one with an indelible pen. Use a piece of graph paper placed on the diagonal to determine the range of focus. Then zoom the microscope to maximum magnification and focus the television image while observing the monitor. By adjusting the distance between the C-mount adapter and the tube face, you can determine the midrange of focus for the television camera. This should be a one-time step in the preliminary setup of the system.

Next the surgeon rotates the oculars on the eyepiece until the image is as sharp as the one on the television monitor. A focusing reticle is important because it allows the surgeon to maintain proper focus in his field of view and on the TV monitor throughout the surgical procedure. Without it, the surgeon might not notice the television image drifting out of focus because his vision can accommodate to small changes whereas the monitor cannot.

The following steps are recommended to obtain a good television image with the operating microscope. During the procedure, the assistant should notify the surgeon when the picture drifts off the point of interest and when it goes out of focus because the surgeon has forgotten to keep the eyepiece crosshairs sharply in focus. Remember, when the surgeon works at lower magnification, the image might cover only about one-fifth of the television screen; therefore, it might be necessary to zoom to higher magnification to fill the screen. This step is important to show detail, since the image on the monitor will be slightly less than 21 to 26 inches, depending on the size of the monitor.

If the video tape is to be edited, let the tape run throughout the surgical procedure. Attempts to edit while recording live are usually not successful, and starting and stopping the tape recorder results in electronic breakup, which in later editing creates extreme difficulty in smoothly assembling sequences.

Video Tape Recorders and Editors

Several tape sizes and formats are used in the television industry, schools, and homes. Video recorders use either tape on reels or in cassettes; for ophthalmology, the 3/4-inch U-format cassette recorders

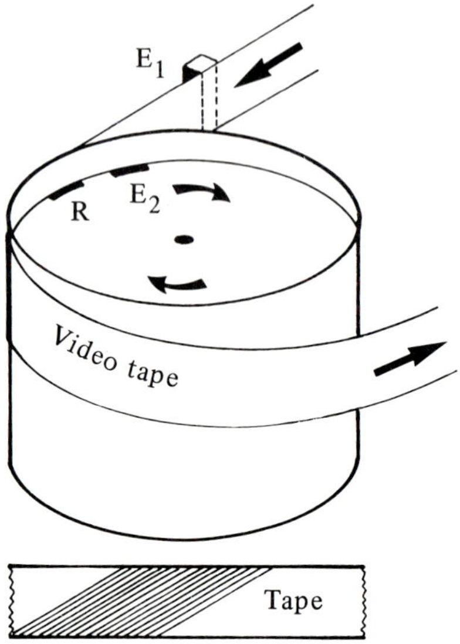

Fig. 22-5. Helical scan (bottom) *and optional erase positions* (top). E_1 = *standard erase head;* E_2 = *flying erase head;* R = *recording head.*

are recommended. They are high quality, reliable, and easily used; only cassettes of this format can be played on any manufacturer's player-recorder.

Other tape formats are:

1. Quadruplex, 2-inch open reel used by the broadcast industry.
2. Helical scan, 1 inch, format A, B, C (incompatible), high quality.
3. Helical scan, 1/2 inch, open reel and cassette. EIAJ tapes are interchangeable. Quality less than 3/4 inch.
4. Helical scan, 1/4 inch, low quality [1].

Cassette housings protect sensitive tape from unskilled hands. The recorder pulls a loop of tape from the cassette and wraps it around the recording drum in a helix; this manner of wrapping, *helical scan,* results in a diagonal recording pathway and allows a great recording amplitude, while the longer scan area gives a more sensitive color picture [1, 5] (Fig. 22-5).

Helical scan offers editing problems on some recorder models. In the simpler recorders, the erase head, which works vertically, precedes the flying recording head, which works diagonally. The result is a small, incompletely erased area on the tape that shows on the monitor as electronic breakup. The solution is an erase head attached to the record

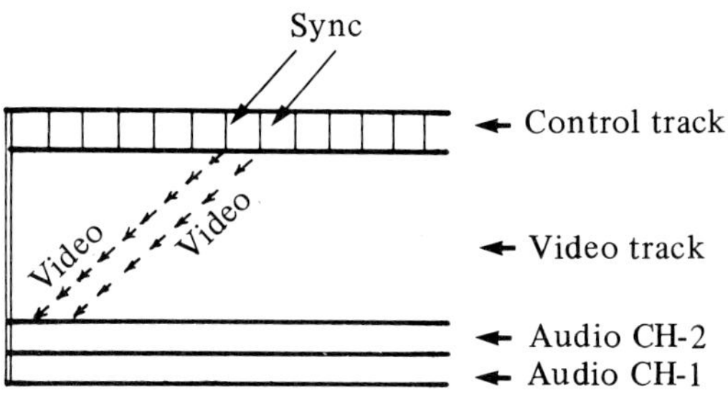

Fig. 22-6. 3/4-inch video tape showing two audio channels, video track, and control track.

head so that the erasure pattern is diagonal and precedes the recorder head. This device, a *flying erase head,* is found on most editing recorders (Fig. 22-5).

In addition to the video track, 3/4-inch tape has channel 1 audio, channel 2 audio, and a control track (comparable to the sprocket holes on movie film) [1, 5]. A prerecorded control track on the tape is required for insert editing, a technique in which new material is placed over previously recorded material. The control track regulates the capstan servo system, which controls variations in tape speed and allows smooth insertions [4, 5] (Fig. 22-6).

Types of Editing

ASSEMBLY EDITING. In assembly editing, new control track is added with each new edit. At the junction of the old and new control tracks, breakup can be noticed, analogous to that found when two film sprocket holes are spliced close together (Fig. 22-7).

VERTICAL-INTERVAL EDITING. This type of editing can be performed on editing tape recorders. The edit point is made when the vertical scan lines are visible on the monitor screen (unless an underscan monitor is used) [5, 7] (Fig. 22-7).

SIMPLE EDITING. This editing is possible with two recorders if one is an editing recorder that is used as the recorder. Both machines are backed up 10 to 15 seconds before the desired edit point and are rolled forward together until the edit is made. This same technique is called a *crash edit* when performed with two nonediting recorders [5, 7]. The analogy of shotgun versus rifle accuracy could be made here.

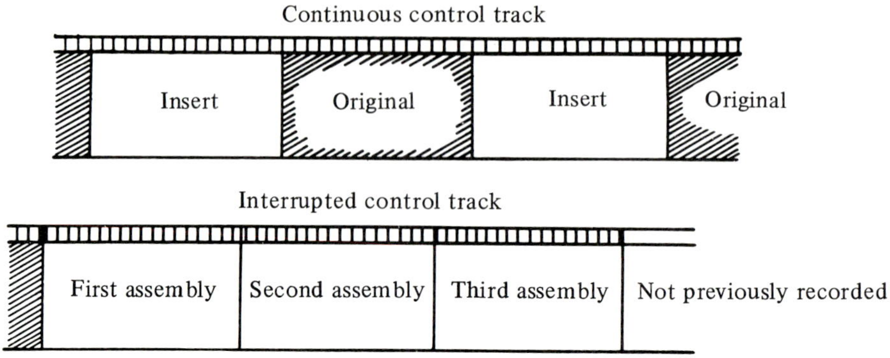

Fig. 22-7. Comparison of insert (top) *versus assembly* (bottom) *editing.*

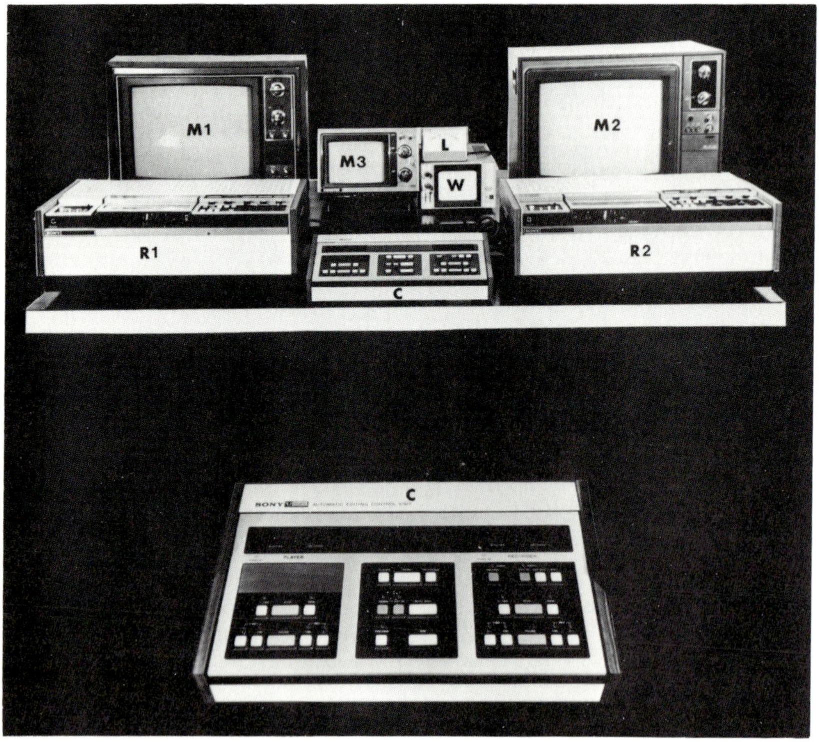

Fig. 22-8. Sony RM430 editing system: player monitor (M1); *editor monitor* (M2); *underscan monitor* (M3); *waveform monitor* (W); *player* (R1); *editor* (R2); *control unit* (C); *AC power line monitor* (L).

TIME-BASE CORRECTION. The most precise editing employs time-base correctors to compensate for the electronic instability found in 3/4-inch video cassette machines; time-base correction is essential if video cassettes are to be used for broadcasting [6].

AUTOMATIC EDITING. Automatic editing control units such as the Sony RM430 system employ digital tape time counters to aid in finding edit points by searching forward or backward at one-twentieth the normal speed. Preview edit points can be rehearsed with this control. Prerolling and the edit are done automatically [4] (Fig. 22-8).

References

1. Bensinger, C. *The Video Guide* (2nd ed.). Santa Barbara, Calif.: Video-Info Publications, 1977.
2. Fishman, M. Television ophthalmoscopy: Ophthalmic photography of the future? In Ophthalmic Photographers' Society, *Scientific Paper.* Chicago: November 2, 1980.
3. Hoerenz, P. The design of the surgical microscope: I. *Ophthalmic Surg.* 4(1) : 40–45, 1973.
4. Hoerenz, P. The design of the surgical microscope: II. *Ophthalmic Surg.* 4(2) : 89–93, 1973.
5. Robinson, J. F., and Beards, P. H. *Using Videotape.* New York: Hastings House Publishers, 1976.
6. Trayna, J., and Owens, N. *The Video Handbook* (3rd ed.). New York: United Business Publications, 1977.
7. Utz, P. *Video Users' Handbook.* Englewood Cliffs, N. J.: Prentice-Hall, 1980.

23

Photographic Filing Systems

BARRETT P. WALKER

This chapter presents some solutions to a problem that most photographers vow to solve as soon as there is a hiatus in their schedule of patients. What is sought is a system that will file, in one location, all of the photographs taken of an individual patient on different dates and with various types of photographic equipment. A method of storage is desired that will protect valuable photographs and slides, either stereos or single frames, from fingerprints and careless handling, and yet will facilitate easy viewing and usage. Once the photographs have been filed, a system of cross-indexing is needed to retrieve them by patient name, date (of the original photographs), and diagnosis (Fig. 23-1).

A simple, effective method of filing patient photographs in chronologic order and retrieving them by patient name and date will be described first. This integrated system of filing and retrieving patient photographs from many sources may then be combined with one of three systems of increasing complexity and completeness for retrieval of patient photographs by diagnosis. The last system described will be a commonly used method for filing and retrieving slides by diagnosis only.

Integrated Patient Filing System

Information is written down when the patient is first seen and photographed on a document called the patient photography card. The information always needed on this card includes the patient's age, sex, race, the name of the referring physician, the type of photograph requested (e.g., external, fundus), and a provisional diagnosis. In some cases a brief history, address, phone number, and insurance information on the patient are also required.

After the films have been processed, the photographs of a particular patient can be identified by referring to a log book, which is used to list the patient's name in the order that the photographs were taken, or by referring to a photograph of the patient's name which is taken at the beginning of the films on each patient. The photography card provides a check on the correct identification of the photographs for each

Appreciation is expressed to Janet and Jim Fierst for programming the KWIC Index. Without their advice, the project would not have been possible.

Special thanks go to Johnny Justice, Jr., for information on his carbon copy retrieval system, and to Ann Bryant for her help in the preparation of the manuscript.

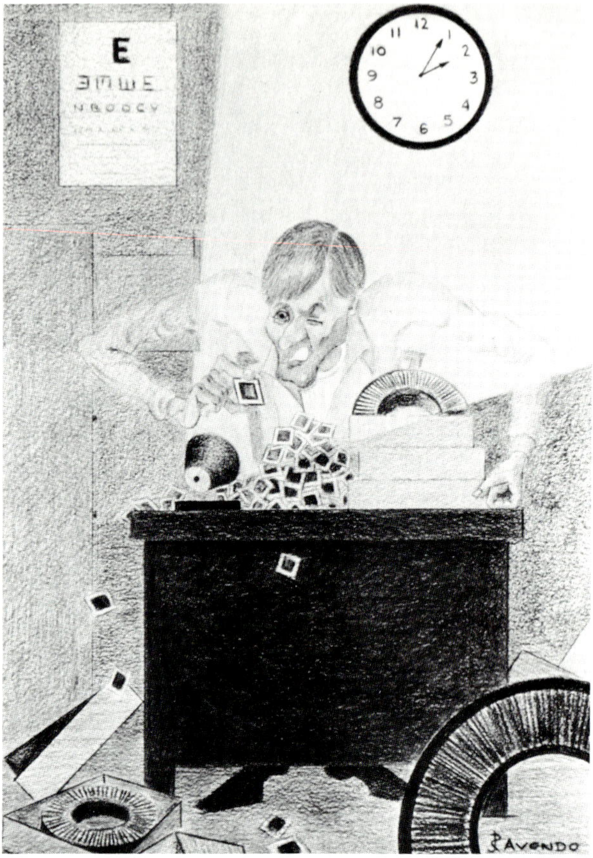

Fig. 23-1. The problem.

patient. After identification of the patient's slides, photography cards are filed alphabetically by name in a standard index card file.

The mounted slides are marked with the date of the photograph, the patient's name, and, when necessary, the letters *LE* or *RE*, to identify photographs of the right or left eye. The slides are then filed in a clear vinyl envelope having twenty slide pockets arranged in four vertical rows of five pockets each. The open sides of the two columns on the left and the two on the right face each other, as shown in Figure 23-2. This feature allows stereo slides to be marked on their adjoining edges, making it easier to identify them as a pair. Single photographs to be kept in a patient's record are placed in the right half of the double column below the corresponding stereo slides, if present. If an extra slide has been made for use by the referring physician or for any other purpose, it can be stored in the left-hand column; thus one can retain the extra slides without keeping a separate file.

It is helpful, but not necessary, to arrange the photographs taken on a particular day by subject, with full face first, then close-up externals; fundus, fluorescein, and surgical slit-lamp photographs; and photographs of test results. If more photographs are taken at a later date, they are added in chronologic order, using as many vinyl envelopes as necessary. If any photographs need to be selected for use in journal articles or for duplication at a later date, an erasable mark can be made with a grease pencil over the appropriate photograph on the vinyl surface of the envelope.

The vinyl folders containing the patient photographs are placed in an open-topped manilla envelope. The date of the first group of photographs is written on the upper left edge and the patient's name on the upper center of the envelope. The envelopes are filed in chronologic order in any standard-size office filing cabinet. Any extra printed test results or patient history information can be dropped into the open-topped envelope along with the vinyl envelopes containing the patient's slides.

Slides can be retrieved directly by date using the integrated patient filing system, since all patient folders are filed in chronologic order. To retrieve photographs by patient name, one must first refer to the alphabetic file of patient cards, note the date on the patient card, and then pull the patient's photographic folder directly from the photographic file by date (Fig. 23-3).

Retrieval by Diagnosis

The most important function of any complete filing system is its capacity for retrieval of photographs by diagnosis without the sacrifice of easy retrieval of slides by patient name and date. The following three systems can all be combined with the integrated patient filing system to provide retrieval by patient information as well as by diagnosis.

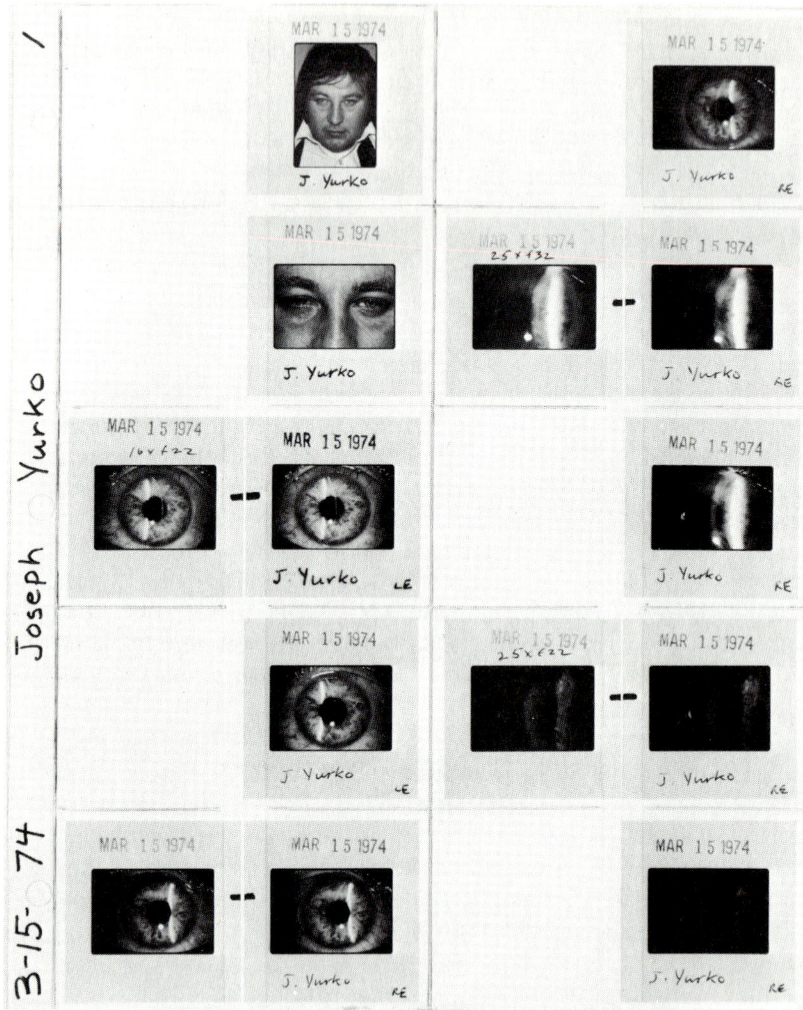

Fig. 23-2. Stereo and single slides are stored in clear plastic envelope.

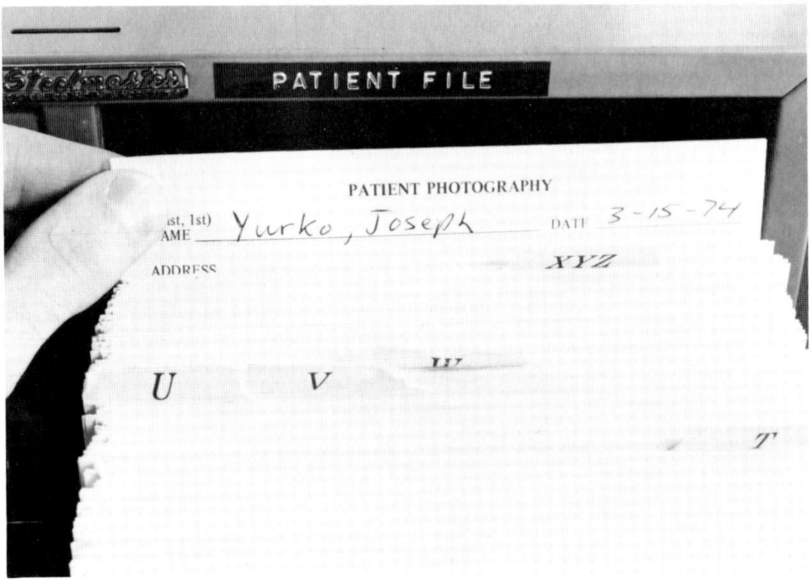

Fig. 23-3. Alphabetic card file by patient name.

Carbon Copy Card System

The carbon copy card system consists of a duplicate patient card form. The first card of the duplicate form is filled out with the name, date, diagnosis, and other necessary information on the patient photographed. The original card is filed alphabetically under the patient's name, and the carbon copy is filed alphabetically by disease name. If more than one diagnosis is needed for a particular patient, then an extra single card for each diagnosis must be filled out in full and filed under the name of the disease listed on the card face.

For a single photographer or physician, a carbon copy indexing system is particularly quick and easy to use. Unfortunately, however, the system is not as efficient when the responsibility for filing or the need for retrieval is divided among several individuals, since the terminology used for specific diseases will vary. The carbon copy diagnostic indexing system works best in an office or institution where the individual responsible for filing must retrieve his or her own slides by diagnosis.

Edge Sort Index

Retrieving slides by diagnosis is considerably more difficult than it might appear, since the terminology used for ophthalmic diseases varies considerably among physicians. However, by describing every disease as an anatomic site affected by a process, one can rapidly develop a common descriptive terminology. A short list of frequently used sites and processes printed on the back of the patient photography cards provides a standard reference vocabulary enabling several ophthalmologists within a department to classify diseases rapidly and consistently.

A single exception to this standard sequence of listing anatomic site, process, and disease name is the large disease category of glaucoma. Glaucoma is listed as if it were an anatomic site coupled with a process and specific name; for example, pigmentary glaucoma would be listed as *glaucoma, degeneration, pigmentary,* while angle recession glaucoma would be listed as *glaucoma, trauma, angle recession.*

The edge sort diagnostic filing system provides a mechanical means for cross-indexing and retrieving patient photographs by diagnosis, anatomic site, and process. A duplicate card form 5 by 8 inches in size with a row of prepunched holes around the entire margin is used for this system. The name, date, diagnosis, and other pertinent information on an individual patient is written on the face of the duplicate form. The original card is placed in an alphabetic file by patient name. The carbon copy duplicate is used to retrieve photographs by diagnosis. To create the cross-indexing feature of this system, one uses a handheld paper punch to punch one or more holes in the top row on the duplicate card. This row of holes corresponds to the anatomic sites listed on the back of the card. One then punches one or more holes along the bottom row to indicate the disease process involved. The duplicate card itself is filed alphabetically by the first word of the diagnosis on the card face. As in the case of the simple carbon copy card system, a separate individual card must be filled out for each specific diagnosis on a single patient.

Information on a diagnosis by anatomic site or process is retrieved by removing all cards from the file drawers, blocking them together in a corner, and running a long steel rod through a hole in the same position on all cards corresponding to the anatomic site or process desired. When the rod is lifted, all the cards that have been punched through the particular hole selected will fall out of the stack onto the table below. The cards that were not punched will continue to hang from the rod until they are replaced in the file and the rod is pulled out. A second search may then be made so that only a small stack of selected cards will remain, corresponding to the combination of a specific anatomic site and disease process. Holes on the ends of the cards may be used to indicate a limited number of specific disease names or research topics of particular interest in the office or institution where this system is used.

The edge sort system (Fig. 23-4) is particularly well suited to situations calling for an average amount of cross-indexing. A moderate

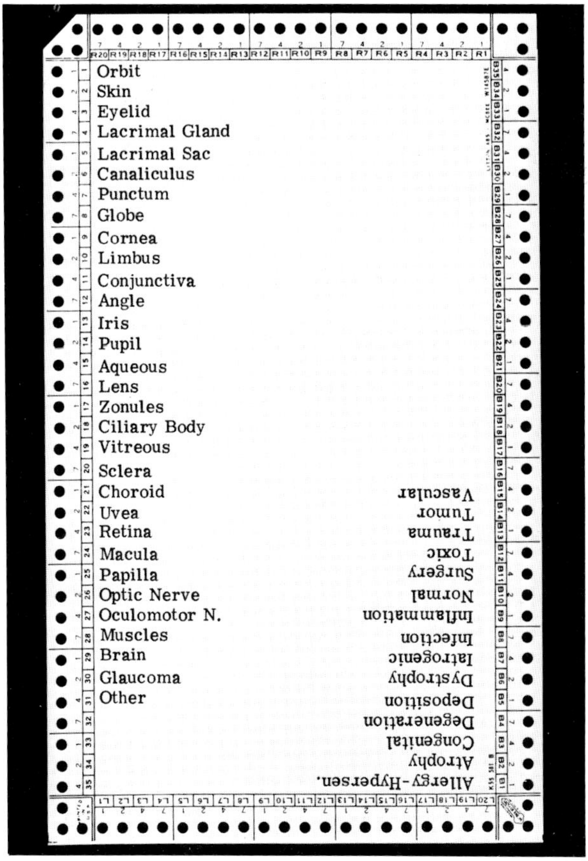

Fig. 23-4. Back of edge sort diagnosis card showing list of anatomic sites and processes.

amount of clerical time is required to search for multiple disease listings, since this mechanical system requires a fair amount of manual manipulation.

Refiling the edge sort cards in alphabetic order after each sort with the steel rod is time consuming because the cards that have fallen out of the stack lose their alphabetic order. If retrieval by specific disease name is not a requirement of the system, a considerable amount of filing time may be saved by keeping the stack of diagnosis cards in random order and using the steel rod to search for the anatomic site, process, and other specific categories represented by the holes along the perimeter of the cards. A large, active photographic department would probably find this system inadequate, since the edge sort cards are damaged by repeated searches and the system becomes cumber-

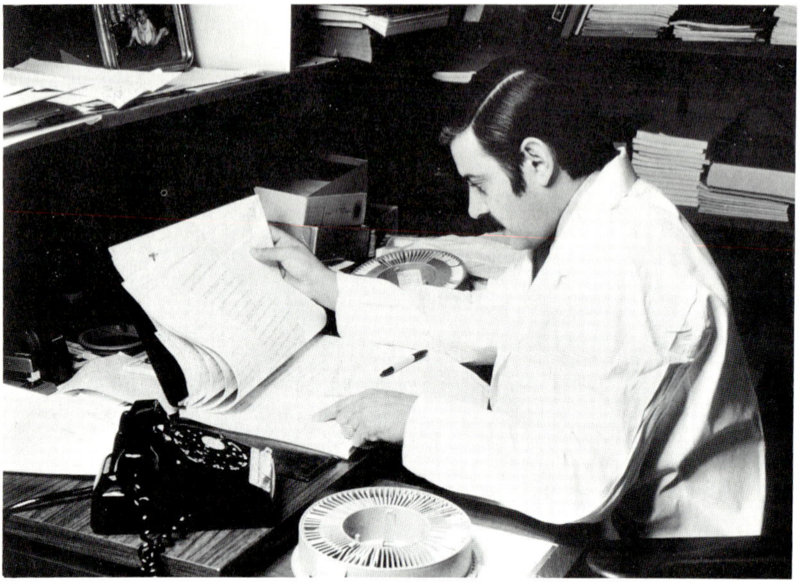

Fig. 23-5. Use of the KWIC Index.

some when the total quantity of cards exceeds about two to three thousand in number.

KWIC Index

The steps leading to the production of the Key Word in Context (KWIC) Index are rather complex compared to the other filing systems described, but the actual use of this index for retrieval is efficient and simple. The index is a computer printout bound in a reusable cover in the form of a book opening from the bottom (Fig. 23-5). It is divided into three sections: patient directory, KWIC diagnosis, and word frequency list.

The first section of the index, the patient directory, lists all patients in chronologic order by the date they were first photographed. The first seven characters of the name (a character is a letter, symbol, number, or space having meaning to the computer) and the complete diagnosis of each patient are listed to the right of the date (Fig. 23-6). Since the actual patient photography folders are filed in chronologic order, the patient directory provides a valuable double listing for checking against the order of the filed photographs in case any photographic folders are misplaced.

The second section of the index is the KWIC diagnosis section. Each page of this section is divided into two broad columns of type with a

03 14 74 SCHULTZ	D	CORNEA DEPOSITION, DYSTROPHY ? ETIOLOGY? (12WF)
03 14 74 DILLMAN	D	CORNEA DEPOSITION, COPPER, KEYSER FLEISHER RING, WILSONS DISEASE (DILLMAN FAMILY TERRY 17WF, PATTY 11WF POTENTIAL WILSONS= MIKE 8WM, ELIZABETH 4WF)
03 14 74 VAN ZYR	D	AQUEOUS TRAUMA, HYPHEMA SURGERY, PHACO=EMUL (12WF HIT BY BLOW DART WITH SUCTION CUP)
03 14 74 DROZYNS	D	RETINA INFECTION, TOXOPLASMOSIS, CHORIORETINITIS MACULA VASCULAR, EXUDATES
03 14 74 PANDOCC	D	RETINA VASCULAR, BRANCH VEIN OCCLUSION (56WF)
03 15 74 YURKO J	D	CORNEA TRAUMA, U=V KERATITIS, PUNCTATE STAINING (29WM EXPOSED TO WELDING FLASH 5 HRS)
03 18 74 FIORAVA	D	THIRD NERVE PALSY VASCULAR, DIABETIC EXOPHTHALMUS (58WM)
03 19 74 WEYANT	D	CORNEA INFLAMMATION, PERFORATION SKIN INFLAMMATION, ACNE ROSUCEA (37WF)
03 19 74 TOBAKOS	D	CONJUNCTIVA DEPOSITION, MASCARA CONJUNCTIVA ALLERGY, COSMETICS (24WF)
03 19 74 CHASTEL	D	PAPILLA DEGENERATION, RETINA DEGENERATION, LEBERS DISEASE (19WM)
03 19 74 BARJACK	D	HYSTERICAL VISION LOSS, NO LEBERS (18WM)
03 19 74 PISTOLE	D	ANGLE CONGENITAL NORMAL, PROMINENT SCHWALBES LINE, PIGMENT PAPILLA CONGENITAL, CUPPING .7 .4 RETINA CONGENITAL, MYELINATION NO GLAUCOMA (28WF SLIGHT MYOPIA)
03 19 74 RUSSELL	D	CORNEA TRAUMA, SCAR (51WM FB 6MO AGO)
03 21 74 HELD L	D	ORBIT INFLAMMATION, ALLERGY NO CELLULITIS (43WF PAINTY?)
03 28 74 LYBARGE	D	LIDS INFECTION, MIXED BLEPHARITIS CORNEA HYPERSENSITIVITY, THINNING, NEOVASCULARIZATION (18WF)

Fig. 23-6. Patient directory section of the KWIC Index.

separating space running down the middle of the page (Figs. 23-7, 23-8). A narrow column on the right-hand side of the page lists patients by date and the first seven characters of their names, with the last name first. To find a particular diagnosis, one scans vertically the alphabetized words on the right-hand edge of the center space until the key word is found. If a complete diagnosis on a patient is desired, the line of type to the left of the patient's date and name is read across the page from left to right. In this way the key word of the diagnosis can be read in context with the complete diagnosis; hence the title *K*ey *W*ord *I*n *C*ontext. On occasion a diagnosis will be so long that the full diagnosis cannot appear on a single line in the KWIC index. In this case, one may refer to the patient directory section using the date and patient name to locate the full listing.

The slides are coded with the diagnosis written in the form of the involved anatomic site, process, and specific disease name. When more than one finding or disease is present for a particular patient, the findings are listed in order of importance by the standard form of anatomic site, process, and specific name. For example, the diagnosis of a patient who sustained a subluxated lens and choroidal rupture in an automobile accident would be listed as: lens trauma, subluxation, choroid trauma, rupture. Additional information such as age, sex, race, and history can be included in the KWIC diagnosis by enclosing it in parentheses. For example, the complete listing on the patient involved

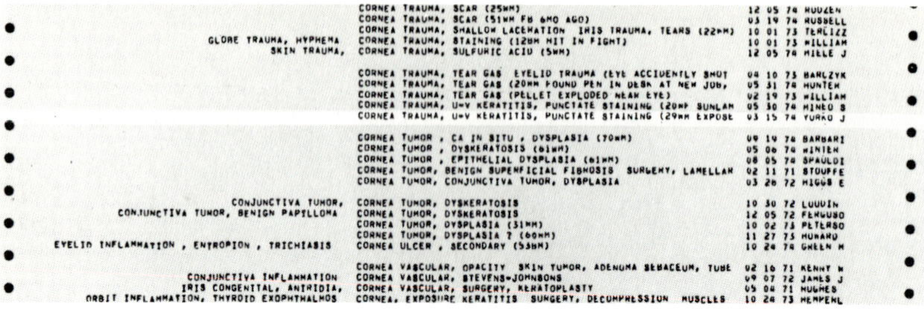

	CORNEA TRAUMA, SCAR (25WM)	12 05 74	RUDZEN
	CORNEA TRAUMA, SCAR (51WM FB 6MO AGO)	03 19 74	RUSSELL
	CORNEA TRAUMA, SHALLOW LACERATION IRIS TRAUMA, TEARS (22WM)	10 01 73	TERLIZZ
GLOBE TRAUMA, HYPHEMA	CORNEA TRAUMA, STAINING (12BM HIT IN FIGHT)	10 01 73	WILLIAM
SKIN TRAUMA,	CORNEA TRAUMA, SULFURIC ACID (5WM)	12 05 74	MILLE J
	CORNEA TRAUMA, TEAR GAS EYELID TRAUMA (EYE ACCIDENTLY SHOT	04 10 73	BARCZYK
	CORNEA TRAUMA, TEAR GAS (20WM FOUND PEN IN DESK AT NEW JOB,	05 31 74	HUNTER
	CORNEA TRAUMA, TEAR GAS (PELLET EXPLODED NEAR EYE)	02 19 73	WILLIAM
	CORNEA TRAUMA, U-V KERATITIS, PUNCTATE STAINING (20WF SUNLAM	05 30 74	MINEO S
	CORNEA TRAUMA, U-V KERATITIS, PUNCTATE STAINING (29WM EXPOSE	03 15 74	YURKO J
	CORNEA TUMOR , CA IN SITU , DYSPLASIA (70WM)	09 19 74	BARBARI
	CORNEA TUMOR , DYSKERATOSIS (61WM)	05 06 74	WINIER
	CORNEA TUMOR , EPITHELIAL DYSPLASIA (61WM)	08 05 74	SPAULDI
	CORNEA TUMOR, BENIGN SUPERFICIAL FIBROSIS SURGERY, LAMELLAR	02 11 71	STOUFFE
	CORNEA TUMOR, CONJUNCTIVA TUMOR, DYSPLASIA	03 26 72	HIGGS E
CONJUNCTIVA TUMOR,	CORNEA TUMOR, DYSKERATOSIS	10 30 72	LUDDIN
CONJUNCTIVA TUMOR, BENIGN PAPILLOMA	CORNEA TUMOR, DYSKERATOSIS	12 05 72	FERGUSO
	CORNEA TUMOR, DYSPLASIA (31MM)	10 02 73	PETERSO
	CORNEA TUMOR, DYSPLASIA ? (60MM)	11 27 73	HOWARD
EYELID INFLAMMATION , ENTROPION , TRICHIASIS	CORNEA ULCER , SECONDARY (53BM)	10 24 74	GREEN M
	CORNEA VASCULAR, OPACITY SKIN TUMOR, ADENOMA SEBACEUM, TUBE	02 16 71	KENNY M
CONJUNCTIVA INFLAMMATION	CORNEA VASCULAR, STEVENS-JOHNSONS	09 07 72	JAMES J
IRIS CONGENITAL, ANIRIDIA,	CORNEA VASCULAR, SURGERY, KERATOPLASTY	05 04 71	HUGHES
ORBIT INFLAMMATION, THYROID EXOPHTHALMOS	CORNEA, EXPOSURE KERATITIS SURGERY, DECOMPRESSION MUSCLES	10 24 73	HEMPEHL

Fig. 23-7. KWIC diagnosis section of the KWIC Index. The key word "Cornea" is alphabetized.

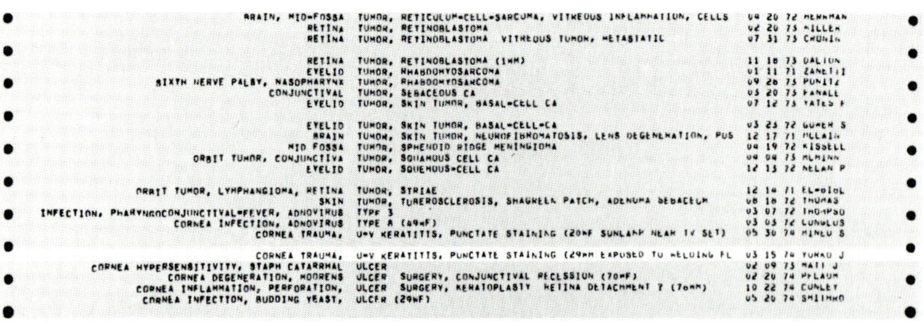

BRAIN, MID-FOSSA	TUMOR, RETICULUM-CELL-SARCOMA, VITREOUS INFLAMMATION, CELLS	04 20 72	HERRMAN
RETINA	TUMOR, RETINOBLASTOMA	02 20 73	MILLER
RETINA	TUMOR, RETINOBLASTOMA VITREOUS TUMOR, METASTATIC	07 31 73	CRONIN
RETINA	TUMOR, RETINOBLASTOMA (1MM)	11 16 73	DALTON
EYELID	TUMOR, RHABDOMYOSARCOMA	01 11 71	ZANETTI
SIXTH NERVE PALSY, NASOPHARYNX	TUMOR, RHABDOMYOSARCOMA	09 26 73	PUNITZ
CONJUNCTIVAL	TUMOR, SEBACEOUS CA	05 20 73	FANALE
EYELID	TUMOR, SKIN TUMOR, BASAL-CELL CA	07 12 73	YATES F
EYELID	TUMOR, SKIN TUMOR, BASAL-CELL-CA	03 23 72	GOMER S
BRAIN	TUMOR, SKIN TUMOR, NEUROFIBROMATOSIS, LENS DEGENERATION, PUS	12 17 71	MCLAIN
MID FOSSA	TUMOR, SPHENOID RIDGE MENINGIOMA	04 19 72	KISSELL
ORBIT TUMOR, CONJUNCTIVA	TUMOR, SQUAMOUS CELL CA	04 04 73	MCMINN
EYELID	TUMOR, SQUEMOUS-CELL CA	12 13 72	NELAN P
ORBIT TUMOR, LYMPHANGIOMA, RETINA	TUMOR, STRIAE	12 14 71	EL-BIOL
SKIN	TUMOR, TUBEROSCLEROSIS, SHAGREEN PATCH, ADENOMA SEBACEUM	08 16 72	THOMAS
INFECTION, PHARYNGOCONJUNCTIVAL-FEVER, ADNOVIRUS	TYPE 3	03 07 72	THOMPSO
CORNEA INFECTION, ADNOVIRUS	TYPE A (49WF)	03 03 72	CONGLOS
CORNEA TRAUMA,	U-V KERATITIS, PUNCTATE STAINING (20WF SUNLAMP NEAR TV SET)	05 30 74	MINEO S
CORNEA TRAUMA,	U-V KERATITIS, PUNCTATE STAINING (29WM EXPOSED TO WELDING FL	03 15 74	YURKO J
CORNEA HYPERSENSITIVITY, STAPH CATARRHAL	ULCER	02 09 73	MATT J
CORNEA DEGENERATION, MOORENS	ULCER SURGERY, CONJUNCTIVAL RECESSION (70WF)	02 20 74	PFLAUM
CORNEA INFLAMMATION, PERFORATION,	ULCER SURGERY, KERATOPLASTY RETINA DETACHMENT ? (76MM)	10 22 74	CONLEY
CORNEA INFECTION, BUDDING YEAST,	ULCER (29WF)	05 20 74	SMITHRO

Fig. 23-8. KWIC diagnosis section of the KWIC Index. The key word "U-V Keratitis" is alphabetized.

in the automobile accident would be: lens trauma, subluxation, choroid trauma, rupture (23 WM, auto accident). The computer will always print the parenthetic information at the end of each diagnosis but will not alphabetize it.

Cases of particular photographic or clinical interest may be marked with an asterisk after the parenthetic patient information. All of these noteworthy cases will be indexed by the computer and listed in the KWIC diagnosis section before the letter *A* as well as alphabetically by diagnosis. This feature is particularly valuable when the selection of the best case examples in a particular disease category is desired.

Production of the KWIC Index begins with the copying of information from the patient photography card onto a standard key punch form (Fig. 23-9). This form consists of horizontal rows of 80 spaces each; the 80 spaces represent the maximum number of characters that may be punched into a 4- by 8-inch computer card. If the patient identification information and diagnosis take more than 80 characters, additional computer cards may be used. Each card is identified by a code letter *D* (diagnosis), followed by the number of the card. Ac-

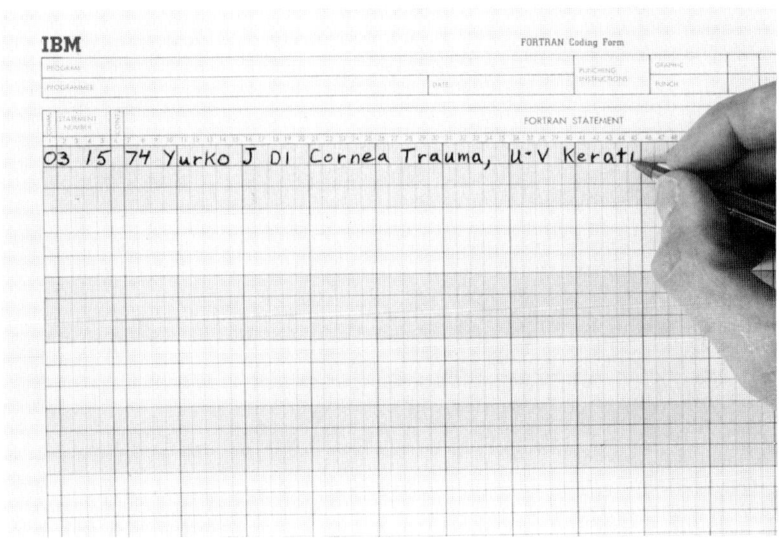

Fig. 23-9. Standard key punch form.

cumulated coding forms are taken to a key punch operator at intervals of one to two months to be punched onto the computer cards. A visibly typed line at the top of each punched card corresponds to the holes below. All of the current computer cards are placed in chronologic order behind the previously punched cards in a file box. If the diagnosis of a previously filed patient has been revised, the old card is removed from the computer card file and replaced by a new card with the revised diagnosis (Fig. 23-9).

Remote stations that will rapidly read punched cards into a central computer are often conveniently located in hospital and university centers. Because the cards that automatically instruct the computer to find and run the KWIC Index master program are located at the beginning and end of the data deck, a clerical person unskilled in computer technology can easily learn to feed patient data into the computer through a card reader. The program is now being modified to permit data to be entered directly into the computer through a terminal with a display screen and a keyboard as well as through punched cards. By the next working day a new KWIC Index will be computed, printed on a line printer, and placed in a mail slot ready for pickup. If desired, an instruction card placed in the data deck will cause the computer to print a second copy of the KWIC Index for circulating use (Fig. 23-10).

If the KWIC Index is run in "batch mode," a considerable amount of money may be saved. This means that an instruction card placed

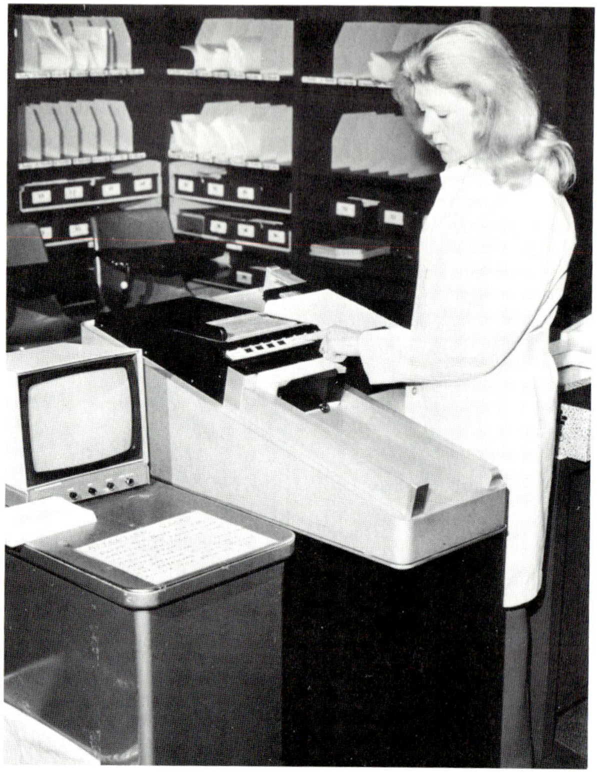

Fig. 23-10. Card reader with shelves for completed printouts in background.

in the data deck is read into the computer indicating that the program may be run on a low-priority basis. Since the computing load is highest during normal working hours, the KWIC Index will be computed and printed at night and be ready for pickup the next morning.

Initially, the computer program necessary to run the KWIC Index retrieval system should be established and debugged by a trained computer consultant. However, once the program has been run, an individual with minimal computer knowledge can use the program as a tool to organize large amounts of diagnostic data.

The basic KWIC Index program was adapted from an existing library sort program in 1972 and refined to its present form in May, 1973. The program uses 32 K of core and requires approximately 26 minutes of computing time with 2000 data cards. The language used is COBOL.

Before initiating the KWIC indexing system, an institution should carefully estimate the projected volume of use. A photography department with infrequent requests for retrieval of photographs by diagnosis or fewer than 1000 patient visits per year should consider the edge sort or carbon copy retrieval system. Computer availability and reliability are other important factors affecting the decision to use computerized retrieval. When patient volume and computer availability favor the use of a computerized system, the KWIC Index should be considered superior to computer systems that retrieve information in real time. A computer breakdown could, at worst, delay the printing of a revised edition of the KWIC Index, but the information stored in a real-time program is completely unavailable during a computer shutdown. At least the old edition of the KWIC Index and the new unindexed computer cards are available until computer repairs are made and a new index can be generated. For additional protection in case of flood, fire, or theft at the computer center, both the data cards and an extra copy of the KWIC Index program in card form are stored within the hospital.

With frequent use, the cost of a real-time retrieval program can become prohibitive, since each search for a diagnosis must be paid for individually. By contrast, the KWIC Index system is relatively inexpensive with increased use, because only one monthly or bimonthly computing charge is paid. Since the KWIC Index is a direct system, reference to and memorization of accession numbers are completely unnecessary. Any individual who understands basic ophthalmic terminology can learn to use the system within a few minutes.

Notebook Filing System

If retrieval by diagnosis only is needed, the complexity of slide filing is immensely simplified. For the simple diagnostic filing system, vinyl envelopes containing slides on general diagnostic topics may be placed in loose-leaf notebooks that are labeled by anatomic site. Individual pages within the notebooks may be labeled on the margin by disease process or specific diagnosis. For example, a notebook might be entitled "Cornea" for a specific anatomic site and subdivided by process into sections such as infection, inflammation, dystrophy, and trauma. This system can be very easily customized to the particular ophthalmologic specialty of the user. For example, a physician interested in oncology could label a whole notebook with the process "Tumors" and divide it into specific diagnoses such as malignant melanoma, retinoblastoma, causes of leukokoria, and pseudotumors.

This simple diagnostic filing system is particularly well suited for the physician working in an academic setting where a department of ophthalmic photography has already established a filing system for retrieval by patient information. A second use of the simple notebook system is in photographic departments where slides are filed by patient name with a cross-reference for diagnosis. To speed retrieval and protect valuable original slides on frequently used disease topics, a duplicate set of slides can be made from the originals and filed in loose-leaf notebooks by anatomic site and process or specific disease name. In this way, a condensed teaching collection duplicated from the best slides in a department's patient files can be made available for general use on a loan basis.

Computerized Slide Retrieval

PAUL R. MONTAGUE

Several systems for retrieval of slides by diagnosis have already been described by Barrett P. Walker (Chap. 23) [6]. This chapter specifically deals with retrieval by computer.

Before slide retrieval systems can be considered, an adequate filing system is mandatory. Walker has described a system through which charts are filed in chronologic order. If hospital or clinic numbers are issued to patients, filing by this number should be considered in order that all patient records can be located with the same number. In any event, alphabetic filing is not advised for an institution whose files grow at a rapid rate, since charts must continually be moved to make room for new charts in the center of the file.

A checkout system for charts must be established and rigidly enforced. The most elaborate retrieval system is rendered useless when records are not returned to the file. Standard checkout cards, which replace the chart in the file, serve the purpose quite well.

Computer Retrieval Overview

Card index systems and other manual retrieval systems provide adequate service to institutions with a small number of photographic cases or limited retrieval requirements. For example, perhaps 10 percent of the patients photographed by a clinic were diabetics. If that clinic had 2000 records on file, a retrieval of diabetics would contain 200 cases. This number could easily be scanned on the index cards and appropriate cases selected. If, however, the clinic had 20,000 records on file, the diabetic list would list 2000 cases. At this point, it would be beneficial to let a retrieval system do some of the work by sorting out only those diabetics who might meet our needs; for example, diabetics with macular edema. The resulting list would, of course, be substantially shorter. The number of retrieved cases can be further reduced if the selection criteria were even more specific. In an extreme case, one might request diabetics with macular edema and proliferative neovascularization, who have had angiograms done, and are under 30 years of age. This selection would be impractical with the cross-index system, but could be accomplished with an efficient computer program in 1/2 to 3 minutes.

About Computers

Computers are machines that can be given a set of instructions and then execute those instructions when programmed to do so. The ma-

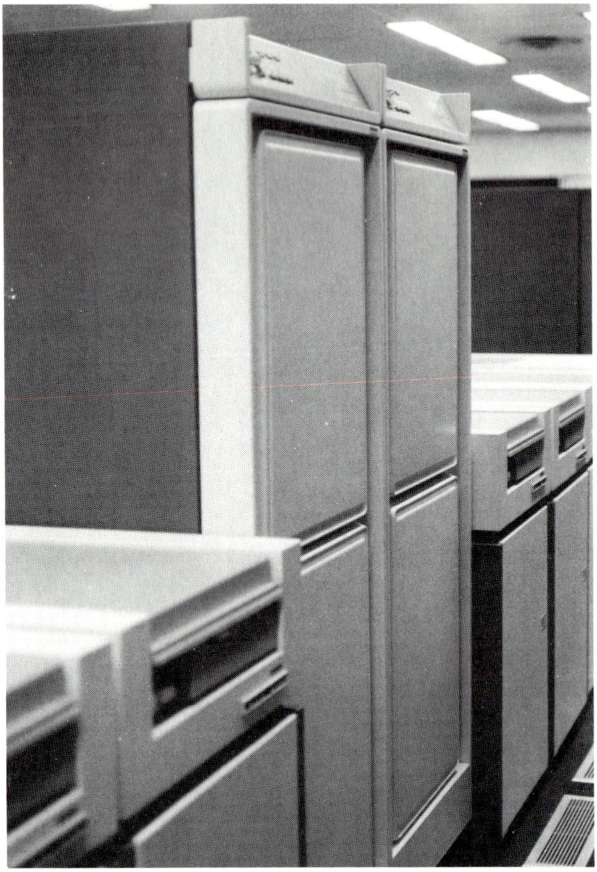

Fig. 24-1. Two Prime 750 computers with disc drives. (Weeg Computing Center, University of Iowa).

chinery, or *hardware,* is the electrical and mechanical gadgetry located in the computer room (Fig. 24-1). Since the machine by itself cannot perform tasks, the manufacturer writes several programs (*software*) for the computer that allow the user to communicate with the machinery in a computer dialect of English. This software instructs the machine to perform functions such as addition, subtraction, multiplication, and alphabetization.

Programmers write systems programs and applications programs for computers in order to serve specific needs of customers. Once the programming is complete, no detailed knowledge of computers is necessary to add records, delete records, or perform any other functions set forth in the program. As Daniel Dern [3] of Prime Computer, Inc. points out, "Just as you don't have to know how an internal combustion engine works to drive a car, you don't need to understand how the computer works . . . to use it."

Computers are available in various models ranging in price from several hundred to well over a million dollars. The main differences among them are the speed at which they carry out functions and the amount of data they can handle at one time.

Computer Retrieval

In order to retrieve information, a computer file containing all the pertinent information about each patient must be made. This file is stored on magnetic tape similar to that used with a common tape recorder (Fig. 24-2A), or a magnetic disc similar to a phonograph record (Fig. 24-2B). When a program is run, the computer is told where to find the file in order that the file can be accessed. The operator, therefore, does not need to know the file's location or how to access it.

The greater the amount of information for each patient, the more costly it can be to store. File size also often affects processing time, so it is advisable to file useful information but not burden the system with unnecessary data. Consider the following patient information:

1. Name
2. Hospital number
3. Contact date
4. Age
5. Sex
6. Weight
7. Race
8. Type of photograph
9. Diagnosis
10. Height
11. Address

The name and hospital number are necessary for chart identification. The contact date is useful in identifying individual patient visits. Age, sex, race, and weight might be considered useful if one ever wished to know their distribution for a given disease group. Height might be considered less important to ocular disease. The type of photograph taken must be known if, for example, only patients on whom angiograms were done are to be selected. Since the main purpose of the system is to cross-reference diseases, diagnosis is mandatory. The patient's address is filed in the patient's hospital or clinic records and should probably be omitted from this data file.

These data options must be considered carefully, and the programmer should be informed about the data to be contained in the file.

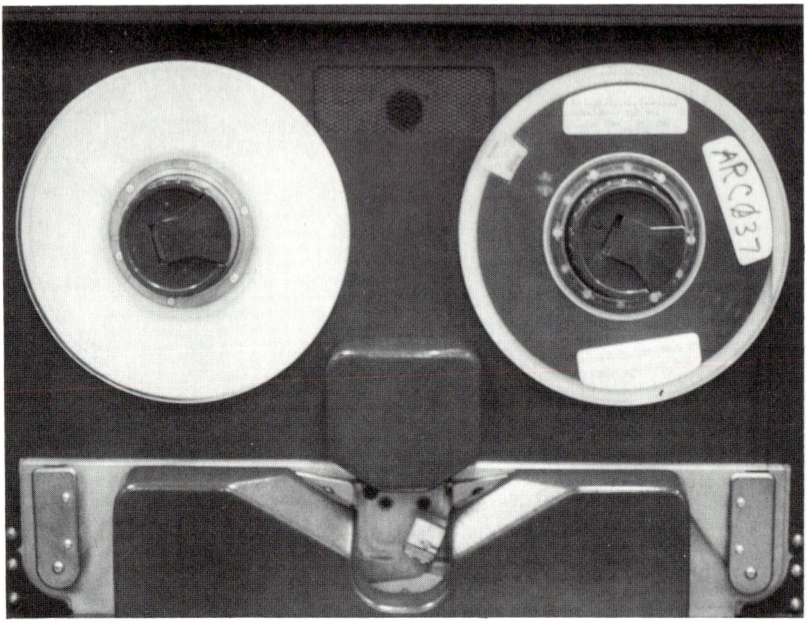

A

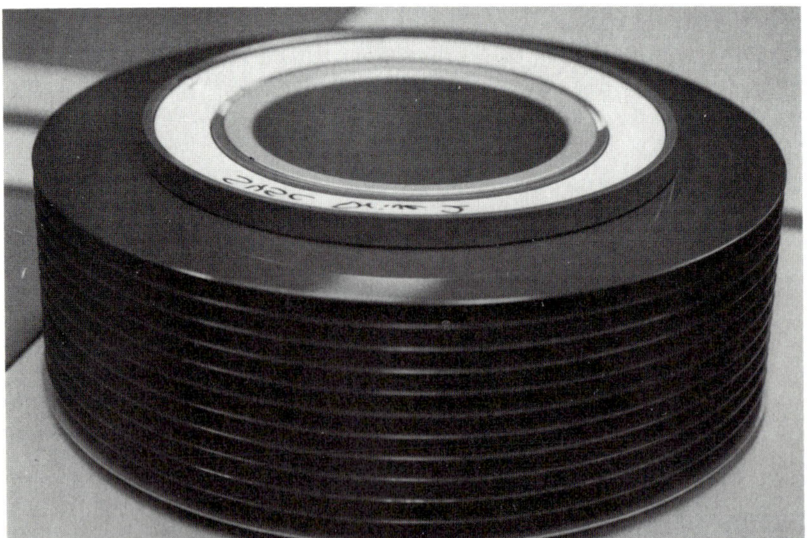

B

Fig. 24-2. (A) *Magnetic tape on a tape drive for input to or output from the computer.* (B) *Disc pack composed of a stack of magnetic discs that are loaded into a disc drive and spun at high speeds. An arm floats a few thousandths of an inch above each surface, reading and writing data on the disc.*

Structuring the file to contain the necessary information is a simple matter, but adding items after the programming is completed can require extensive reprogramming efforts.

The programmer will want to know how the data is to be retrieved. All patients with a particular disease, but not necessarily all patients of one sex, need to be retrieved. Reasonable primary retrieval criteria includes a (1) specific disease, (2) specific name, and (3) specific hospital number. Other information can then be used to qualify these basic groups. List all patients with a specific disease and of a certain:

1. Age
2. Sex
3. Height
4. Weight
5. Race
6. Type of photograph

All the above information is entered and retrieved fairly easily with the exception of the disease entry. Sex is designated *M* or *F;* age can be represented as a three-digit number. Diseases are more difficult to enter because a patient might have several simultaneously. Thus, provision must be made for including several disease processes per record. If the diseases are stored by their English names, such as "nevus," some would be short, while others, such as "acute posterior multifocal placoid pigment epitheliopathy" would be very long. Diseases and procedures can be represented by key words, numbers, or alpha-numeric codes.

Coding Schemes

The purpose of converting the disease name into a code word or number is threefold. First, the information is presented in a uniform format that can be more easily manipulated by the computer. Second, coding can ensure that all synonyms for a disease receive the same value in the data file. Third, the information is condensed to a few letters or numbers, or both, requiring less storage space on the magnetic tape or disc. As stated by Dr. Colenbrander [1], "Classification and coding schemes are the link between the vocabulary of the computer and that of the human user."

Coding Lists

It is beyond the scope of this chapter to present actual coding theories, but an overview is in order. All schemes require a list of disease processes and surgical procedures organized in such a way that a process or procedure can be located at will. Their arrangement might be alphabetic, anatomic, hierarchic, or some combination of these. Associated with each name in the index is the appropriate code for that item. Some prepared coding lists that are commercially available follow.

CURRENT PROCEDURAL TERMINOLOGY (CPT). This list uses five-digit numbers issued sequentially to identify the procedures that are grouped by body systems and by procedure within each body system [2].

INTERNATIONAL CLASSIFICATION OF DISEASES (ICD). This classification uses a base of three-digit numbers; the first two always identify groups of related diseases [4]. Addition of a fourth or fifth digit gives the system greater specificity [1].

UNIVERSITY OF IOWA DATA RETRIEVAL SYSTEM. This classification is based on lists furnished by Mary Lou Louis, M.D., at Bascom Palmer Eye Institute in Miami, Florida [5]. It is organized alphabetically by procedure. Codes are divided into three sections: basic disease group, subclassification group, and anatomic location. The categories to describe neovascularization could be listed as follows:

		N002	Neovascularization
	01	N002	Idiopathic neovascularization
SR		N002	Subretinal neovascularization
SR	01	N002	Idiopathic subretinal neovascularization

In choosing a coding scheme, the organization of the list (e.g., alphabetic or hierarchic) is more important than the actual code values. If the individual who will be converting diagnosis to code is familiar with ocular disease processes and procedures, a hierarchic list might be best, but if the coder has no medical knowledge, the alphabetic variety would be a more practical choice.

Because of my familiarity with the system, the remainder of this chapter will be based on the University of Iowa scheme, although any of the other systems could be applied through the same practices.

Implementation

After one has decided what information is to be stored and which coding system seems most practical, the computer programmer must be consulted. The programmer will establish instructions for the machine so that it will perform the required functions.

There are two basic ways to enter information into the computer. One method is to have the data typed or punched onto data cards, then to submit the cards to the computer through a card reader. The second is to enter the data from a computer terminal equipped with a television screen upon which a form is drawn (Fig. 24-3); the terminal can be located anywhere and connected to the computer by phone line.

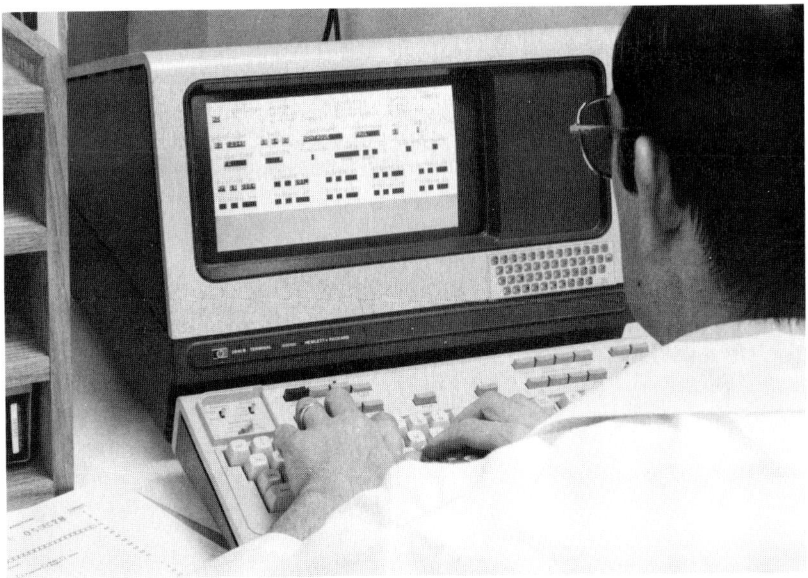

Fig. 24-3. Data are entered through a terminal connected to the computer by a telephone line.

This method is most effective with an interactive computer that allows users to supply data through the terminal while the program is executing.

Once the programming is completed and the terminal installed, data entry can begin.

Coding Practice

A system must be established to ensure that each patient is entered in the file. The following excerpt describes the coding practice at the University of Iowa.*

Photographs are processed, sorted, and placed in charts identified by hospital number. Patient name, hospital number, age, sex, contact date, and slide type are entered on a data sheet by a clerk and filed with the photographs.

The charts are grouped according to ophthalmic subspecialties (retina, strabismus, cornea, etc.), and checked out to staff physicians in those areas. Diagnoses are written on the front of the photo chart. Physicians are encouraged to be as specific as possible in their disease descriptions, and to use common terms whenever possible. For example, the diagnosis of diabetic retinopathy is too inclusive to permit accurate retrieval of specific disease processes. A complete description of the disease state is more helpful:

* From P. Montague et al., Iowa Ophthalmic Data Retrieval System. In R. Greenfield and A. Colenbrander (Eds.), *Computers in Ophthalmology*. New York: IEEE, 1979. Reprinted with permission.

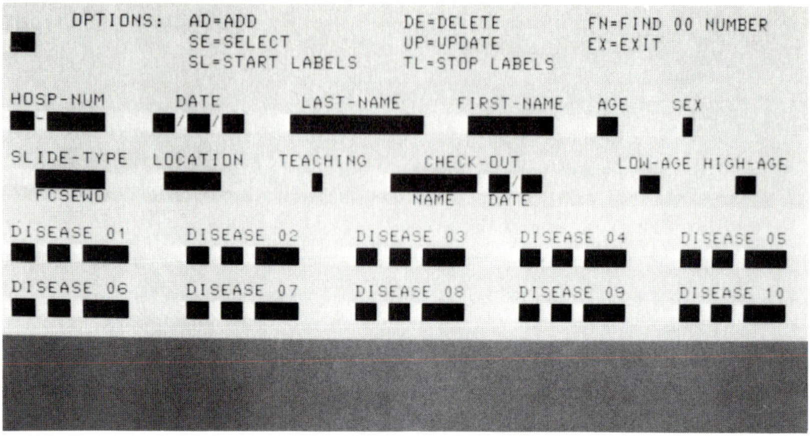

Fig. 24-4. This form, drawn on the screen of the computer terminal, acts as a guide to data entry. Information can be typed only in the black boxes. The screen is drawn and data entry is controlled by the application's programs.

1. Proliferative diabetic retinopathy
2. Macular edema
3. Optic disc neovascularization
4. Microaneurysms
5. Hard exudates
6. Post argon laser photocoagulation

Once the diagnosis has been entered the photo charts are returned to photography for coding. A technician who is familiar with ocular disease locates the disease groups in the alphabetic Disease Index, and records the corresponding codes on the data sheet. Clerks then enter the data from the data sheet into the computer through the interactive computer terminal.

The data sheets are filed with the photo charts to serve as the ultimate back up system. If the data file and all back up files were somehow destroyed (perhaps by some disaster at the computer center) the sheets could be removed and sent to keypunch to regenerate the file.

Retrieval

Records can be retrieved from the system by (1) hospital number and contact date, (2) hospital number only, (3) last name, or (4) disease group. Disease group can be qualified by any combination of:

1. Teaching cases
2. Age group
3. Other disease groups
4. Type of photo
5. File location
6. Sex

```
47-06929    01/06/78             FILE LOCATION:    P            CHECKED OUT TO:

     LAST NAME: ########    *           C              *     01 R018   DIABETIC RETINOPATHY
    FIRST NAME: BLAIR F     * - - - - - - - - - - - - - - - *
           AGE: 45          * F=FLUORESCEIN  C=COLOR FUNDUS *
           SEX: M           * S=SLIT LAMP    E=EXTERNAL     *
                            * W=WIDE ANGLE   O=OTHER        *


49-02830    04/07/77             FILE LOCATION:    P            CHECKED OUT TO:

     LAST NAME: ####        *           C              *     04 R018   DIABETIC RETINOPATHY
    FIRST NAME: MARGARET    * - - - - - - - - - - - - - - - *
           AGE: 45          * F=FLUORESCEIN  C=COLOR FUNDUS *
           SEX: F           * S=SLIT LAMP    E=EXTERNAL     *
                            * W=WIDE ANGLE   O=OTHER        *


49-13389    10/07/77             FILE LOCATION:    P            CHECKED OUT TO:

     LAST NAME: ########    *           S              *     04 S005   CATARACT
    FIRST NAME: PHYLLIS     * - - - - - - - - - - - - - - - *       V011   VITRECTOMY
           AGE: 55          * F=FLUORESCEIN  C=COLOR FUNDUS *       L007   LENSECTOMY
           SEX: F           * S=SLIT LAMP    E=EXTERNAL     *    04 R018   DIABETIC RETINOPATHY
                            * W=WIDE ANGLE   O=OTHER        *


51-05293    03/20/78             FILE LOCATION:  LIB            CHECKED OUT TO: MONTAGUE

     LAST NAME: ########    *           FC             *     02 R018   DIABETIC RETINOPATHY
    FIRST NAME: GERARD      * - - - - - - - - - - - - - - - *       H025   DOT AND BLOT HEMORRHAGES
           AGE: 50          * F=FLUORESCEIN  C=COLOR FUNDUS *
           SEX: M           * S=SLIT LAMP    E=EXTERNAL     *
                            * W=WIDE ANGLE   O=OTHER        *



 ########## LAST NAMES OMITTED


 SAMPLE OUTPUT GENERATED BY REQUESTING PATIENTS WITH DIABETIC RETINOPATHY (R018).
 THE OFFICE IN WHICH THE FILE IS LOCATED IS INDICATED BY 'FILE LOCATION:'  (P = PHOTOGRAPHY, LIB = LIBRARY).
 IF THE CHART IS CHECK OUT A NAME FOLLOWS 'CHECKED OUT TO:'.
```

Fig. 24-5. Sample output from a retrieval of all patients with diabetic retinopathy.

All selections are made by typing *SE* in the option box (Fig. 24-4) and then filling in the spaces on the screen that correspond to the selection parameters.

Hospital number and contact date selections identify one record within the file, which is displayed in the form on the screen. *Hospital number only* selects all contact dates for that hospital number, and the records are displayed on the screen without the form. *Last name* selects all records with a particular last name. Again, the records are displayed on the screen without the form. *Disease group* selects all records that meet all the criteria requested; any number of the disease fields can be filled in. The computer then locates those patients having all these simultaneous disease processes. If "low age" or "high age" are both filled in, only patients in that age group will be reported.

Brief information is displayed on the screen, as above, but all the information is listed by the printer in readable form on termination of the session (Fig. 24-5).

Conclusion

A computerized retrieval system can be viewed as a bank of information initiated and maintained in order to be available when needed. Data entry and retrieval can be performed by office personnel with a minimal amount of operational training.

References

1. Colenbrander, A. Classification and Coding in Ophthalmology. In R. Greenfield and A. Colenbrander (Eds.), *Computers in Ophthalmology*. New York: IEEE, 1979.
2. Current Procedural Terminology (4th ed.). Chicago: American Medical Association, 1977.
3. Dern, D. *The New Users Guide to Editor and Runoff*. Framingham, Mass.: Prime Computer, Incorporated, 1978.
4. *International Classification of Diseases* (9th revision). Ann Arbor: Commission on Professional and Hospital Activities, 1968.
5. Montague, P., et al. Iowa Ophthalmic Data Retrieval System. In R. Greenfield and A. Colenbrander (Eds.), *Computers in Ophthalmology*. New York: IEEE, 1979.
6. Walker, B. Photographic filing systems. In J. Justice, Jr. (Ed.), Ophthalmic Photography. *Int. Ophthalmol. Clin.* 16(2) : 221, 1976.

The Founding of the Ophthalmic Photographers' Society

JOHNNY JUSTICE, JR.

The following is a personal historic review of the founding of the Ophthalmic Photographers' Society and its subsequent success. My first view of an ocular fundus came shortly after I was hired as a medical photographer trainee at Duke University Medical Center in July, 1957. I managed to escape from the photographic darkroom long enough to look over the shoulder of Raymond L. Howard, medical photographer, while he was photographing a patient's eye. He was using a strange-looking instrument called a Zeiss-Nordensen fundus camera. What an incredible view of the retina! Although I was thoroughly impressed, it never occurred to me that one day I would be taking photographs of the eye on a full-time basis.

Two years passed quickly and, as fate would have it, Leonard M. Hart moved from the Chicago area to accept the position as Chief of the Medical Illustration Service at the Veterans Administration Hospital in Durham, North Carolina. When Mr. Hart offered me the position as Assistant Chief Photographer, I eagerly accepted, recognizing it to be a tremendous opportunity to gain some experience at last as a clinical photographer. Little did I know that I was making a direct move toward ophthalmic photography.

As it happened, Dr. Noble J. David, then Chief of Neurology at the V.A. Hospital had recently read an article by Novotny and Alvis entitled, "Photography of Fluorescein Dye Circulating Through the Retinal Vessels." Before his arrival in Durham, Mr. Hart had modified an old Bausch and Lomb fundus camera by replacing the carbon arc light source with an electronic flashtube. At Dr. David's request, Mr. Hart placed the appropriate excitor-barrier filters in the modified Bausch and Lomb fundus camera. Incredibly, his first attempt at fluorescein angiography was successful, and soon, under Mr. Hart's guidance, I too was performing fluorescein angiography. In retrospect, it is difficult to relate the excitement and apprehension felt as I anticipated the perfusion of dye through the central retinal artery. At that time, one of the primary uses of fluorescein was in determining arm-to-retina circulation time. It was critically important to obtain high-quality angiograms of the initial appearance of dye in the central retinal artery. Be-

This chapter is reprinted in part from the *Journal of the Ophthalmic Photographers' Society* 1(1) : 5, 1978.

cause of the slow recycling time of the electronic power supply (only 1 flash every 6-8 sec), one can imagine how difficult it was to document the early filling phases routinely while performing fluorescein angiography.

Shortly after our success, Dr. Edward W. D. Norton, Professor and Chairman of the Bascom Palmer Eye Institute in Miami, Florida, became interested in using fluorescein angiography to investigate diseases affecting the retina and choroid. Mr. Hart was offered the task of establishing a fluorescein laboratory at the institute. Fortunately for me, Mr. Hart declined the offer and, as a second choice, I was offered the position. Without any reservations, I accepted the challenge and, on January 3, 1963, became a full-time ophthalmic photographer. Since that title had not yet been created, however, I was still classified as a medical photographer. The record clearly shows that investigators such as Dr. E. W. D. Norton, J. Donald M. Gass, and others at the Bascom Palmer Eye Institute took an early lead in establishing fluorescein angiography as an aid in evaluating the pathophysiology of the retina and choroid. Although unaware of it at the time, I can now appreciate the unique educational opportunity that I faced: learning alongside giants such as Norton and Gass as they and other faculty members unraveled the complexities of angiographic interpretations. After performing more than 35,000 angiograms, I think it is safe to say that my career as an ophthalmic photographer was launched on a "sea of fluorescein."

Shortly after arriving at the Bascom Palmer Eye Institute, I began to hear the name Lee Allen repeated in conversation. It was obvious that, although I had not met him, Allen was a legend in his own time. He enjoyed an outstanding reputation not only as an ophthalmic photographer but also as a medical illustrator and ocularist. Finally, I had found someone with whom I could correspond regarding common problems and new techniques. I became curious; surely there were others who specialized in photography of the eye. The popularity of fluorescein angiography rapidly spread worldwide, with a subsequent need for photographers in this specialty. This need for medical photographers brought names such as Choromokos, Frazier, George, Lancaster, Magli, Tomer, Cader, and Wong to the forefront. More recently, others, far too many to enumerate, have shown enormous enthusiasm and interest in furthering ophthalmic photography.

In April, 1969, I proposed establishing an association of ophthalmic photography to several people in the field at the Association for Research in Vision and Ophthalmology (ARVO) meeting in Sarasota, Florida. The overall reaction was very gratifying and led me to believe that the establishment of such an association would be advantageous not only to ophthalmic photographers but also to ophthalmology. At that time, Don Wong had several suggestions and ideas that I included in my original letter. Most of them, including his suggestions to publish a professional journal and establish certification testing for ophthalmic photographers, have become realities.

On October 15, 1969, an informal meeting of the proposed Ophthalmic Photographers' Society convened at the Palmer House in Chicago. In attendance were L. Allen, E. Choromokos, O. Frazier, Y. Magli, M. Manella, T. L. Tomer, W. Stenstrom, A. Wiley, D. Wong, and myself. I opened the meeting by reporting the enthusiastic response to my letter from people in the field of ophthalmic photography. Following discussion by others in attendance regarding organizational matters, Lee Allen was nominated and unanimously elected interim President. Mr. Allen then appointed me interim secretary-treasurer and program chairman until the society had its first formal election of officers.

On July 13, 1970, the Ophthalmic Photographers' Society (OPS), Inc. became a formal reality. Our society has grown from an original group of 10 to an international group of more than 500 members. We can be proud of our growth, but we cannot rest on our laurels. Since its formative years, many individuals have, through their efforts, kept the society moving on an upward course. Some names in particular come to mind. John L. Johnson has done an outstanding job as Editor of the OPS *Newsletter* and was primarily responsible for the design of our current OPS exhibit. Csaba L. Martonyi, OPS President, has followed the early lead of Don Wong in establishing our now excellent certification program. Don Wong and the editorial committee have successfully published the *Ophthalmic Photographers' Society Journal* since its inception in October, 1978. Terrance L. Tomer is primarily responsible for instituting the instructional courses held annually at the OPS meeting. Barrett P. Walker has successfully upgraded the quality of education by establishing a comprehensive course in opthalmic photography. Earl A. Choromokos has for many years been the senior instructor at the American Academy of Ophthalmology annual meetings. International members who have been productive include Albert Aan de Kerk of the Netherlands and Sadao Kanagami of Japan.

The following have been elected honorary members of the Ophthalmic Photographers' Society: Lee Allen, Leonard M. Hart, Drs. David L. Alvis, Pierre Almaric, Gerard W. Crock, David D. Donaldson, J. Donald M. Gass, Milton Flocks, W. M. Haining, Harold R. Novotny, Emanuel S. Rosen, and Koichi Shimizu, and Jessica Eichrodt, my secretary during the planning and founding of the society.

The Ophthalmic Photographers' Society is indeed fortunate to include such distinguished individuals among its members. If we proceed on our present course, I foresee nothing but continued growth and improvement of the professional image of our members and for our society.

Index